Situating religion and medicine in Asia

Manchester University Press

SOCIAL HISTORIES OF MEDICINE

Series editors: David Cantor, Anne Hanley and Elaine Leong

Social Histories of Medicine is concerned with all aspects of health, illness and medicine, from prehistory to the present, in every part of the world. The series covers the circumstances that promote health or illness, the ways in which people experience and explain such conditions, and what, practically, they do about them. Practitioners of all approaches to health and healing come within its scope, as do their ideas, beliefs and practices, and the social, economic and cultural contexts in which they operate. Methodologically, the series welcomes relevant studies in social, economic, cultural and intellectual history, as well as approaches derived from other disciplines in the arts, sciences, social sciences and humanities. The series is a collaboration between Manchester University Press and the Society for the Social History of Medicine.

To buy or to find out more about the books currently available in this series, please go to: https://manchesteruniversitypress.co.uk/series/social-histories-of-medicine/

Situating religion and medicine in Asia

Methodological insights and innovations

Edited by

Michael Stanley-Baker

Manchester University Press

Published by Manchester University Press
Oxford Road, Manchester M13 9PL

www.manchesteruniversitypress.co.uk

British Library Cataloguing-in-Publication Data
A catalogue record for this book is available from the British Library

ISBN 978 1 5261 6001 0 hardback
ISBN 978 1 5261 9112 0 paperback

First published 2023
Paperback published 2025

EU authorised representative for GPSR:
Easy Access System Europe – Mustamäe tee 50,
10621 Tallinn, Estonia
gpsr.requests@easproject.com

Typeset by Newgen Publishing UK

In memory of Nathan Sivin
who throughout his career challenged the
'Awesome Taboo' of comparing religion and science.

Although the origins of illness are many, they all concern deviants. As for deviants, they have improper causes. ['Deviants'] refers to those forces which antagonize the constant principles of the human body: wind; cold; summerheat; damp; hunger; fullness; exhaustion; idleness – these are all deviances, not just ghost *qi* and plagues.

Tao Hongjing 陶弘景, Preface to the *Collected Annotations to the Materia Medica*

[M]edical cognition differs in principle from that of scientific cognition. A scientist looks for typical, normal phenomena, while a medical man studies precisely the atypical, abnormal, morbid phenomena... . There exists no strict boundary between what is healthy and what is diseased... such is the cognitive task of medicine. How does one find a law for irregular phenomena? – this is the fundamental problem of medical thinking.

Ludwik Fleck, 'Some specific features of the medical way of thinking 1927' [1986], 39

Situated knowledges are about communities, not about isolated individuals. The only way to find a larger vision is to be somewhere in particular... . Its images are not the products of escape and transcendence of limits (the view from above) but the joining of partial views and halting voices into a collective subject position that promises a vision of the means of ongoing finite embodiment, of living within limits and contradictions – of views from somewhere.

Donna Haraway, 'Situated Knowledges', 590

One must see then that the daunting double task of translation of cultures and their comparative study raises not only the question of the mentality of us and other peoples, but also ultimately the issue of '*rationality*' itself, and the limits of western 'scientism' as a paradigm.

Stanley Tambiah, *Magic Science and Religion and the Scope of Rationality*, 3

[This account of the real] eschews the picture of a given foundation and its symbolizing, instead having worlds, with their objects and subjects, as accomplished in collective going on... . Worlds emerge all of a piece... [with no] a priori separation of the symbolic and the material... .

Helen Verran, *Science and an African Logic*, 37–38

Curing is always and everywhere the cutting edge of religion.

Sivin's Fourth Law

Contents

List of illustrations ix
List of contributors x
Foreword by Dagmar Schäfer xv
Acknowledgements xviii

Introduction – Michael Stanley-Baker 1

Part I: East Asia

1 Religion and health care in middle-period China – Nathan Sivin 61
2 Religion and medicine in premodern Japan – Katja Triplett 94
3 Female alchemy in late imperial and modern China – Elena Valussi 128

Part II: South Asia

4 Religion and medicine in Sanskrit literature: the *Rāmāyaṇa* and the politics of an epic plant – Anthony Cerulli 165
5 From 'medical men' to 'local health traditions': the secularisation of medicine in portrayals of health care in India – Helen Lambert 198
6 Sound medicine: towards a nomadology of medical *mantras* in seventeenth to twentieth-century Bengal – Projit Bihari Mukharji 219

Part III: Himalayas, Southeast Asia

7 Sowa Rigpa, Tibetan medicine, Tibetan healing – Geoffrey Samuel 257
8 Homeopathy and Islam in Malaysia: encounters of religion and complementary medical traditions in a modern Asian multi-ethnic society – Constantin Canavas 305
9 Questioning the boundaries between medicine and religion in contemporary Myanmar – Céline Coderey 341

Index 379

Illustrations

Figure 0.1	Group photo of the Bellagio Symposium on Taoism, 1968. Courtesy of the Needham Research Institute.	xvii
Table 7.1	The field of Tibetan healing practices	259
Map 9.1	Map of Myanmar and its divisions. Aotearoa/ Wikimedia Commons, CC BY SA 3.0.	342

Contributors

Constantin Canavas holds a Diploma in chemical engineering (National Technical University of Athens, Greece) and a Dr.-Ing. in system dynamics and control (University of Stuttgart, Germany). He has been Professor at the Hamburg University of Applied Sciences, Faculty of Life Sciences in the fields of control, technology assessment, as well as history and philosophy of technology, since 1993. He has taught History of Technology at the University of Athens and the National Technical University of Athens, as well as Arab History and History of Islam at the University of Crete (Greece). A major part of his teaching and research concerns the history of science and technology in premodern and modern Islamic societies. A special focus is on medical systems and healing practices in Muslim communities and multi-ethnic societies. The methodological approach combines questions of health technology assessment with the perspective of historical anthropology.

Anthony Cerulli is Professor of South Asian Studies in the Department of Asian Languages and Cultures, and Director of the Center for South Asia, at the University of Wisconsin–Madison. He teaches courses on the histories of religions and medicines in South Asia, and his research combines ethnography and philology to explore the intersections of premodern and modern literary cultures at sites of ritual healing, and in institutions of medical education, in south India. He is the author of *The Practice of Texts: Education and Healing in South India* (2022) and *Somatic Lessons: Narrating Patienthood and Illness in Indian Medical Literature* (2012), and co-editor of *Time, Continuity, and Rupture: Medicines and*

Memories in South Asia (2020), *The Gift in India in Theory in Practice* (2018), and *Medical Texts and Manuscripts in Indian Cultural History* (2013).

Céline Coderey is a Lecturer at Tembusu College and a Research Fellow in the Science, Technology, and Society Cluster at the Asia Research Institute in the National University of Singapore. She received her MA and PhD in Anthropology from the University of Provence, Aix-Marseille 1 (France). Her field of expertise spans from medical anthropology and anthropology of the body, to anthropology of religion, but also to questions of identity in relation to artistic and cultural practices, heritage making and temporalities. Her research is mainly focused on Myanmar and neighbouring Southeast Asian countries, with a recent expansion also to Papua New Guinea and the Marquesas Island in French Polynesia. Among her main publications is the book *Circulation and Governance of Asian Medicines* (2019), and the articles 'Myanmar Traditional Medicine: The Making of a National Heritage', *Modern Asian Studies* (2021), 'Healing the Whole: Questioning the Boundaries between Medicine and Religion in Rakhine, Western Myanmar', *Journal of Southeast Asian Studies* (2020) and 'Immortal Medicine: Understanding the Resilience of Burmese Alchemic Practice', *Medical Anthropology* (2018).

Helen Lambert (D.Phil) is Professor of Medical Anthropology in the Department of Population Health Sciences at the University of Bristol, UK. She has been carrying out ethnographic and interdisciplinary health-related research in India and other parts of Asia for over three decades, with a particular focus on medical pluralism, treatment-seeking and vernacular therapeutics. Other principal research interests are antimicrobial resistance (AMR) and sociocultural dimensions of infectious diseases including COVID-19 and HIV. She has published over 100 articles and has co-edited two books: *Social Bodies* (2009) and *How to Live through a Pandemic* (2023). Among numerous advisory roles, Helen serves on the MRC Applied Global Health Research Board and is a member of the UK–India Advisory Council to the UK Foreign Commonwealth and Development Office.

Projit Bihari Mukharji is Professor of History of Science at the University of Pennsylvania. His work focusses on issues of marginalisation in and through medical and scientific knowledge. He is the author of three monographs: *Nationalizing the Body: The Medical Market, Print and Daktari Medicine* (2009); *Doctoring Traditions: Ayurveda, Small Technologies and Braided Sciences* (2016) and, most recently, *Brown Skins, White Coats: Race Science in India, 1920–66* (2022).

Geoffrey Samuel is an Honorary Associate at the University of Sydney, Australia and Emeritus Professor at Cardiff University, Wales, UK, from which he retired in 2014 after an academic career in the UK, Australia and New Zealand. His PhD was an anthropological study of Tibetan Buddhism in India and Nepal. His books include *Mind, Body and Culture* (1990), *Civilized Shamans: Buddhism in Tibetan Societies* (1993) and *The Origins of Yoga and Tantra* (2008). His current research interests include Tibetan yogic health practices, Tibetan medicine, and the dialogue between Buddhism and science.

Nathan Sivin contributed studies across the sciences and medicine of China, throughout imperial and modern history, and comparative studies of these fields in China and Europe. After he obtained his doctorate with a dissertation published in revised form as volume 1 of Harvard Monographs in the History of Science, he taught at MIT from 1965 to 1977, founding what is now the Science, Technology, and Society program. The Chinese Academy of Sciences made him an Honorary Professor. He taught at the University of Pennsylvania with appointments in eight departments and programs, until 2006, when he retired. He continued to publish prolifically, including volumes on Yuan dynasty astronomy, *Granting the Seasons* (2009), and on the Song dynasty medical marketplace, *Health Care in Eleventh-Century China* (2015). His research interests included the social relations of Chinese medicine, combining the conceptual tools of history of science with cultural and social anthropology and sociology; the intellectual biography of Shen Kua 沈括 (1031–1095); and the theoretical structure of alchemy. A set of translations of key documents for a source book of Chinese science and medicine is forthcoming.

Michael Stanley-Baker is an Assistant Professor in History at the School of Humanities, and of Medical Humanities at the Lee Kong Chian School of Medicine, at Nanyang Technological University, Singapore. He is currently a vice-president of the International Association for the Study of Traditional Asian Medicine (IASTAM), and sits on the Daoist Studies committee of the American Academy of Religion. An historian of Chinese medicine and religion, particularly Daoism, Michael also holds a licentiate diploma in the practice of Chinese medicine. He works on the early imperial period as well as contemporary Chinese speaking communities, is co-editor of the *Routledge Handbook of Chinese Medicine* (2022), and head of the *Polyglot Asian Medicine* project, which uses digital humanities tools and datasets to investigate the migration of medicine across spatial, temporal, intellectual and linguistic domains in Asia. He is currently completing a monograph on the emergence of medicine and religion as related genres of practice in early imperial China.

Katja Triplett, PhD, was Professor of the Study of Religions at Göttingen and is currently based at Leipzig University. She is Affiliate Professor of the Study of Religions at Marburg University. Her doctorate in the Study of Religions is from Marburg University, where she also studied Japanese Linguistics and Social and Cultural Anthropology. Triplett held a postdoctoral research fellowship at the Centre for the Study of Japanese Religions, SOAS, University of London, in 2004/2005. From 2007 to 2012 she was Associate Professor and curator of the Museum of Religions at Marburg University. Her main fields of interest are Buddhism; religion and medicine; and visual and material culture. She has published widely on religions in Japan including with a focus on medicine and medical history. Among her publications is *Buddhism and Medicine in Japan: A Topical Survey (500–1600 CE) of a Complex Relationship* (2019).

Elena Valussi received an MA in Chinese Studies from the University of Venice, and an MA and PhD in Chinese History and Religious Studies, from the School of Oriental and African Studies, London. She is a senior Lecturer in the History Department at Loyola University Chicago. She has been a visiting scholar and researcher at the University of Venice, at the Chinese University of Hong

Kong, and at the University of Erlangen-Nuremberg in Germany. Professor Valussi's research interests and publications revolve around the intersection of gender, religion and body practices in Late Imperial Daoism, and Republican period discourses on gender and religion. She is co-editor of a book on the history and practice of spirit writing in China. She is co-directing a project on religious diversity in Sichuan with Professor Stefania Travagnin, funded by the Chiang Ching-Kuo Foundation. Valussi was the co-chair of the Daoist Studies Group at the American Academy of Religions and a member of the editorial group for the International *Daozang Jiyao* Project. With Professor Natasha Heller, she is co-founder of Wisar, a website that showcases the work of women scholars in Asian Religions. She is also currently the Vice-President of the Society for the Study of Chinese Religions.

Foreword

Dagmar Schäfer

This comparative study of Medicine and Religion tackles how health was desired or restored in Asia historically, placing healing practices into the hands of the actors who wielded the practices, materials, tools and spirits of healing and their lore. It foregrounds the diversity of actors and communities who had a stake in healing bodies and souls. Health care, as the contributions in this book illustrate, functioned because it operationalised means and methods across the boundaries that are so prevalent in global health regimes today. In Japan, China, Tibet, India, Myanmar and Malaysia, historical therapies included rituals, bodily exercise and drug lores, sacred and secular cures. While some of it has survived regionally, it has taken new forms in national adaptations or imaginaries of traditional medical knowledges, such as Ayurveda or Traditional Chinese Medicine (TCM), often invoked in juxtaposition to modern biomedical approaches to health and healing.

A meeting in 2016 at the Max Planck Institute for the History of Science (MPIWG), Berlin, brought together specialists working on how and what therapeutics were related to eschatology, soteriology, canon and orthodoxy, sectarian identity and access to divine beings. Twentieth-century historical analysis attests to strong emphasis on 'fields', such as science, religion or medicine, as well as regional and cultural distinctions marked by ideals of twentieth century nation-state debates operating in binaries of medicine and religion, truth and superstition, global or local or traditional versus modern. By the twenty-first century, research within the context of social science and anthropology had moved away from a rigid polarisation to enquiries about the mutual impulses, contradictions and changes. Some historians of science and technology and religion pinpointed a similar historical conundrum, namely that the Western dominance in global accounts produces similar methodological difficulties in both fields.

Situating Medicine and Religion in Asia shows through a series of nuanced case studies how much religion really mattered in everyday life, and that health and medical practice are thus often a quite local story and individualisable. Religion, like medicine, was subject to trends of consumption and thoroughly involved in power struggles as well. Commercialisation, economic and geographical expansion and the mechanisation of the world have been much more powerful factors changing the measures to combat illness and bring about health. This volume could not be more timely also in the way that it rethinks the historical sources of healing and how historians can approach them. Digital Humanities, but also a thorough inclusion of objects and the environment into the historical purview, have revealed a diverse and complex world of religion and medicine that goes beyond easy distinctions between Buddhism or Daoism, pharmacological or therapeutic history, and invites collaborative efforts from specialists in multiple disciplines: anthropology, botany, biochemistry, philology, traditional medical theory, medical history and religious studies.

An enormous asset to rethinking religion and medicine as is done in this volume has, therefore, been the initiative of Michael Stanley-Baker and began as an infrastructural initiative about 'Drugs across Asia' at MPIWG but has since developed into a truly global community initiative. Critically engaging with drug lore variances, therapeutic methods and health ideals across the sources and resources of history reveals a multitude of epistemic communities: doctors, monks, individual holy people and their lineages, cultic shrines, folk practitioners and local families. Middle Chinese, Tibetan, Khotanese, Old Turkic, Uyghur, Sogdian and Sanskrit are some, but not the only, languages used to convey healing practices. The historical realities of plant identification, local terminology (mis)representation, adaptation, and substitution in Asian health and healing cultures are attested to in medieval and more recent sources, as well as modern ethnographies. The epistemic shifts in these material and linguistic transformations pose serious problems for claiming equivalent material 'identities' across these diverse linguistic, intellectual and social divides. This collection is an important step to expand Ludwik Fleck's framing of scientific knowledge as an inescapably historical and social phenomenon; offering critical analysis and new methodological insights it allows more fine-grained, and more extensive accounts of what it means to be healthy and live in a healthy world.

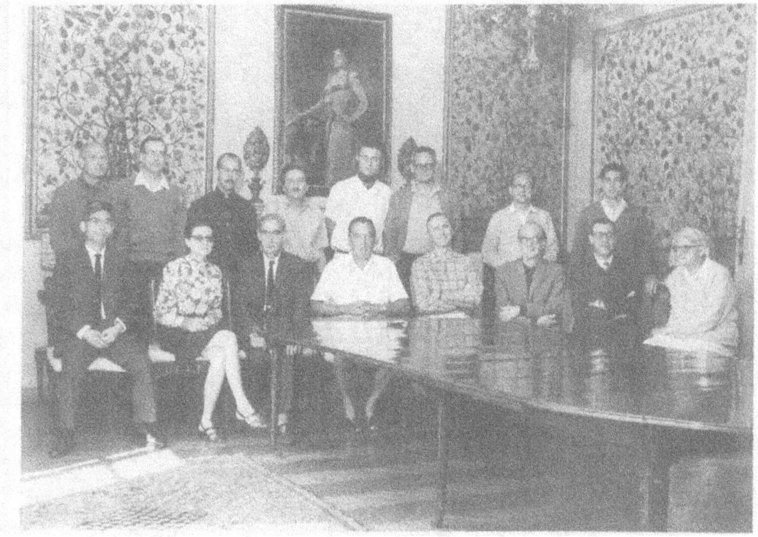

Figure 0.1 Group photo of the Bellagio Symposium on Taoism, 1968. In attendance were, from left to right:

Arthur Link	Richard Mather	Kristofer Schipper	Nathan Sivin	William Doub	Angus Graham	Ho Ping-yoke	Michael Saso
Miyuku Mokusan	Anna Seidel	Max Kaltenmark	Arthur Wright	Edward de Bary	Mircea Eliade	Holmes Welch	Joseph Needham

With thanks to John Moffet and the Needham Research Institute.

Acknowledgements

Just as the final manuscript was submitted to the publishers, we lost one of the leading lights in the history of science and religion, Nathan Sivin, who also contributed to this volume. He was one of the first people we invited to the Berlin workshop, but could not attend as he was caring for his dear wife. Nevertheless, he contributed a sterling chapter, and continued to work on perfecting it up until his final days. He was assisted by Professor Marta Hanson, who carried the love and support for Nathan from the wider research community with her as she helped him in all manner of ways. For this, we are truly thankful. Nathan entrusted her with a substantive collection of translations for a forthcoming source book on Chinese science, and so he continues to contribute prolifically to the field.

Nathan's work has been exemplary for the field and for the enquiry in this volume. Not one to step away from controversy, his first book, *Chinese Alchemy* (1968), published in the same year as the Bellagio Symposium pictured opposite, challenged fundamental assumptions about the history of Chinese science and Daoism. Through close reading the alchemical work of the fabled medical author, Sun Simiao 孫思邈 (581?–682), as well as scrutinising retrospective catalogues which attributed to him dozens of texts, he conclusively called into doubt Sun's identity a Daoist in any way beyond perfunctory affiliations, as well as disproving dozens of retrospective attributions that were assigned to him by later bibliographers and historians. These insights raised questions about the status of Daoism as a broad-brush term, and as an institution, that shaped the field of Daoist Studies to come. One of his most frequently cited essays, 'On the Word "Taoist" as a source of perplexity' (1978), now required reading for generations of students of Chinese religion, points out the ambiguous and careless use of the use of the word 'Daoist' in traditional and modern scholarship. It introduced an entirely new level of clarity and precision that has shaped not only our understanding of the relationship between different historical sects, but has shaped the practice of scholarship on Chinese religions. While not all agree on a single definition of what constitutes 'Daoism', and Nathan himself even developed new positions later in his career (2010), all scholars have, since his 1978 paper, learned to carefully situate their historical actors and sects in relationship to known movements of their time.

These two studies are just a sample from among the hundreds of his books, papers and critical reviews on the history of Chinese science, religion and medicine, which range from religion to medicine, astronomy to mathematics and the history of science at large. His comparative work on religious and medical actors in Song dynasty China (2015) inspired us to invite him to the workshop, and I invite readers to see his chapter in this volume. They closely situate historical actors within what he later termed the 'cultural manifold' of their time (Sivin 2005), paying close attention to their ideas, language and motivations, contrasting these with the categorical assumptions and academic conventions of later scholarship. Their influence on the field demonstrates that being willing to read beyond seemingly settled history and accepted convention can produce entirely new historical insights, and lead to new avenues of investigation. Nathan poked fun at the inertia of unwittingly inherited categories, and misguided notions of scholarly professionalism by referring to them as an 'Awesome Taboo', which prevented scholars of China from reading works on science, technology or medicine (2000). It is for these insights into the power of close reading, his spirited refusal to take accepted norms at face value, and his commitment to closely interrogating how actors thought, wrote and acted within the currents of their own time and place, that this volume is dedicated to his memory.

In terms of the production of this volume, Pierce Salguero deserves the deepest thanks. His friendship, encouragement and constant intellectual engagement have been present throughout the many stages of producing the initial workshop and this volume. The many conference panels and late-night conversations on this topic, wherever we might be around the world, led to our co-organising the workshop in Berlin in 2016, titled Sacred Cures for want of a better name. Taking on the volume as co-editor, he handled the organisation, reviews and contract negotiation, while I focused on the intellectual questions and argument structure of the volume. As reviews came in, and all was running smoothly, he bowed a grateful exit, removing his name as co-editor. A great colleague, confidante and comrade-in-arms, a truer and kinder friend would be hard to find indeed.

The volume has had institutional support from many quarters. Dept III of the Max Planck Institute for the History of Science, generously supported the initial workshop, titled Sacred Cures, in Berlin in 2016. Many attended the workshop and contributed very important reflections, but did not end up in the volume, including: Donald Harper described an important shift towards more religious forms of cultivation in the Eastern Han dynasty; Katharina Sabernig pointed out important overlaps and comparisons between the subtle and the physical bodies in Tibetan anatomy; Michael Slouber introduced broaching the notion of Tantric medicine as a critique to the secularised representations of Ayurveda and South Asian medicine more generally; Leslie DeVries explored textures at the interface of scholarly *ru* 儒 (sometimes translated as 'Confucian') medicine and religion both within Chinese and Vietnamese medical literature; Elisabeth Hsu explored the temporality of bodily transmission of techniques documented in the *Yijin jing* as 'sedimented' in the body; and Joey Hung and the late Tu Aming presented used corpus-level analysis of the Buddhist Canon to identify the Six Dynasties period in China as the height of the medico-religious market. Insightful overviews were provided by Vivienne Lo, Angelika Messner and Mona Schrempf. Judith Farquhar and Kenneth Zysk gave keynote speeches which profoundly shaped future research: Farquhar's summative insights formed key guidelines for the later volume, and Zysk's call for more fundamental, basic work on identities, objects and names is at the heart of my current digital work on *Drugs Across Asia*. Judith has been a constant inspiration for this project, from introducing me to Ludwik Fleck, invitations to Vitalities events, and continued advice and consultation.

The Max Planck Institute for the History of Science (MPIWG) is truly a rare place, and the comparative approach in this volume, the focus on knowledge practices and the relationship between positionality, or situatedness, of knowledge are certainly products of the happy years I was able to spend there as a researcher. Support by the Berlin Centre for the History of Knowledge during my initial years, and then by Department III, allowed me to conceptualise and implement the workshop, and then follow through with the initial stages of publishing the volume. More than material support, the social and intellectual fabric of the institute was consequential. Seminar debates, insightful conversations, research tips and readings shared so generously by colleagues there were fundamental to the insights in this volume. Philologists like Sonja Brentjes and Martina Siebert emphasised the need for balance between textual rigor and theoretical approaches. Martina Schlunder, Nina Lerman and Francesca Bray debated finer points of how technology, assemblage, tacit knowledge and Denkstyl contribute to the production, form, transmission and negotiation of knowledge. Martina introduced me to Helen Verran's work, and also to Verran personally when she came to visit, which was deeply influential on my writing and thinking. Working closely with Terri Chettiar and Rohan deb Roy to convene a workshop on 'Life' as an object of knowledge was both a pleasure, and a great source of learning.

The opportunity to meet, and sometimes to host, world-class scholars like Volker Scheid, Judith Farquhar, Pamela Smith, Angela Leung, Sean Lei and others, directly impacted how I conceived this volume, or shaped my vision of the broader conversations in which this volume is imagined. Chen Kaijun, Marten Söderblom Saarela, Alina-Sandra Cucu, Hong Hong Tinn, Harun Küçük, Victoria Lee, and many others shared their camaraderie, support and insight while we navigated that indeterminate space beyond the PhD. Stewart Allen was a stalwart companion, offering good humour, fine drinks and a place to rest my head after the last commuter train departed for Sachsen-Anhalt. Chen Shih-pei and Brent Hao-yang Ho welcomed me into the world of Digital Humanities, sharing tools, opening networks, writing grants, giving papers and developing major projects which have enabled me to 'situate' medicine within Chinese religious corpuses. Without their generosity and eagerness to share what they knew, my work in this field could not be possible. Gina Grizmek, Karin Weninger and the beloved Nuria Monn were kind and generous guides through the administrative side of the workshop and my time at the institute. One of the most influential contributions was the seminar held by Dagmar Schäfer, where we investigated 'Planning' as 'emergent processes by which actors develop, enact and stabilize or transform strategies for "making things work"'. This vision of emergence and the processes by which practices to make life itself work become stabilised into 'religious' or 'medical' frames lies at the heart of the volume.

The Forschungsgruppe for Multiple Secularities at Leipzig University generously hosted me several times in Leipzig as a Senior Fellow while editing these chapters and writing the introduction. Seminars here on the boundaries of religion honed the volume further, focusing more on institutional actors, broad social patterns, and the different ways these shape boundaries in contrast to epistemological definitions. The working group and seminar on religion and medicine in Asia hosted by Christoph Kleine, Katrin Killinger and Katja Triplett, who also joined this volume because she was invited to and delivered a paper to the original Sacred Cures workshop, was an important counterpoint, and this volume should be seen in dialogue with their special issue of *Asian Medicine*. Both Kleine's and Monica Wohlrab-Sahr's support of the project, from afar during the COVID-19 pandemic, and also participating in a seminar in Singapore long distance, have continued to bolster the thinking and critical focus of the introduction.

The School of Humanities at the Nanyang Technological University in Singapore funded copyediting and a subvention under SUG Grant M4082222.100. Faizah Zakariah, a friend and interlocutor about many things including a class on medical and religious therapeutics, kindly offered last minute comments on a chapter. The focus group on Religion, Society and Trust let by Justin Clarke and Chistopher Trigg has further allowed me the opportunity to refine my thoughts on the introduction. Nicholas Witkowski, Katherine Hindley and Graham Matthews have been thoughtful interlocutors on the theme of medicine and religion.

I am indebted to Sally Stewart and Dolly Yang for their organisation, attention to detail and generosity as they shepherded the copyediting of this volume through its final stages. I am very grateful for their continuous efforts at many stages of the volume. I also wish to express my thanks to the two anonymous reviewers whose comments sharpened the chapters and the introduction, and to David Cantor and Meredith Carroll at Manchester University Press for shepherding this through peer-review and publication.

Since the inception of this project, Dr. Jennifer Cash and Geoffrey and Rowan Stanley-Baker have given me freedom to travel and time to work, and they have always welcomed me in loving embraces on my return. You are ever my heart and home.

Bibliography

Sivin, N. (1968) *Chinese alchemy: preliminary studies*, Cambridge: Harvard University Press.

Sivin, N. (1978) 'On the Word 'Taoist' as a Source of Perplexity: With Special Reference to the Relations of Science and Religion in Traditional China', *History of Religions*, 17.3–4: 303–30.

Sivin, N. (2000) 'Book review: Christoph Harbsmeier, Science and Civilisation in China, vol. 7, The Social Background, Part 1: language and logic in traditional China', *East Asian Science, Technology, and Medicine*, 17: 121–33. https://www.jstor.org/stable/43150592

Sivin, N. (2005) 'A Multi-dimensional Approach to Research on Ancient Science', *East Asian Science, Technology, and Medicine*, 23: 10–25. http://www.jstor.org/stable/43150669

Sivin, N. (2010) 'Old and New Daoisms', *Religious Studies Review*, 36.1: 31–50. https://doi.org/10.1111/j.1748–0922.2010.01355.x

Sivin, N. (2015) *Health care in eleventh-century China*, New York: Springer. https://doi.org/10.1007/978–3-319–20427–7

Introduction

Michael Stanley-Baker

The terms 'medicine', 'religion' and 'Asia' influence our understanding of the world in important ways. They organise intellectual, social, institutional and economic priorities and orient selves and bodies within the world. Studying the confluence of these three topics, as we suggest in this volume, speaks to larger orders of the ways in which individuals, bodies and things come into relation with each other, with institutions, states and with the world around us. These three carry broad implications about other terms, such as rationality, faith and self. Even while they have shaped the study of Asia for centuries, recent years have seen a new confluence of these interests. People of diverse ethnic, national and political orientations seek individual and collective self-definition through bodily treatments, practices and cultivation techniques that are labelled, in some way, 'Asian'. Attention in the public sphere ranges from the multi-billion dollar 'wellness' industry, to the geopolitical negotiations and national policies of China's and India's national medical institutions, to the ways in which those markets and policies are shaping anew the status, practice and self-understanding of practitioners from those regions. At the same time, humanistic research in the academy has also seen a burgeoning of individual studies, collective works and state-funded research projects. This volume takes stock of recent developments in the field, outlines some theoretical frameworks and ways to understand these issues, and suggests methods and directions for future research.

Why religion and medicine?

Why examine religion and medicine as a 'field' or shared locus of inquiry? Surely the humanistic study of medicine is well-established, as is the study of religion. Shouldn't it be sufficient to note inter-disciplinary studies in those fields? When these two subjects are further refracted through their nuances in Asia, a particular focus comes into view. Medical anthropologists and historians of religion and medicine in the region have long pointed out that practices, which might be considered religious, are involved in therapy and bodily treatments: incantation, prayer, visualisation, rituals, meditation, sacred objects and more. Recent years have seen many of these methods circulate in Western countries under rubrics such as 'alternative', 'complementary' and 'integrative' medicine, and more recently as 'wellness' – labels markedly distant from religion. Many of these methods have been closely or more distantly associated with 'spirituality' movements – another calculated distinction from 'religion', with clear genealogical ties. Conversely, cognitive science and neurology have placed core religious practices, such as meditation and mindfulness, squarely within high-end biotech research labs.

It is undeniable that the terms 'medicine', 'religion' and 'Asia' are not singular nor universal nor stable categories with definite boundaries. The analogues of these terms vary in different times and places, and the actors in these contexts disagree on their boundaries. No attempt is made in this volume to answer the questions: 'What is religion?' or 'What is medicine?' in the abstract. These issues are answered within the histories of those disciplines, where more often than not the response is to point to established local traditions and institutions: genealogies of texts, practitioners and methods. Rather, the focus here is on how religion and medicine have been produced in relation to one another in different times and contexts, and how such boundaries between the two have come to be construed or elided. The question is whether the scholarship on various regions and time periods across Asia has made assumptions about how they were distinguished, and how better to recover the terms and motivations of earlier, regional actors.

This interest in intersections, in rifts, and how actors situate themselves within them, is informed by Helen Verran's (2014) term 'disconcertment', that indistinct sense of rift or disconnect in a given moment of coming-together, and the intellectual work to unpack that epistemological 'itch' to reveal variances in deeply held tacit assumptions about the world and how things work. The unpacking of this sense of disconcertment and what causes it is 'a crucial tool for moving beyond the metaphysics, the subjectivities, and the institutional organisational forms that reproduce hegemonic Western knowledge traditions' (Law and Lin Wen-yuan 2010: 135). The space of encounter, in the interstices of these fields, provides a view onto how people live their lives, how they experience, evaluate and respond to the world at large, and the kinds of authority they rely on. It mediates critical questions about authority, sovereignty, selfhood and the possibilities for being in the world. In these 'epistemic borderlands', moments and spaces where styles of knowing and domains of authority meet and encounter, we see how the boundaries of knowledge are negotiated by the actors who inhabit them.

Why Asia?

Once we cease to accept the historical relationship of the Church to the sciences as a base against which to compare non-European civilisations, or as foundational to our concepts of 'religion', 'science' and 'medicine', the frames of reference for these knowledge forms become much more open-ended. Since the wave of Arabic translations of Greek science and philosophy crashed on Europe's shores in the tenth century and revitalised classical knowledge, the ensuing debates about natural philosophy, theology and medicine have transformed the legitimation, institutions and transmission of medicine in Europe. By the thirteenth century laws appeared in various institutions prohibiting the admixture of clerical and medical learning or practice, and the major European centres of learning began to form discrete faculties for law, theology and medicine (Ziegler 1998: 1–34). The institutional separation of medicine and religion had already begun to take shape, and consistently did so in dialogue with the contours, boundaries and knowledge forms of religion, within parameters set by ecclesiastical institutions. Yet, it is not clear that parallel legacies applied equally in Asia or, if so, how.

Asia forms a distinctive region within which to examine these questions. Historical connections across the region go back at least two thousand years, as shown by the longue durée exchange of goods, art objects, ideas and religion, travelogues and geographic treatises. Monks, traders and envoys have long been circulating along the multiple land and sea routes collectively referred to as the Silk Road (von Richthofen 1877; Waugh 2007; Hansen 2017). They brought medical and religious ideas, materials, texts and practices as demonstrated in a number of landmark works in the last twenty years. Medical knowledge and products were an important ingredient in regional exchanges, and a critical medium for that was religious networks (Lo and Cullen 2005; Despeux 2010; Salguero 2014, 2017; Yoeli-Tlalim 2021). Similarities in biospiritual physiology – the internal structures of the body, which conflate simple differentiations between body, mind and spirit – have drawn the attention of researchers and practitioners over the years. These include the parallel, but subtly different, notions *prana* and *qi* 氣,[1] and the potent locations through which they flow, be they chakras, channels (Ch. *mai* 脈, Skt. *nāḍī*), abstract general fields, specific regions or acupuncture points. The notion of the 'subtle body' has been used as a common lens to encompass these (Samuel and Johnston 2013), and it may be evinced through practices such as meditation, yoga, breathing exercises, visualisation, stretching, incantation and talismans. As Samuel (2013: 250ff) points out, the Chinese, Indian and Tibetan models of the subtle body much more closely correspond with each other than with those from other parts of the world.

These continuities and the histories of their transmission motivate the contours of 'Asia' in this volume, a regional term which means different things to different peoples. In Germany it begins just east of the Bosphorus, whereas in the UK it often refers simply to South Asia. This volume's focus on East, South and Southeast Asia and the Himalayas is not intended to defend an idealised definition of Asia, but rather as to enquire into the kinds of comparability that reflects not only the transmission of *qi*/*prana* ideas and regional trade routes, but also the history of European contact, and the impact of Europhone ideas on scholarship and local administration of the region. While more Westerly Asian medical traditions such as Greco-Arabic Unani are referenced peripherally here in styles of

Bengali mantra as well as the framework of 'Prophetic medicine' in which homeopathy circulated in Malaysia, there is no reason why it should not receive more focus in future comparative studies. Yoeli-Tlalim (2021), for example, describes extensive networks and means of transmission from Europe throughout Asia, and invites the reconceptualisation of region-bound notions of medical knowledge.

The focus on historical continuities across these regions also reflects a recent critical turn in Asian Studies. Collectively, these exchanges invite us to ask whether broader similarities exist in how religion and medicine were configured across the region? Scholars have already begun to work towards decentralising European and American interests in historiography and social theory, and examining regional centres of theory. Chen Kuang-Hsing's *Asia as Method* (2010) has provoked a great deal of commentary, a work which recapitulates Yoshimi Takeuchi's 竹内 好 (1961, 2005) lecture, asking intellectuals in East Asia to think about theory, culture, modernity and progress in terms which are referential not just within distinct nations, but within interrelated regions. Chen's twenty-first century revitalisation of Yoshimi's ideas builds on a swelling tide of publications that preceded his own. To mention a few, Yamashita Shinji *et al.* (2004) track the history of anthropology and ethnography in different nations of East Asia, and describe a sophisticated relationship to theory production, ethnicity and reporting audience. Elman (2005) examines the production of scientific knowledge in the nineteenth and twentieth centuries in ways which privilege the agency of local Chinese actors and institutions, and steps away from a diffusionist model of the transmission of scientific knowledge. On South Asia, the Sanskrit Knowledge-Systems project has produced multiple studies, primary resource databases and a multi-authored volume (Pollock 2011), which examines the vernacularisation of scientific knowledge in 1500–1800 in South Asia. Fu Daiwie (2007), Grace Shen (2007) and Fan Fa-ti (2012) all ask what it would look like, and why it is important, to perform Science and Technology Studies of East Asia that focus on local agency and eschew a European dissemination model of historical change.

Within the study of religion, the concern with representing local actor categories has a genealogy that pushes at the category of religious studies itself, as scholars have wrestled with perennial questions about the identity and intellectual agenda of the discipline, and sought to identify and escape Christo-centric frameworks which still dominate that academy (Masuzawa 2005). One scholar in particular, Robert Campany (2003, 2005, 2009, 2010, 2012, 2018), has persistently asked whether or not the modern category of religion viably reflects the intents and schemas of actors from early imperial China, and Krämer (2013) and Kleine (2013) interrogate the category of religion (*shūkyō* 宗教), imported to Japan only in the nineteenth century. While work on decolonising South Asian religions has been a driving force in studies for some time (King 1999; Mandair 2009; Nicholson 2010), it was only by 2019 when Natasha Heller announced the goal to 'de-colonise Chinese religion' at a workshop titled *Critical Terms for Chinese Religious Studies*, convened by herself, Mark Meulenbeld and others at the Hong Kong Polytechnic University and the Chinese University of Hong Kong. The goal of the workshop was to consider a cluster of terms from Chinese religions as a resource for critical thinking about religion more widely and thereby to develop a gaze on world religions from the perspective of China. Studies such as those above consider religions from *within*, the terms by which they are constructed and emerge. In this volume the perspective is to consider them from the viewpoint of what they are *not* – when do religions become marked as distinct from medicine, vice versa, or are they elided?

As Chen Kuang-hsing (2012: 323) states in his summary of Yoshimi Takeuchi's lecture, 'With the economic rise of India and China, "Asia as Method" has increasingly become an inescapable demand. It has been elevated to be an issue of subjectivity in dealing with the globe'. The focus on medicine and religion in this volume is a reminder that the formation of subjectivity is deeply informed by both scientific and religious praxes – both deserve attention, and as we shall see, boundaries between them are often quite blurred, and are hotly negotiated.

Anxiety and autonomy

Asian religions and medicines speak to multiple aspects of the ways we order things. It is widely accepted that science is part of the very fabric of modernity, the cloth out of which nation states are created and legitimised. Experts do not, however, agree on what the definition of 'science' or 'scientific method' actually is (Shapin 2007). Science is perhaps most particularly fluid at the level of practice as Mol (2002), for example, demonstrates by showing how atherosclerosis is not understood to be the same *thing* by patients, clinicians, lab technicians and hospital managers.

Geopolitically and economically, the world is moving away from a US-centric geo-political formulation. With China and India large on the global horizon, it is imperative for institutional habits of thought to become more flexible, to cope with multiple ways of knowing. Such flexibility is vital for social justice, to address the failure of hegemonic institutions and value norms to accommodate diverse individual and minority-group experiences. It is also important that providers understand, and take into account, in contexts of medical care, the ways that individuals build their worlds of meaning and the significance of their experiences do not match up to the statistical measures which are increasingly the basis of evidence-based medicine. Insight into the ways whereby patients engage in polymedicine is also relevant to anticipating their health-seeking behaviour better. The recent popularisation of traditional Asian medical and spiritual practices has burgeoned into a multi-billion dollar 'wellness' market spanning bodily and spiritual practices.

Modern actors who engage with 'traditional', 'Asian', 'medicines' and 'religion' participate in a kind of modernist shell game, which tacitly negotiates critical issues of selfhood – be they 'modernity', 'rationality' or 'subjectivity'. Practitioners and participants must also navigate the tricky problem of how to retain authority and autonomy, and not surrender one's singular, irreducible experience to reductive quantification, the assimilative power of science, which allows technocrats to wield vast swaths of knowledge about the world and bodies and people themselves. This anxiety is not just personally felt, it takes political forms as nation states attempt to capitalise on such knowledge in governance, while at the same time preventing technical experts from becoming the only authoritative, decision-making voice. The tricky goal here is to keep expertise 'on tap' without its becoming 'on top' (Shapin 2007).

This anxiety, this disconcertment, informs the rise of the wellness industry today and the reach for praxes outside the biomedical, such as Asian medicine, both through scientised means and in resistance to scientific determination. It is that concern to preserve and affirm value systems wherein people can prevent their sense of self from being reduced to data points in someone else's algorithm. This anxiety of reducibility is the essence of Sartre's park bench metaphor. In *Being and Nothingness* (1956: 254–302), Sartre describes the difference between being alone in a park – free to take in its beauty in all the ways one likes, a world with one's self at the centre – and the terrible switch when another person enters the scene and gazes upon one, reconstructing the world in ways that place the 'other' at the centre, and in which the first man's entire system of meaning becomes valueless. In that moment, he must confront the terrible potential of his own reducibility, the reduction of his selfhood to an insignificant feature of someone else's version of the universe. It is telling that the culmination (1956: 302) of Sartre's extensive reflection comes down to his body: 'What then is my body? What is the body of the Other?' This question, arguably, is refracted in the Western turn to Asian body practices and rejection of the alienation of biomodern reductivism, in a search for a fundamental ground of being.

Tensions with Asianness, otherness and existential being percolate at the boundaries of the Western quest for existential being. To portray Sartre's work as 'indebted' to Buddhist thought would be simplistic, but numerous scholars have debated whether nineteenth century portrayals of Buddhist philosophy played a part in his intellectual genealogy, leading him to phenomenologists like Heidegger and Husserl (for an overview, see [Franklin 2012]). Camus' (1946 [1942]) existentialist novel *L'Étranger*, written roughly ten years earlier than *Being and Nothingness*, culminates in the killing of an Arab (cf. the orientalised 1980 pop song 'Killing an Arab', by The Cure). The tale makes painfully clear that the 'Oriental' or 'Asian' other is a powerful part of that imagination of modernity, selfhood and otherness, and that those relations are filled with the potential for violence.

Although the examples above are European/American, patterns of identity, autonomy and sovereignty around these questions are widely felt, and at many different levels of society. It is no coincidence that the rise of the Indian ministry for traditional medicines, the Ministry of Āyurveda, Yoga, Naturopathy, Unani, Siddha, Sowa-Rigpa and Homoeopathy (AYUSH), was coeval with the resurgence of the Hinducentric nationalism and the rise of the Bharatiya Janata Party (BJP) in India. Formed in part to prevent patenting of Indian-origin medical knowledge by foreign concerns, a modern form of earlier colonial extraction and appropriation of cultural goods, AYUSH is part of the same broad phenomenon of this negotiation of modernities, identity and authority (Chaudhary and Singh 2012). In a curious refraction of Shapin's (2007) point above about the widespread emphasis on science, despite ambiguities about what science actually *is*, China's large-scale state backing of Chinese medicine began with Mao's policy to promote it as a 'national treasure', even though Mao himself reportedly did not use it (Li Zhisui 1994; Taylor 2005). Religion, Medicine and Asia do not refract simply personal, local or regional concerns, they are felt at international levels. The World Health Organization (WHO) (2019) introduced Chinese disease terms into the *International Statistical Classification of Diseases and Related Health Problems*, and a standardised set of technical terms (2022), opening the way for traditional medicines to be included within science-determined techno-polities around the world, to mixed reception by the international community (Editorial 2019; Lam *et al.* 2019). The religious aspects of some concepts are muted, but nevertheless present: the term for spirit (*shen* 神) is largely treated as a synonym for state of mind, and the notion of correspondence theory (天人合 – *tianren heyi*) which has described the relations between gods and humans, is given as 'Unity of humans and nature' (2022: 45).

The history of modern knowledge production has traditionally been dominated by the history of 'science' cut loosely as a Western- or European-origin praxis, so that scholars working in areas across Asian regions have been at pains to justify and define the terms of the inquiry. The inherent hierarchies and biases implicit in terms such as 'rationality', 'science', 'oriental', and 'belief', have been well documented (Tambiah 1990; Good 1994). Needham's monumental *Science and Civilisation in China* series was a major contribution not only for China but for Asian sciences more generally, and the study of Asian medical systems came into its own with Charles Leslie's (1977) *Asian Medical Systems*, and the founding of the International Association for the Study of Traditional Asian Medicine (IASTAM).[2] Despite the long history of this work, recent ethnographies continue to underscore the problems of this language. Mei Zhan (2009: 119–42) describes how the notion of the 'miracle cure', when used to represent Asian medicines, is compromised by a self-orientalisation which at once exoticises and alienates. Documentaries, such as Giles' and Finch's (2006) BBC programme on Traditional Chinese Medicine (TCM), still blithely characterise practitioners of these medicines as those who 'believe', and scientists as those who 'discover' and who 'know', to say nothing of the orientalising tropes used to disparage Chinese medicine during the COVID-19 pandemic (Palmer 2020; Lawson 2022).

Such concerns not only surround practices circulating in the global wellness market, but also the ways in which traditional Asian medicines are promoted or resisted by national organisations, having repercussions in turn on the ways practitioners in the countries of origin perceive and engage with their heritage. As China and India play larger roles in the global economy and geopolitical relations, humanistic scholars have increased their efforts at decolonialising, at re-evaluating the history of knowledge in those regions and decentralising European historical and epistemological priorities. Scholarly research on religions and medicine plays a part in the cosmopolitics of knowing (Stengers 2010) that are being negotiated at multiple levels on the world stage.

Situat*ing* knowledge

Examining how actors situate religion and medicine brings our attention to the fact that practitioners often negotiate their positions within multiple fields at the same time, as they organise the hierarchies and relationships between those different kinds of knowledge. As Haraway (1988) pointed out in her paper on the power relations inherent in the way different kinds of knowledge are positioned vis-à-vis each other, knowledge is always 'situat*ed*'. The term calls attention to the ways in which cultural categories and forms of knowing emerge and shape ourselves, our action, our worlds, and how people inhabit those categories through specific practices. By placing seemingly static and isolated knowledge within a web of social, power and material relations, the term 'situated' brings that knowledge to life, and emphasises its processes and its changing dynamics. This further aligns with a move in science studies away from representational depictions of scientific knowledge.

Representational theories portray science as a theoretical mirror of reality, which takes the form of laws and theories. These laws have no space or time: they exist in an abstract consciousness, a nameless subjectivity akin to Cartesian pure consciousness. Because human understanding of nature is forever flawed, scientists struggle to continue to improve it so that it matches more closely the real world, but can never fully represent it. In science studies and actor-network theory, the image of science is that of a processual engagement, a set of actions performed by specific historical actors who engage with the world on the basis of certain assumptions and, over time, gradually adjust their assumptions and expectations. This interaction takes place between humans and the world mediated by material, institutions, knowledge forms, tools, technical practices and many other factors (Latour 2007). Such an analytic shifts 'knowledge' from the realm of thought to the social, from that of abstract ideas to material (and social) practice. In line with Haraway's (1988) paper, knowledge becomes embedded in social and material networks. This moves from a focus on epistemology (how one knows) to ontology (what is known, or what constitutes knowledge). In this perspective, knowledge is never permanently fixed or situated. Rather, we encounter different moments of actors situating their worlds, and themselves within those worlds, and the positions are dynamic and changing. This ontological take is reflected in the title of Department III of the Max Planck Institute for the History of Science – 'Actions, Artefacts, Knowledge' – which generously hosted the workshop which began this project. A specific agenda of the department is the inclusion of non-European knowledge forms in the history of science, as this book does.

'Situat*ing*' could be used to describe not only the work of local actors which we study in their times and locations, but also the intellectual work of scholars who write about them. They too keep busy situating actors, action and knowledge, not only in relation to their local environs, but also within the space they occupy in modernity, through their use of 'medicine' and 'religion' as scholarly, categorical terms. Whether scholars adopt nineteenth-century frameworks that orientalise, that bifurcate 'rationality' and 'reason' from 'faith' and 'superstition', or whether they advocate for marginalised voices – all these choices are based in relations of power. They are always bound up in situating knowledge, jostling them up in a world order of authority. The chapters in this volume apply the same lens to both secondary scholarship – situated in modern academies and time periods and contexts of relation between Europe and Asia – and primary sources – be they catalogues, manuals, bureaucratic records or stories of informants. Medicine and religion serve as actor categories for academics. Scholars and practitioners are not separate communities; categories matter and we all participate in them.

Embodiment

As these moments are situated within local relations, they are also inescapably material and embodied, and not infinitely open to cultural inscription. The body is at once the locus and genesis of selfhood and subjectivity, while it is also defined and shaped by the systems which describe it and embed it in ideologies. Put another way: we live in bodies, and also through them; our experience and expression are shaped by our bodies and how they are described, while the body is itself also resistant to discursive reduction – it has its own material reality, its own life, which goes on regardless of the cultural system in which it exists. Whether we are talking about interior meditation practices, exercise, diet, acupuncture, rituals, incantations, visualisation, massage, surgery, herbal formulas or other methods, these practices participate in world values and systems of habit that shape and configure the individual, to which they can shape themselves, and which also embody truths in the world.

The history of studies of the body and embodiment are far too broad to summarise here, but it is useful to situate the perspectives discussed here in relation to a few genealogies of inquiry. Lévi-Strauss (1963: 167–85) was interested in borderline, periphery figures, like the shaman, because he thought the ways in which their behaviour was afforded extra-special status, which might be taken for madness in other cultures, indicated the structural value systems of a society. While latent social and intellectual forces are still a goal to tease out in current research, scholars do not now take for granted that such systems hold ubiquitously throughout a society, or manifest an abstract philosophy, or cultural universal cultural grammar, linking to reality. It is the processes and relationalities, rather than structures, that are of interest.

Where Foucault (1978 [French edn. 1976], 2012) was perhaps the most articulate about power and its expression through medical knowledge and practice, the strong sense of the hegemonic in his writing is not assumed here. Power is manifest through knowledge of the body, through institutions and practices, but individuals also wield it, and are not solely subject *to* it. Rather than individuals being subject to biomedicine, power is variously negotiated through the relations, hierarchies and forms of knowledge. Whether this be through China and India asserting the value of traditional medicines on the national or international stage, through local politicians appealing to myth structures and religious tropes, or to scholarly collectives which assert the equal and comparative value of studying non-European sciences, Asian religions and medicine serve as vehicles through which power and epistemic authority are actively negotiated.

The late eighties and early nineties focus on 'the' singular body is perhaps exemplified by the collected series published by Zone (Feher *et al.* 1989). A broad, diverse collection of multiple ways in which bodies are encultured, this series moved towards the statement that 'the' body is not unitary. With this foundational assumption in place today, chapters in the present collection do not display a panoply of embodiments, but rather present a narrowly focused examination of ways in which embodied cultures are negotiated, compared and evaluated, attending to comparable historical 'moments' and their possible continuities. The goal is not to demonstrate diversity, but to begin to collect a working vocabulary of methods of how these come to be, to provide a palette of working tools for research.

Arthur Kleinman's (1980; Kleinman and Benson 2006) concept of 'explanatory models' is extremely useful for focusing on the ways that people understand and relate to the processes of disease independent of physicians' disease concepts. Kleinman's end goal was to improve medical care and improve the patient–physician interaction, and it matters less how the patient gets to her model than it does to understand clearly what model she has. The interest of chapters in this volume is decidedly ontological – asking how do clusters of ideas/practices/people come into being, how are they negotiated? Therefore, while explanatory models are key to understanding these clusters, the terms and conditions by which they are formed are the primary focus.

Annemarie Mol's (2002) study of a Dutch atherosclerosis unit is exemplary in two ways. Firstly, in the careful but explosive way she teases out radically different epistemologies and relations to the disease across different actor communities – patients, physicians, lab technicians and hospital administrators. Secondly, her steady rejection of the claim to the God's-eye view that is asserted by theoretical abstraction, and her commitment to remain close to terms relevant to the action at hand. These create a mediated space between participant observation and abstract philosophy, a space where the patterns of the moment reach out beyond the immediate context yet remain indeterminate. She teases out the latent patterns, the implications and epistemologies at play in a given moment which point beyond, out towards something more, something that might be transcendent, but refrains from ever making absolutist claims about these abstractions. Absolutist claims take part in a power game, and deny the emplacement, the situatedness of the scholar within the creation of discourse and power. The current volume also invites readers to pay attention to the power inherent in the terms scholars use, the gazes they adopt.

Judith Farquhar's (1994; Farquhar and Wang Jun 2011) insight into the absence of epistemological reflection in Chinese medicine, and the ways in which it manifests in training, genealogies and practice, has been informative for Asian medicine more widely, and for all the authors in this volume. Her contribution to the field of Asian medicine and to the workshop that produced this volume in particular has been substantial, as we will see below.

Bourdieu's (1977, 1990, 1991) notion of the 'field' is central to the understanding of 'religions' and 'medicines' as social contexts of competition in which actors seek to position themselves in relation to one another. His interest in 'practice' and 'habitus' is vital for understanding how bodily habits embed, or situate, actors within those fields – taking on specific habits, practices, tastes and values embeds one in a nexus of social relations. These are foundational for understanding the social value and valence of religio-medical practices.

State of the field

With these theoretical approaches in mind, it is useful to situate this volume within the broader context of scholarship on medicine and religion in Asia. While it is impossible to provide a comprehensive review here, I will point out some major landmarks, research questions and frameworks that have been at play in conferences, special issues, funded research projects and new journals over the last twenty years, which have collectively brought the conversation to a new place.

Linda Barnes' (2011) methodological overview of religion and healing is a good place to begin. Her paper, in over 80 pages, spans a wide range of materials that do not normally get associated in the same conferences, journals or departments, providing short histories of the fields of religious studies, medical anthropology, cross-cultural psychology and biomedical clinical care. She typologises ways in which multi-modal praxes of religion and healing are studied, such as in different religious, regional or ethnic traditions, and then turns to applied medicine and biomedical approaches – whether through psychology, applied anthropology, different forms of clinical care, medical chaplaincy, or the development of theoretical models, such as the biopsychosocial. She lays out histories of important theoretical problems that fields like anthropology and religion have wrestled with, such as the constructedness of the term religion and the problem of establishing universal categories of comparison. The breadth of literature is so wide, especially between the history of religion and applied clinical psychology, that it becomes apparent that these fields and discourses are *not* in conversation, but Barnes argues that they *should* be, and the paper brings these together in important ways. Of note is her response to the failure of 'universal categories', such as medicine and religion, to encompass the wide varieties of practice, with a list of comparative categories of action in which religion and medicine intersect:

- Ultimate Human Possibility
- Suffering and Affliction
- Personhood/Self
- Illness
- Healers

- Health-Seeking Behaviour
- Interventions
- Efficacy

In general, the breadth of this paper, underscored with hundreds of references, make this foundational reading for any graduate or advanced undergraduate seminar.

Focusing more narrowly on religion and medicine in Asia in particular, is Vargas-O'Bryan and Zhou's (2014) edited volume, which gathers studies from across the region to consider the confluence of disease, healing and religion. The considerable overlaps in the chapters reinforce the sense that there is a particular set of conversations about these themes that is common to Asia, and that work needs to be done to tease out what they are. Topics range widely. Paula Arai's (2014: 155–69) study of the neurological benefits of socio-ritual practices like bowing in Japan shows a correlation of these practices to lower aggression and higher conflict resolution. Ivette Vargas-O'Bryan (2014: 122–45) considers the contrasts between purified, non-ritual presentation of Tibetan healing in urban settings and rural practitioners' free mixing of the role of geomancy, local spirits and social forces in their explanatory models of disease and corresponding treatments. Both papers articulate a tension between narrower and broader notions of medicine, located in an urban/rural divide in Tibet for Vargas-O'Bryan, and for Arai's elderly Japanese women Zen practitioners, between two notions of healing. Arai articulates bowing within a wider praxis of what she calls the 'Way of Healing', an attitudinal adjustment to suffering as a way of transforming their life experience into Buddhist praxis. While they regard this approach as *iyasareteiru* 癒やされている (to gratefully be healed), they distinguish this from a more self-centric *iyashi* 癒やし (to heal). Vesna Wallace (2014: 101–21) identifies Chinese medical theory clothed in syncretic garb in Mongolian medicine, where Yin and Yang theory are translated as wisdom and method; and Mark Greene (2014: 54–68) demonstrates how even though a Wong Tai Sin 黃大仙 temple in Hong Kong has replaced mediumistic treatments with TCM dispensed by trained physicians, participants still feel that the influence of the god improves treatment efficacy.

Anthony Cerulli (2014: 86–100) draws on medical humanities and medical anthropology approaches to argue that the medical adaptations within Ayurvedic literature of literary, mythic and religious narratives can be fruitfully read as narrative medicine.[3] Some practitioners, despite being disconcerted by the need they feel to square a dichotomy between spiritual and material forces and treatment methods, provide narratives which are nevertheless richly informative, and reflect well Kleinman's (1980: 107) breakdown of five areas of explanatory models: aetiology; onset and type(s) of symptoms; pathology; severity of sickness; and treatment.

Daniel Cohen (Vargas-O'Bryan and Zhou 2014: 69–84) also pays attention to explanatory models in a Hindu context, describing the work of a medium who dispels ghostly-caused disease in Varanasi. He presents one complex case of a priest's unpacking of individual and community experiences of accountability, suffering loss and blame, and how he prescribes rituals to untangle these knotted relations, with the end result that after years of effort, the couple are able to have a child. Helen Lambert's (2014: 9–21) examination of north Indian subaltern medical practices sets out to counter the dominant portrayal of Asian therapeutic methods as predominantly secular, and as other chapters in the volume do, to elide any boundaries between 'medicine' and 'religion', offering instead modes of 'collision' and 'convergence' as conceptual tools with which to think. Taken together, this volume comprises a methodological toolset and, as I have intimated here, the potential for an emergent typology of *ways* in which actors situate themselves in relation to medicine and religion.

Just recently, in a series of Terry Lectures at Yale, the anthropologist of Chinese medicine, Judith Farquhar (2020: 14), shared her own position on the relationship between religion, science and Chinese medicine. Arguing that 'medicine is the field of human endeavour that most challenges the idea that religion and science are different things', she invites readers to appreciate and bear witness to how 'an East Asian science joins its unique powers for knowing and intervening in the patterns of human life and human suffering with the virtues of the myriad things that make up the vast flow of the spontaneous cosmic Way' (2020: 180). This position piece responded to the endowment for the lecture series, which expressly calls for 'the building of the truths of science and philosophy into the structure of a broadened and purified religion' (2020: v). While Farquhar distances herself from the progressivism of the endowment's founder, which presaged Needham's own vision of an ecumenical, unified sea of science, she finds common ground in denying a hard binary between science and religion. She argues that there are multiple ways of knowing – and thus of being in – the world, that are accessible through traditions like Chinese medicine. These multiple modes of inhabiting the world, and the move to elide science/religion binaries, is one of the approaches to religion and medicine written about by the authors in this volume.

While the three volumes discussed above stand as important landmarks within the field, it is also important to sketch out overall currents within which these works should be understood. While the conversations in scholarly communities have been mainly contoured by region and language, the discussion below shows common directions in representing the intellectual legacies within each region.

South Asia

Looking to the changing patterns of research on Asian knowledge over the past twenty years or so, it is worth recalling how they have been anticipated by the great ritual scholar, Fritz Staal, in his 1993 inaugural lecture at the International Institute for Asian Studies at Leiden. Scholars have, he argued, been blinkered to science in South Asia because 'Europeans Discovered China during the Enlightenment and India during the Romantic period. We are therefore predisposed to find in China science and in India religion' (Staal 1993: 21). The dynamics of medicine and religion are not uniform across Asia, not only do they have their different regional characteristics, our understanding of them is also impacted by varying styles of Western scholarly attention to those regions. It is thus important to take stock of what has been done in various regions in recent years.

The explosion of yoga scholarship in the last twenty years can hardly be encompassed in this brief overview, but it has seen conversations about embodiment, consciousness, religion, healing and knowledge transmission move from esoteric academic discourse to mainstream public consumption, through numerous high-quality translations and historical studies. A tiny selection of works might include the following, but should be taken as a starting point rather than a comprehensive overview: White (1996), Feuerstein (1998), Alter (2004), Richard (2009), Mallinson (2010), Newcombe (2019), Newcombe and O'Brien-Kop (2021).

Major research projects have also focused on embodied and epistemic practices. The ERC-funded *Haṭha Yoga Project* (Mallinson 2015–2020), based at SOAS in London, has gathered together world-class Sanskritists, practitioners, ethnographers and art historians to participate in a multi-modal historiographic and modern study of yoga, generating large amounts of scholarship (http://hyp.soas.ac.uk/). The AYURYOG project (Wujastyk, 2015–2020), also funded by the ERC, headed by Dagmar Wujastyk and based in Vienna and Alberta, has generated a large number of publications, exhibitions, workshops and physical demonstrations of alchemical recipes that are changing the conversation on Āyurveda, yoga and alchemy, drawing out the interrelated knowledge and history of these three fields (www.ayuryog.org/).

On South Asian sciences more generally, the journal *History of Science in South Asia* (Wujastyk *et al.*) was founded in 2013, affording a new locus for conversation about the domain, scope, methods and principles of science more extensive than knowledge of European origins. It takes science to be broadly conceived, to include all forms of rigorous intellectual activity that adopt at least to some extent a quantitative and empirical approach, as in the German 'Die Wissenschaft', that covers most forms of academic scholarship. The editors set a curriculum that engages with principal terms, methods and ideas in the history of science, inviting scholars to engage with logical, empirical and quantitative thought also in South Asia. They propose a reading list of Grant's *History of Natural Philosophy* (2008), Latour's *Laboratory Life* (1979) and Netz' *Shaping of Deduction* (2011), alongside critiques against the fetishisation of science in modernity (Shapin 2007).[4]

This journal and its intellectual directions are informed by the earlier *Sanskrit Knowledge-Systems on the Eve of Colonialism* project which sought to affirm the rigour and outline the contours of core South Asian sciences between 1550–1750 across major regional complexes in South Asia and Tibet, work which has been downplayed by legacy scholarship from earlier generations (Pollock *et al.* 2001–2005). Those contours are defined in the project as '*vyākaraṇa* (language analysis), *mīmāṃsā*, *nyāya* (logic and epistemology), *dharmaśāstra* (law and moral philosophy, broadly speaking), *alaṅkāraśāstra* (poetics), *āyurveda* (life science), and *jyotiḥśāstra* (astral science)' (Pollock 2011: 6). The relationship with religion and their interplay with innovative and bold position statements have come out of this project, including the journal, and also the collected volume *Forms of Knowledge in Early Modern Asia* (Pollock 2015: 2011), an important salvo at pains to correct the unequal heritage called out by Staal (1993). This volume introduced early modern scholars and intellectual movements that had been little studied, which deserved more light in their own right. Religion appears little as an operative term in these pages, and as these intellectual directions become more understood, it would perhaps be useful to enquire in the vein of the *Multiple Secularities* project (see section below) about the contours of these disciplines' relation to religion, although Gyatso's chapter stands out (Gyatso 2004 [2011]). Since the *Forms of Knowledge* volume, studies of South and East Asia are coming into closer conversation, as witnessed by the recent comparative volume on historiography of both regions (Elman and Pollock 2018).

Himalayas

Research on Tibetan medicine, or the de-nationalised term *sowa-rigpa,* has also burgeoned dramatically. The ERC-funded project Re-Assembling Tibetan Medicine RATIMED (Kloos 2014–2019) studied the translocal industrialisation of *sowa-rigpa* medicine across Himalayan regions, a necessary feature of which was the stripping away of religious and ritual elements, and the resignification of treatment and transformation of disease terms, among other material and institutional changes. Sienna Craig (2012) enquires into the notion of efficacy, and how the very framework of the question reduces Tibetan medicine to something other than itself, excluding patients' lived experience. Adams *et al.* (2011) collected together a host of chapters examining the multiple worlds that are inhabited by, and created with, Tibetan medical practice, and examined the ways in which religious practice is not simply foreshortened by biomedical frames, but also how Tibetan medicine exerts a transforming force on hegemonic forms of knowledge as they are adapted when deployed in local contexts. They note the overall framework in which Tibetan medicine is situated with regard to religion and to science, which connects residents of the Tibetan highlands seeking IV injections and syringes, and American practitioners interested in meditation and spirituality, both are turning to Tibetan doctors. Frances Garrett's (2008) study of Tibetan embryology engages the religion/medicine dichotomy during the twelfth to the fifteenth century, arguing that because spiritual cultivation takes place within and through the body, and the philosophical questions about matter arising from nothingness, embryology was a religious matter and site for philosophical reflection. The discussion about embryology over this period also demonstrates the gradual emergence of writing concentrated on medical matter.

Looking to the latter end of this period, Janet Gyatso (2015) argues that medicine was the site of a conflicted relationship between empiricism and religion, and of a 'mentality' (2015: 91) that knowledge can be revised and improved based on empirical evidence, which set medicine apart from other forms of knowledge. Notably this took place within the bounds of state-supported literate medicine. Geoffrey Samuel (Ch. 7) responds to her study on this topic in this volume. William McGrath's (2019) volume, *Knowledge and Context in Tibetan Medicine,* squarely confronts dichotomies between religion and medicine, with half of the contributions addressing this conceptual divide in the context of humoral versus demonic aetiologies, divination versus channel examination, spirit possession and the industrialisation of modern pharmaceuticals. Theresia Hofer's (2014) Rubin Museum of Art exhibition and edited volume, *Bodies in Balance*, bring together the visual, the experiential and the epistemological, making these domains more accessible to the public, as did the exhibit of the Lukhang Temple at the Wellcome Museum by Baker and Garde (2015–2016). Baker (2019) calls on historical, anthropological and biological research to outline the spiritual physiology of Tibetan yoga and situate the practices within both biological and soteriological frames.

East Asia

Looking to East Asia, new foci and topics have emerged. Early on, Joseph Needham (Needham and Wang 1956: 161) argued that Daoism contained 'the elements of political collectivism, religious mysticism and the training of the individual for a material immortality, developed many of the most important features of the scientific attitude'. This claim was initially influential, but came be refuted in Western scholarship, in particular by Nathan Sivin (1995a, 1995b), although it is still popular in East Asian histories (Gai Jianmin 2001; Jiang Sheng and Tang Weixia 2002, 2010 – see below). On the back of subsequent developments in the histories of Daoism, technology and medicine in China, new attempts have been made to fine tune our understanding of the ways and means by which Daoism and medicine have or have not converged. Two research groups have emerged in Germany in recent years, including Department III of the Max Planck Institute for the History of Science, directed by Dagmar Schäfer. While not limited to East Asia, the department's research networks and impetus to bring Chinese sciences to the table of the history of science as a non-subaltern partner have made it an important port of call for historians of science from East Asia. The *Reclaiming Turtles All the Way Down* project (Onaga *et al.* 2020), looks at Asian cosmologies and their reception in Europe. *The Body of Animals*, also based in Department III, looks at the ways in which humans know and configure animals, and challenges the framework of the laboratory or natural history as endpoints of that knowledge, and has produced papers such as Schäfer and Yi's (2018) foray into Song dynasty veterinary medicine. *Visualization and Material Cultures of the Heavens* (Brentjes 2018) examines Eurasian and North African texts, images and objects representing the heavens. My own *Drugs Across Asia* project, initially funded by Department III, examined the circulation of *Materia medica* across early imperial medical, Daoist and Buddhist writings (Stanley-Baker 2018; Stanley-Baker *et al.* 2018), before I relocated to Nanyang Technological University in Singapore, where I have published digitally tagged editions of early medical texts by Daoist authors (Stanley-Baker *et al.* 2020a, 2020b; Xu Duoduo and Stanley-Baker 2021). Further work comparing Chinese and Malay primary sources and linking them to modern botany, biodiversity and biochemistry databases is available at www.polyglotasianmedicine.com/ (Stanley-Baker *et al.* 2021).

The International Consortium for Research in the Humanities *Fate, Freedom and Prognostication* directed by Michael Lackner at Erlangen-Nürnberg University focusses on premodern East Asia in comparison with European predictive regimens and technologies.[5] Deliberately not contouring to 'science' as an analytic, it focused on methods and the frameworks in which they emerge, giving voice to the means for organising knowledge on East Asia that do not intuitively fit within older rubrics of 'science'. Many scholars of Daoism, Buddhism and East Asian medicine have developed publications while there. Most notable is their volume on prognostication in the Chinese literary imagination (Lackner *et al.* 2020).

The term 'Daoist Medicine' has arisen as a historical topic in Chinese scholarship, inspired in particular by Gai Jianmin (2001), prompting calls for nuance in the ways in which 'Daoism' is used to qualify early actors. I argue (Stanley-Baker 2009, 2019) that the pivot to Daoist medicine as a form of science is situated within contemporary politics and institutional funding inside China. A major project on Daoist Science at Jinan University has sought to document Daoist Science as a distinct genre of knowledge, producing periodised histories of developments within medicine, alchemy, divination and assorted technical arts (*fangshu* 方術) (Jiang Sheng and Tang Weixia 2002, 2010). Inspired by studies (Garrett 2008) in Tibetan embryology, Andreeva and Steavu (2015) have collected a number of chapters on embryological theory in East Asia, articulating the way sexual cultivation, embryology and cosmogenesis cohered as common fields of enquiry among Buddhists and Daoists in China and Japan. While the influences of Tantric yoga which were dynamic in Tibetan embryology were felt in Japan, Daoist cosmogenetic practices were home-grown, emerging from the earliest phases of Han dynasty (209 BCE–220 CE) Daoism, where salvation involved transformation of the interior subtle and physical bodies.

It should be pointed out that the convergence of personal and bodily well-being and salvational goals are tacit in the titles of works on the early imperial period such as *In Search of Personal Welfare* (Poo Mu-chou 1998) and *Imperilled Destinies* (Verellen 2019), which deliberately cover wide ranges of concern for those actors who bridge what are now considered as secular or religious fields. I argue (Stanley-Baker 2013, forthcoming) that cultural categories were in flux over this time, as shown by the imperial bibliographies at either end of the Six Dynasties (220–589 CE) when medicine and religion emerged as related, but increasingly distant, cultural categories over this period. Elsewhere, I have argued that *qi* 氣 forms a cohering substrate, which brings together epistemic practices that take part in very different ontologies, spanning the gamut of the sciences, religion and governance (Stanley-Baker 2021). Practices such as *daoyin* 導引 (guiding and pulling exercises) were adopted by religious sects during the Six Dynasties and later re-medicalised in the unified Sui dynasty, under the aegis of the court medical academy (Yang 2018, 2022). These practices are cognate to Indian and Tibetan yoga, and while no direct textual links exist to prove it, many scholars suspect these practices were influential on the South and Central Asian traditions (Yang 2023). Dominic Steavu (2015) argues that both religion and medicine were subject to the same processes of domestication by the state, and that bureaucratisation served as an important epistemologically defining force. Not all scholars of Imperial China narrate a convergence of medicine and religion, however. Paul Unschuld consistently pits a hard line of empirical rationalism within medical writings against those who 'have truck with spirits' (Unschuld 2009, 2010), and argues (2003: 324) that the same motivations were shared between first-century Chinese physicians and eighteenth- and nineteenth-century Western naturalists and physicians.

Looking towards Japan we find a strong epistemological control exerted by Buddhists, and backed by the state, which prevented the explicit transmission of Daoist ritual techniques (Richey 2015), but did mean that Chinese medicine, exported to Japan, was practised equally by physicians and monks (Triplett 2019a, 2019b, 2021). As pointed out by Triplett in this volume, the discipline of medicine was defined by legal codes, but practice was diversified across secular and religious actors. She argues for the 'interplay' of medicine and religion, and her volume (2019) identifies this as a 'complex relationship'. A diverse range of healing rituals were practised by monks. Special attention has been given recently to studies of obstetric and pediatric rituals (Andreeva and Steavu 2015;

Lomi 2014, 2017, 2018). The topic of Buddhism and religion in Japan has become so rich that it is now a section of Oxford Bibliographies (Andreeva 2018).

Transregional approaches

While each region has its own conversations and historiography, these are not siloed from one another; related methodological approaches are employed by scholars across Asian studies. Whether through critical philology, de-colonisation and cultural reappropriation of ethnic practices, whether nation-states nationalising their indigenous medicine, whether it be Europeans and Americans expanding their cultural horizons through Asian health and wellbeing practices, there is a common fabric that all participate in. One example is the publication of three books on poisons in the same year: Liu Yan's (2021) *Healing with Poisons* on the multi-valent notion of *du* 毒 in medieval China, Barbara Gerke's (2021) *Taming the Poisonous* on toxic minerals in Tibetan medicine, and Alisha Rankin's (2021) *Poison Trials*, which documents early modern experimentation in Europe on poisons and toxins. Read together, the three works make an excellent case study for the different configurations of religion, medicine and epistemic authority across Eurasia.

Some programmes have focused specifically on these similarities across Asia: the Anthropology Research Group at Oxford on Eastern Medicines and Religions, headed by Elisabeth Hsu, focuses explicitly on the family resemblances between religions and medicines across South and East Asia and the Himalayas.[6] Hsu's (1999) work on religious and medical dimensions of Chinese healing should be taken as germinal for the group, which has hosted a wide variety of projects, seminar series, conferences examining religion and medicine in popular settings, in institutions and in transnational diaspora. Topics have covered blood, women's bodies, self-cultivation, Chinese *materia medica*, ethnic minority religions, classical literature and many more. The scholarship produced through the Group is a significant cornerstone of the field.

The International Association for the Study of Traditional Asian Medicines (IASTAM) is also an important intellectual forum for researchers to compare scholarship across Asia. A practitioner-scholar society, it brings together historians, anthropologists and practitioners from across the region, with foci on traditions from East and South Asia and the Himalayas. It regularly hosts conferences, gives senior and junior academic prizes, publishes the journal *Asian Medicine* and practises outreach through social media via www.asianmedicinezone.com/ and the Facebook group of the same title. Publications, prize-winning papers and conference submissions regularly reflect religious kinds of therapy, and address the problematics of Western-category bifurcation of contiguous streams of therapeutic practice. Many of the authors in this volume are members of IASTAM, and the conversation this book takes part in is an ongoing current within the society.

Multiple secularities

Another important development in the last decade is the work of the Kolleg Forschungsgruppe 'Multiple Secularities' at Leipzig University.[7] Rather than a study of secular*ism* (loosely defined as an anti-religious position, promoting empiricism and science instead), this project examines modes of secular*ity*, that is the ways in which societies, cultures and institutions mark boundaries between religious and non-religious domains (Wohlrab-Sahr and Burchardt 2012; Burchardt and Wohlrab-Sahr 2013). Beginning with premodern Asia, they examine how different societies contour the religious and the non-religious, in order better to understand the match or mismatch of boundary markers adopted during or after European encounters (Kleine and Wohlrab-Sahr 2016; Wohlrab-Sahr and Kleine 2021). They 'seek to identify the respective epistemes and cultural predispositions, the social and epistemic structures that existed prior to the introduction of Western knowledge regimes and generated certain path-probabilities, in order to account for the multiplicity of secularities in the present world' (Killinger *et al.* 2019: 236). Their special issue of *Asian Medicine* includes a series of papers analysing emic categories of distinction in Japan, India and Tibet. Of note is their introduction of the sociological frameworks favoured in the project, namely Weber's attention to intended primary purposes, Niklas Luhmann's (2013) systems theory for analysing social structures, and Bourdieu's notion of social fields. The editors note the challenges of distinguishing social structures once one descends from the meta-level of general structures to the meso-level of institutions, where actors of all stripes are engaged in healing, be they priests, family members, literati, government appointees or otherwise, and suggest that a number of analytical tools can be found at the level of epistemes where religion and medicine become distinguished (Killinger *et al.* 2019). These include ends and purposes; means and methods; framing and interpretation; competence or charisma; function or service; and sources of authority and legitimacy.

Buddhist medicine

Buddhist medicine has recently come to the fore as a second-order category which traverses all three regions of the Himalayas, South and East Asia, foregrounding the translation of practices and knowledge in different regional contexts (Salguero 2014, 2017, 2020; Salguero and Macomber 2020). Dozens of translated primary sources and critical essays cover themes and topics as diverse as figures of healers; monastic discipline; doctrinal issues; healing rituals; meditation cures and illnesses; hybridity and interaction with medical traditions.

Some have pointed out that Buddhist medicine was never a historical actor category, an intellectual device used by actors in the past to organise knowledge, and that it has only recently been invented (Gyatso 2017). I have levelled an analogous critique about the term 'Daoist medicine', a term of art that is a novel intellectual concept with no precedent before the twentieth century (Stanley-Baker 2019). I differ from Gyatso, however, in that I do find that such anachronisms are useful as analytical etic concepts, they simply need to be used with nuance and precision, in order to carefully distinguish actor categories from modern notions. Used without caution, the novel term could artificially homogenise quite varied cultural practices, and impose continuities at times when practitioners were very vocal about their differences – something

Salguero scrupulously avoids. Such categorical frameworks can be used fruitfully to outline a wide swath of related cultural materials, for considering the ways in which they are related. On this point, also see Salguero (2022).

Salguero and I have also used another term in earlier work, namely the 'religio-medical marketplace' in early medieval China (Stanley-Baker 2013; Salguero 2014). This metaphor refers to the comparison, critique, borrowing and repackaging of each other's therapeutic and salvific practices engaged in by actors in medieval China. There were known tropes or genres of activity, which were more related to each other than to others, such as herbal medicine; exercises; incantations and spells; visualisation and meditation; the healing power of charismatic figures; explanatory models for disease and others (Stanley-Baker 2013: 41). Practitioners clearly competed with one another in varying ways, and a great deal of negotiation of authority took place.

An excessive focus on the economic aspects of the metaphor, and the construct of a singular market is distracting, and projects too much homogeneity, transactionalism and capitalism. The contexts of comparison were non-homogeneous, and took place in a wide variety of disparate contexts, which were not determined by a singular currency, physical location or even notions of capital (including subtler forms of financial, social, medical or religious capital) (Bourdieu 1986). The terms and conditions of these contexts of negotiation each deserve detailed, close situating, and then comparison with one another, before claims about larger patterns and rules can be made. This is the approach used in this volume.

Medicine and Islam

Narratives about the spread, adaptation, influence and localisation of Greco-Arabic and Prophetic medicine across South, Central and Southeast Asia have, since the mid-2000s, come to be 'refigured'. (Attewell 2007). Scholars have sought to look beyond the impact/response narratives of colonial and postcolonial renderings of 'it' as a coherent 'system', which could be 'reformed' or 'purified', and to account for the complex transformations and relations of *Unani Tibb* (Greco-Islamic Medicine) and *Tibb-ul-Nabi* (Medicine of the Prophet) in the various locales where it has come to thrive. Attewell's study situates the complex relations among its own practitioners, with Islamic doctrines, and with regional practices and traditions – be they folk, state, Western or Ayurvedic. Projit Mukharji (2011) explores the differences in institutionalisation of *Tibb* during colonial and postcolonial rule, with particular reference to the absence of institutionalisation in Bengal, with one of the highest population densities of Muslims in the world. Scholars looking to the Islamic and Mongol world as a point of assemblage of medical traditions, study the polymath Persian Jewish vizier Rashid Al-din (1247–1319) and his gathering of medical experts and translators from around the world in his court in Tabriz, Persia. They have noted his conversion to Islam, and its influence on his medical corpus, the *Tansūqnāma* (Buell 2008; Lo and Wang Yidan 2018). Recent years have also seen an expansion of resources and studies of Islamic medicine in Southeast Asia, particularly with reference to magic, religion and medicine as evident in manuscript collections that are coming to light (Yahya 2016; Ibrahim and Shah 2020). The admixture of material and spiritual methods is also a focus of the digital project, *Polyglot Medical Traditions in Southeast Asia*,[8] which is digitising corpuses of Malay and Chinese manuscripts and documenting scientific names of ethnopharmaceutical plants (Stanley-Baker *et al.* 2021).

The studies in this volume

The chapters are episodic and non-linear. They are scattered across East, South and Southeast Asia and the Himalayas, and taken from different time periods – classical/medieval, early modern and contemporary. These are geographic concepts and temporal frames that have their genesis in a European gaze, and are not germane to these regions or moments. Nevertheless, they have come to be used by scholars of those regions for different reasons, grounded in a comparative history that gives voice to local motivations and historical processes (Pollock 2011; Salguero 2014; Gyatso 2015; Bian 2020). This diversity should remind the reader that each chapter describes ephemeral and contingent moments where relations between medicine and religion are produced. The volume is not intended to be comprehensive nor assert universal claims about essential categories. Rather, the interest is in patterns, and what continuities may or may not be sustained across individual moments. In so doing, the goal is to challenge our expectations of what medicine and religion are, to tease out tacit Eurocentric assumptions we may still attach to those terms, and come to a better vocabulary and critical apparatus for understanding how they come to be defined in their particular 'moment'. Each 'moment' described in these chapters is a different mode of 'worlding', the coming-together and sorting out of different forms of existence – material, discursive, social and ecological (Anderson and Harrison 2010: 8; Haraway 2016: 12–16; Palmer and Hunter 2018; Zhan 2009).

Despite the eclectic spread of the 'moments' covered, the chapters share a common structure that is designed to allow better comparison of the ways in which religion and medicine are figured. The authors have composed their chapters in a regular and specific way, which forms a consistent argument structure across each chapter. This enables readers to compare the similarities and differences of each temporal and geographic area, how scholars of previous generations have approached the topic, and what new methodologies can be applied, perhaps across multiple regions. Each chapter begins with a background to the time period and major issues, and then provides a literature review of the main scholarly approaches used so far. They then discuss the primary sources available for that period/region, the kinds and genres of sources, the contours of the archive, and how these influence the ways in which religion and medicine are framed. Recipe texts, government policies, liturgies and practice manuals operate in dissimilar contexts, transmitting different kinds of knowledge to different kinds of actors. 'Sources' here refers to each scholar's 'archive', whether that be manuscripts, received literature or ethnographic interviews. The 'sources' sections of the papers are reminders that the structure of the archive itself exerts a shaping force on the formation of medicine and religion (Bowker 2005). Authors then perform an analysis or intervention, interrogating the legacy scholarship and asking whether or not scholarly categories have misrepresented the sources. Where legacy scholarship impairs readers' access to actor categories, I have asked authors to propose more suitable approaches and methodologies. These interventions are the intended contribution of the project: to alert us to key methodological concerns in the study of medicine and religion. Taken together, the chapters offer a set of critical tools and research directions for the next generation of researchers.

During the initial workshop for this project, Judith Farquhar gave a keynote speech, in which she offered a number of guidelines for authors, and which are useful for scholarship generally. She invited us all to pay attention to the following:

- Dyads: Dichotomies such as 'text vs. practice', 'knowledge vs. practice', 'religion vs. medicine', etc. are problematic and never as simple as they may at first appear.
- Texts and practices: Attend to how textualisation and institutionalisation (both by actors and scholars) turn practices into stable knowledge.
- Terminology and translation: How do translation and terminology (both by actors and scholars) place knowledge into new discursive contexts?
- Methodology: We define our field by choosing what we study. We must be self-reflexive about our own methods, and be willing to be explicit about methods used, so that we can learn from one another.
- Category interrogation: We are stuck with categories 'religion' and 'medicine', but should explore how these categories shape the archive and what we read. Just blurring the boundaries is weak, but showing the emergence of the categories is a stronger approach.
- State and market: Let us not forget that states are always invested in knowledge production, enabling and constraining actors and styles of knowing.
- Political, economic, institutional: What about our own political commitments and entanglements? We are each situated in our own political and institutional contexts, nationalisms, etc., and need to be explicit about it. What are the politics of canon formation, and nationalist historiographies? What things do they bring into our consideration?

East Asia

Nathan Sivin's chapter (Ch. 1) on middle-period China outlines three main genres: medical, Buddhist and Daoist writing. He points out that the distinctions between physicians, Daoists, Buddhists and folk healers are not easily drawn when we read the sources closely.

He argues that the state and the body formed two distinct but parallel microcosms, and that physicians treated the body within the framework of a larger, natural cosmology. Three different kinds of sources reflect three different approaches to therapy. Elite writings accept the value of medicine and sophisticated explanatory models. While they made universal claims about its efficacy, they ignored the fact that this medicine was restricted to a small, elite, literate and very privileged clientele. Writings by bureaucrats hold varying levels of esteem for Buddhist and Daoist forms of healing, depending on their status and experience. All the written sources tend to disparage popular religion, and see it as the practice of individual charismatic figures, rather than an enterprise rooted in communities. In his analysis, Sivin asks three primary questions, pointing out directions for future research. The first is whether or not we can take seriously the efficacy of spiritual therapy, and the utility of frameworks like Moerman's (2002) reframing of placebo as 'meaning response'. The second is what do we know, or can we know, about the varieties of religious curing. And the third is that, given that little was written down and that elite sources are prejudicial, what can we know about popular religion? How can we usefully compare written documents to ethnographic study?

Katja Triplett (Ch. 2) introduces textual and visual sources from eighth- to seventeenth-century Japan that reveal the diverse sectors and practices involved in treating disease. Noting that Buddhist monks were the dominant force behind the circulation of medical knowledge and practice, the chapter advocates reading against the grain of rationalist approaches to medicine, and for paying close attention to the wide variety of admixture which such reading reveals. Triplett reviews positions by a number of mid-twentieth century scholars, who have approached the Buddhist history of medicine in Japan, comparing their work as 'medicalisation', 'historicising' and 'interplay' of medicine and religion, opting for the latter as the most representative approach. She suggests a number of means by which medicine and religion were distinguished or organised in premodern Japan, drawing on methodologies used in the Kolleg-Forschungsgruppe 'Multiple Secularities', and Niklas Luhman's (2013) systems theory, which focuses on cultural binaries.

Triplett notes that Buddhism provided a number of important epistemes, or culturally transmitted patterns of perception and interpretation, which allow healing to be figured as a transcendent or an immanent goal. She also considers *means and methods* by which to tease out differences in conceptual distinctions. *Kaji* 加持 (Sanskrit: *adhiṣṭhāna*, 'assistance'), or healing rituals, assert healing as a transcendent goal. *Materia medica*, on the other hand, were used widely by monks, physicians and cult members, such as *Shugendō* 修験道 ascetics. Rituals, which activated unseen spirits or other forces, also failed to distinguish religious from secular practitioners, given that they were used by ascetics, monks and physicians alike. Other approaches she suggests include the ascription of *charisma*, based on training, kinds of authority, as well as competencies or skillsets. While religious experts were oriented towards providing salvation, they also had means of curing at their disposal. She notes, however, that it was often very hard to draw clear binary lines between religious and secular actors and activities. She further points out that there is still a dearth of studies on women and animals in relation to medicine and religion in medieval Japan.

Elena Valussi's chapter (Ch. 3) on female alchemy, a late imperial form of Daoist cultivation for women, tracks shifting contours of gender representation across medical and religious writing. Where earlier forms of 'non-gendered' inner alchemy prioritised the conservation of 'essence' (*jing* 精), which should not leak out of the body in its masculine form as semen, female alchemy focused on the cessation of menses (*jing* 經), the female form of essence. When contained within the body, essence can be transmuted into *qi* and then 'spirit' (*shen* 神). Menses and menstruating women were perceived to be impure and polluting of sacred spaces and objects, and thus prohibited from ritual grounds, as in most religious traditions around the world. Valussi argues that such negative portrayals of female sexuality and physiology obscured a woman's generative and social power, if not making it invisible. A primary motivation within female alchemy is recovery from this subaltern position. Valussi tracks the shifting contours of gender amidst religious and secular notions of women's bodies in alchemical and medical literature of the Ming, Qing and

Republican eras. Late Ming texts on health cultivation written by doctors mark the female body by physiological ideas, gendered disease and related practices. These medically oriented texts used gendered practices to ameliorate disease and discomfort. The Qing dynasty saw medical literature turn towards a non-gendered medical body, while women's practices migrated to alchemical literature, which framed these curative practices within the goals of immortality and spiritual transcendence. Male alchemy literature of this period is mute with regard to disease and impurity, and the contrast effectively marks the female body as polluted and weak. The Republican Era scholar, Chen Ying-ning 陳櫻寧, an egalitarian-minded Daoist cultivator who advocated for gender equality and scientific methods, denied the divine origins of alchemical practices, and medicalised the self-cultivation tradition, downplaying its soteriological foundations.

Valussi situates female alchemy within a wider set of female body practices and physiological ideas across early modern and medieval Europe and India. A methodological approach of writing about 'life inside the body' (Duden 1991) serves to highlight the ways that male knowledge separates women from their own bodies, defining their organs and experiences in terms not accessible to, or expressive of, female experience. The intersectional conflux of cosmology, embryology and clinical observation in Ayurvedic literature (Selby 2008) has analogues in female alchemical writing. Similarly, the fascination with sex-specific bodily manifestations, including the stopping of bodily secretions, such as lactation and menstruation, in European monasticism and ascetic practice (Bynum 1987), bears some similarity to Daoist female cultivation. Certain driving questions about female physiology are shared across European and Chinese medical circles, such as the contribution of the mother to conception and to the sex of the child, the contrast of feminine cold and damp to male activity and warmth, the relationship between pleasure and reproduction, and the polluting effects of menstrual blood (Cadden 1993). Taking these together, Valussi shows how female alchemy articulates a religious vision of the female body as a site of transcendence of mortality and also of gender, in contrast to the inherent subjugation in the medicalised female body across a number of regions.

South Asia

Anthony Cerulli (Ch. 4) approaches South Asian medical literature transtemporally, discussing the relationship of medicine and religion in a number of periods and genres. Early medical writings appear as oblique references within the Vedas and the Buddhist *Tripiṭaka*. Around the turn of the first millennium, three major Sanskrit medical corpuses were compiled, and form the foundation of Āyurveda. The *Carakasaṃhitā* (*Caraka's Collection*), considered the oldest among the three, distinguishes between three different kinds of healing: that which occurs through the divine, by physicians, and by the patients themselves. The first category includes the most obvious convergences of medicine and religion, practices which would be seen in the Vedas: mantras, austerities, ritual, sacrifice, pilgrimage and so on. Cerulli notes that, while the *Collection* makes hard distinctions which would be familiar to modern readers – such as divine and non-divine, botanical and non-botanical medicines, and between religious and empirical claims about the world – these distinctions are not sustained through the text. These healing modalities are 'contiguous', 'imbricated' and sometimes blurred. As with middle-period China, this occurs especially so when knowledge is situated within larger cosmological frameworks, which incorporate knowledge of physicians and priests within the same broad set of ideas about reality.

Cerulli extends his investigation beyond the Sanskrit canon to include vernacular tales and epics, in particular the *Rāmāyaṇa*, in its many varied and vernacular forms. Following the move in literary studies to explore vernacular works beyond the hegemony of Sanskrit texts, Cerulli examines the medical narratives within the *Rāmāyaṇa*, in multiple variations, in particular Hanuman's iconic search for a medicinal herb, *saṃjīvanī*. This extends not only to literary and theatrical forms, but also the outplay of this myth in contemporary cosmopolitical debate – the search of a local politician for the herb in his native province. The chapter allows us to play out the political epistemology of Indian medicine and local mythography in the contemporary wellness market, the pharmaceutical bioprospecting market, and the advocacy for traditional local knowledge within an international biopolitical sphere.

Helen Lambert (Ch. 5) and Projit Mukharji (Ch. 6) both attend to sources and practices which have not been enfolded within elite Sanskrit genealogies with long textual heritages such as Āyurveda, Unanni or Siddha medicine. The position of these medicines on the periphery of scholarly attention, until only recently, affords a critical vantage point from which to view the construction and centralisation of those more celebrated traditions. In particular, their enfranchisement within national medical institutions, such as AYUSH, positions them as emblematic of a broader continuity between the current right-wing government and a celebrated, Sanskritic past.

Lambert draws our attention to the role of governmental and academic research categories in her depiction of medical institutions in nineteenth- and twentieth-century Rajasthan. She shows how categories of medical governance changed under different regimes, and drew different boundary lines between various styles of practice. During the arrival and early settlement of the British forces, local practices were largely ignored. By the late nineteenth and early twentieth century ethnological surveys of so-called 'primitive' peoples noted a diverse range of therapeutic activities across four classes of practitioners, but did not distinguish between religious or secular forms of practice. Little attention was given to understanding these practices until independence, when ethnology began to focus on the 'village' as a social unit. As development began to influence ethnology in the fifties to seventies, culture was deemed a 'barrier' to 'English medicine', and more focus was given to aetiological concepts and therapeutic actions. Surveys of afflictions, healing rituals and possession, bound as they were in folk cosmology, bore a great deal of overlap with ritual studies. These were distinguished as 'little traditions' from the 'great traditions' of Sanskritic Hindu beliefs, and treated as religion, not as medicine. As it became clear that economics and not ideology were the main cause for lack of uptake of biomedical care, more ethnographies were done on the biomedicine formation of health services.

The eighties and nineties saw debates emerge about epistemic authority and personal sovereignty, over terms like illness and disease, curing versus healing, and medical pluralism. As these forms of activism began to voice indigenous medical traditions, and subjective, interpersonal patient perspectives in contrast to biomedical knowledge, these had the effect of ceding 'medicine' as a category entirely to biomedicine. Within this discourse, there were also distinctions made between the codified systems with textual legacies, such as Unani, Siddha and Āyurveda as great traditions, in contrast to the other localised practices, and anthropologists began to pay attention to the legitimation practices of these 'Great Traditions'. These categorical, hierarchical differences fed directly into the formation in 2003 of AYUSH, which selects out the great traditions.

Lambert's own fieldwork in Rajasthan, which sought to define a 'medical system', found that, in fact, the medical pluralism there is very unsystematic, although there are common cultural logics that circulate among the varieties of therapeutic means. In her intervention, Lambert argues for not using terms like medicine, healing, belief and ritual as these smuggle in assumptions and hierarchies which impose a tacit normative agenda. She notes that the focus of scholarship on 'Indian medicine' privileges the state's modernist narrative, and fails to account for the diversity of lived medical practice, and that the term 'medicine' has come to stand in for 'systems' amenable to rationalist and naturalistic logics, and aid the progressive erasure of vernacular therapeutics. In focusing on the terminology used, the institutions which use it, and the effects of inclusion and circumscription that these names have on lived practice and social reality, she follows the 'Oxford School' of social anthropology (Ardener 1982; McDonald 2017). Lambert advocates for 'therapeutics' as a neutral term, since it does not contain the tacit epistemological weighting of others, not solely within her own writing, but implicitly in all of ours, because of the larger ramifications these terms have on local lives.

Mukharji (Ch. 6) examines mantric therapy in late-nineteenth- and early-twentieth-century Bengal through little-studied manuscript and print archives of late-eighteenth- and early-twentieth-century mantric texts. The mantras incorporate Buddhist, Islamic, Hindu and Christian motifs in multiple languages and non-translatable syllables, which raise questions about the kind of communication or 'meaning' they might contain. Mukharji approaches the topic with an array of methodological tools, regarding the untranslatable sounds as a form of material religion, a form of communicative therapeutic practice, which does not lend itself immediately to rationalisable ritual logics. The defiance of linear, logical and rational logics that is given full expression in the act of reciting unintelligible, but still meaningful, mantras, is a motif that permeates the other methodological approaches Mukharji adopts, weaving them together in what he terms a 'nomadology', that is a tracking of material practices across boundaries of genre, class, sect, language and culture. The opening gambit for this approach is the cultural history of the Bengal region itself, which he situates within a nexus of historical cultural migrations over centuries that have introduced layered linguistic, religious and political cultures to the region. This situation beggars attempts to construct longue-durée isolated 'traditions' or 'heritage' dating back millennia, and points towards the processes of cultural assimilation and common cultural logics that allow such heterogeneous material to be incorporated.

This methodological point is not forwarded simply as a means for approaching Bengali mantras, but as a much more probing critique of the factors behind their marginalisation and the lack of scholarly attention up until now. Noting the force of selectivity that is involved in defining and isolating an archive for research, Mukharji levels a critique of legacy scholarship on Sanskritic 'medical' literature, that sectioned off the first-millennium Ayurvedic classics as an empirical, rationalised, departure from therapeutics that were previously scattered throughout the 'religious' writings of the Vedas. Scholars in the early seventies wrote about this distinction as one of 'liberal and rational ideas' freed from 'mysticism, restrictions and rigidities of rites and ceremonies', which prepared room for a 'rational system of medicine'. The tacit politics of this interpretation, which has held sway in certain circles since, have changed over time. Early on these were aligned with an anticolonial sentiment, legitimating Indian civilisation in a retrospective apologetics that equated Indian knowledge with Western science. Marxist historians used the distinction to critique religion as a means for elite classes to maintain class power, within certain stages of historical advancement.

Banu Subramaniam (2000) refers to this equation of ancient knowledge with modern science as 'Archaic Modernity', and points out two important effects: firstly it domesticates science into a Hindu nationalist narrative, secondly by creating an epistemological equivalence between ancient Indian knowledge and modern science it removes the possibility of critique, papering over differences and blending Hindu nationalism with scientific modernity. The construction of the archive in this way, argues Mukharji, performs a 'denial of coevalness' (Fabian 2014), by excluding mantras as primitive and retrogressive, even before the study has begun, simply through the circumscription of the archive. Such exclusion has political consequences in the present. The denial of the possibility of religious forces acting on the body to cause disease or secure health, silences these ambiguous powers over human subjects, and renders their labouring bodies more amenable to integration into a disenchanted world that is governed by the rationality of production systems and the state. A world of mantric therapies and lively spiritual forces would make these bodies unpredictable, and interrupt the flows of power and production. Furthermore, argues Mukharji following Subramaniam, the equation of archaic Hindu rationality with modern science allows for non-Hindu minorities, lower castes and heterodox Hindus to be derided and ignored by right-wing Hindu nationalists.

On the flipside, however, while mantras have been excluded from the study of medicine, they have been included in the study of religion, but under the aegis of 'traditions'. Mukharji points out that these notions of 'tradition' are often artificially circumscribed to suit scholarly interests and ability, whereas the approach of material religion allows for the migration of corporeal practices and material objects across these doctrinally defined boundaries, which Mukharji amply demonstrates through his collections of multilingual, trans-sectarian, 'low-brow' materials. Mukharji points out two primary methodological strands that converge to support the study of these mantras: material religion and subaltern medicine. Both approaches attend to the ways in which practices migrate across so-called 'traditions', 'genealogies' and 'rational, coherent doctrines' that are imagined to be cut from whole cloth, as it were.

Both Lambert and Mukharji make clear that the politics of representation in the present affect the conceptual grounds of seemingly distant studies of the long past. We cannot ignore the fact that contemporary actors, and the terms and habits of categorisation they use, have important effects on the ways in which we access and think about the past. In order to study medicine and religion we need to attend not only to actors in the past and analogous terms for our present concepts, but we must also see how contemporary scholars, through whom we access and think about the past, are busy situating medicine and religion, just as much as early actors did.

Himalayas and Southeast Asia

Geoffrey Samuel (Ch. 7) takes up a thread about empiricism and religiosity that has been debated in the field of Tibetan medicine, with reference to two volumes in particular which came out in the last decade. Samuel sets this up with examples of how the twelfth-century *rGyud bzhi* (Four Tantras), the foundational work for *sowa-rigpa* or Tibetan medicine, includes a number of hybrid concepts, that draw on both materialist Āyurvedic and Tantric cultivation literature. This allows him to contrast the fundamental positions underlying Janet Gyatso's *Being Human* (2015) and the edited volume by Adams, Schrempf and Craig, *Medicine between Science and Religion* (2011). Gyatso's study of the production, reception and epistemic authority of the *Four Tantras* emphasises the epistemological rift, painting a picture of religious commitments in conflict with empirical observation which, she argues, is much more of an epistemic good in medical writing than in Buddhist meditation theory. The debates that promoted this in medical writing were a concern of the *sDe srid* (Regent) of Lhasa in the seventeenth century, and formed an important part of his state-building projects. This epistemic rift would eventually lead to the much more empirically based medicine seen today. By contrast Adams *et al.*'s (2011) edited collection of ethnographic and some historical and textual studies, seeks to deprivilege biomedicine as a primary analytic, and promote a '*sowa rigpa* sensibility', which treats religious and medical healing practices as epistemological equals. By sidelining the tricky question of biomedical efficacy, they open up room for an analytic, one which focusses entirely on patient 'illness' – the subjective experience of their situation – rather than biomedical notions of 'disease' – conditions which are ultimately arbitrated by doctors. This acknowledgement allows for the greater weighting of religious practice and experience as important factors in people's experience of their own wellbeing or illness and offers more voice to practitioners and their subjective experience, in a world which is predominantly ordered by the biomedical. Gyatso, writing for audiences from religious studies and the history of science, foregrounds contrast and difference, whereas Adams *et al.* (who are anthropologists) are engaged in the activism for *sowa-rigpa* against attacks from the biomedical world.

Samuel adroitly demonstrates the point made above, that situating issues of religion and medicine in Asia cannot simply draw conclusions from primary sources, but must also take into account the positions and interests of scholars who report on them, and the communities for whom they write. All the different actors within the historical layers of a text and its reception are involved in negotiating the boundaries of medicine and religion within their own time and place. Furthermore, this activity speaks to larger concerns that span the range of the self and the body, institutions, epistemological authority, state-building and cosmology.

The chapters by Constantin Canavas (Ch. 8) and Céline Coderey (Ch. 9) concern modern Southeast Asian nation-states, and rather like in the South Asian chapters, reveal the strong role of the state in defining hierarchies and increasingly sharp differences between religion and medicine.

Focusing on the integration of homeopathy in Malaysia, Canavas portrays the gradual emergence of Traditional, Alternative and Complementary Medicine (TACM) as a category of governance of non-biomedical therapies. The epistemic and political position of homeopathy was negotiated within the currents of an emerging Islamic state, via changing categories over time. Although traditional Malay medicine, Islamic medicine, Chinese medicine and Hindu or Ayurvedic medicine have been practised largely along ethnic lines, there is also a great deal of syncretism and use of polymedicine across these different communities. With Malaysia's increasing independence, and then identification as an Islamic state, different TACMS came to be described in different apologetic terms at different times. During the late colonial period of the 1940s and 50s, the model of a tolerant Islam was described, one which could absorb foreign elements, such as animist nature-spirits and even Hindu deities as *jinn*. Later medical anthropology during decolonialisation in the 1970s and 80s focused on the national health system, and a model of medical pluralism which incorporated 'vigorous systems of traditional beliefs and practices' (Chen 1976: 171). By the 2000s, statistical surveys of usage of traditional medicines substituted earlier investigations into cultural meaning and explanatory models within the different health practices. Islamic beliefs around disease causation became more common, and practices like homeopathy came to be justified with apologetic quotations from the *sunna* literature and the Qur'an. The primary proponent of homeopathy was one Dr. Burhanuddin Al-Helmy, who in addition to founding the homeopathy movement in Malaysia, was also a highly active political figure in political Islam. While he himself did not claim that homeopathy was a prophetic medicine, this claim was taken up by his disciples and proponents of the next generation of homeopathy. We see this practice bound up in the changing politics of Islam in Malaysia, the increasing need for Islamic styles of representation, and association with a charismatic political figure during its early inception in the region.

Coderey also finds in postcolonial Myanmar that medical hierarchy is bound up with religious, political and institutional allegiances. Prior to the introduction of *ingaleik hsay* (English medicine) more widely in the late nineteenth century, religious and medical practices were not clearly differentiated. Noting that in Burmese, the term for 'religion' or *pada*, is a metonymy for *Buda pada*, or Buddhism, the national religion, Coderey demonstrates how Buddhist-affiliated traditional medicine institutions have come to dominate the epistemic landscape of post-independence Myanmar. The styles and limits of orthodox Buddhism are constrained by the state, which has engaged in purification campaigns against heterodox practices, such as *weikza* (alchemy, talismans, mantra and other remedies), that are considered politically dangerous. Prior to the twentieth century, the main types were traditional herbal medicine (*beyndaw*) combined with astrology and mantra recitation for natural disorders, *weikza* for supernatural disorders, divination and spirit-mediumism.

Since independence, state-authorised traditional medicine has privileged traditions from primarily Buddhist provinces, and excluded *weikza* practices, which Coderey argues augments the other political and religious purifications. This study is undertaken against a backdrop of legacy scholarship on the region which has argued, on the one hand, that Buddhism is a distinct religious system of another order than supernaturalist practices, while others, with whom Coderey agrees, have maintained that regardless of scholarly categories, for citizens of Myanmar, all the varieties of practice constitute parts of a synthetic whole. The separation by the government of medical traditions along religious lines does not reflect the preferences or traditions of locals, but rather of political elites. Coderey argues that even while schisms over astrology as epistemically discrete from *nibbanic* salvation have occasionally punctuated the intellectual history of Buddhism from time to time, the Myanmar state has capitalised on these to produce wholesale schisms at national and institutional scale not before seen, and closer to the needs of the state than the people.

Conclusion

While time and place differ, the chapters share common touchstones. Legacy scholarship has often, although not always, taken European notions of medicine for granted, privileging textually oriented traditions, rationality and empiricism. This is consistent with colonial powers in South and Southeast Asia, and postcolonial powers have often built on those categories even more. A good deal of blurring is to be found in earlier sources, and the chapters in general follow a track of increasing categorisation. Once categories are created, they remain in the intellectual fabric, even when practitioners choose to conflate them.

Of note is the strong role of the state in producing distinctions about what counts as religious or medical – this occurs not only in societies during or after British colonial rule, but also in early modern Tibet, for example. Medieval Japan may have allowed physician and Buddhist monks to perform the same spread of therapies, but they did so within what Killinger *et al.* (2019) describe as 'meso-level institutional' roles, which are defined by the state. The same is true for Daoist, Buddhist and medical practitioners in China. At the level of practice, there is much more of a mixture – studies as geographically and temporally wide as medieval China and Japan and modern Malaysia note that categorical distinctions are not adhered to – practices circulate across intellectual and sectarian boundaries. This seems to indicate that parties who are 'interested' in such distinctions operate at an elite level of textual production, institutional practice, and state policy. Distinctions between religion and medicine appear to be more concerned with the organisation of knowledge and communities of knowers than with its application.

Charismatic figures also serve either to polarise debates, or to generate strong coherence across multiple knowledge styles. Two examples are worth comparing: the Desi of Dharamsala who wrested greater authority in empirical argumentation for the medical community against religious sectarian arguments, and the cultural innovator Burhanuddin Al-Helmy, whose outspoken Islamic political views and innovative practice of homeopathy led later followers to elide the two and regard homeopathy as prophetic medicine. In both examples we see how the personality of individual figures enacts lasting epistemic force, in concert with Killinger *et al.* (2019). Both figures inserted new epistemic contours into the organisation of knowledge, but these changes did not consistently lead to rationalisation and disenchantment by later followers, in the manner suggested by Weber (1978: 246–554), but can lead to greater religiosity.

Few of the studies attended closely to personal, patient narratives – how do the sick frame their relationship to disease and treatment? This is partly to do with the privilege of sources – Coderey and Lambert are the sole authors who drew on ethnographic interview data. That more anthropologists were not included in the project is partly a matter of happenstance, others were invited to participate, but for various reasons were unable, but it may also be due to tacit privileging by the editor/organisers – Salguero and I are historians of medieval Chinese texts, after all. Elite records far outnumber individual diaries from earlier period. Mukharji's investigation of 'low-brow' mantra pamphlets performs an important corrective to this bias in administrative and scholarly rubrics, and demonstrates from the outset of the study design a self-awareness of how the contours of the archive shape the eventual study, and also the claims made from them – some of which have political currency today.

Attention to the power of names, and how they structure and condition policy, practice and individual experience is an explicit theoretical intervention by Lambert, who draws to our attention Edwin Ardener's 'Oxford School' of social anthropology (Ardener 1982; McDonald 2017). Notably, all four papers dealing with colonial and postcolonial rule followed a common trope of tracking changing institutions, terms and definitions over time, and yet the simple attention to categories is at the heart of each of these papers. During the initial conference Elisabeth Hsu made the comment that, as a collective, we shared a strong interest in 'marginal' or 'periphery' medicines. This is quite apt. Many of the papers describe quite clearly the processes, both emic and etic, by which certain therapeutics become central or are sidelined by hegemonic interests. Names and categories are central to this. Notably, none of the papers focus on empiricism, rationality, efficacy, and the other epistemological hallmarks of the enlightenment, except as a form of critique, or to situate how other authors have couched debates in these terms. Sivin, for example, points to the changing discourse around placebo and the potential for future focus on the 'meaning response' to religious therapies (Moerman 2002). The tenor of the chapters is much more about reflexivity around the discourses in which religion and medicine are negotiated, rather than making direct claims about the traditions in those terms.

Gender emerges as a focus of interest for Triplett, who points to studies of obstetric and post-partum therapies, and the need for further study of the role of gender. Valussi describes the category shift of female cultivation from health-based *yangsheng* in the Ming to alchemical *nüdan* in the Qing, and how this conceptual change reflects new emphasis from the female body in Ming medical theory to a non-gendered body in the Qing.

With this array of reflections on how medicine and religion have been situated in Asia, across time and region, we offer a tool kit, as it were, for research into this theme going forward, and hope to lay some conceptual groundwork for comparative work in the field.

Notes

1 Libbrecht 1990; Stanley-Baker 2022; on *qi* as a measurable gas, Schäfer 2011: 175–202.
2 The activities and history of the society can be found at https://IASTAM.org, accessed 30 May 2022.
3 On narrative medicine in general as a primary method within medical humanities, see Charon (2008).
4 See also Shapin's (2010) critique of the idea of science as a 'pure' form of knowledge.
5 www.ikgf.uni-erlangen.de/, accessed 20 August 2021.
6 www.isca.ox.ac.uk/argo-emr#tab-418981, accessed 20 August 2021.
7 www.multiple-secularities.de/, accessed 20 August 2021.
8 www.polyglotasianmedicine.com/, accessed 31 May 2022.

Bibliography

Adams, V., Schrempf, M. and Craig, S.R. (eds) (2011) *Medicine between Science and Religion: Explorations on Tibetan Grounds*. New York, NY: Berghahn Books.

Alter, J.S. (2004) *Yoga in Modern India: The Body between Science and Philosophy*. Princeton, NJ; Oxford: Princeton University Press.

Anderson, B. and Harrison, P. (2010) *Taking-place: Non-representational Theories and Geography*. London; New York: Routledge.

Andreeva, A. (2018) 'Buddhism and Medicine in Japan', *Oxford Bibliographies*. https://doi.org/10.1093/obo/9780195393521–0255.

Andreeva, A. and Steavu, D. (2015) *Transforming the Void*. Leiden: Brill.

Arai, P. (2014) 'Healing Zen: Exploring the Brain on Bowing', in I.M. Vargas-O'Bryan and X. Zhou (eds) *Disease, Religion and Healing in Asia: Collaborations and Collisions*. Abingdon: Taylor & Francis, pp. 155–69.

Ardener, E. (1982) 'Social Anthropology, Language, and Reality', in D.J. Parkin (ed.) *Semantic Anthropology*. London: Academic Press, pp. 1–14.

Attewell, G.N.A. (2007) *Refiguring Unani Tibb: Plural Healing in Late Colonial India*. Hyderabad: Orient Longman.

Baker, I. and Garde, R. (2015–16) *Tibet's Secret Temple: Body, Mind and Meditation in Tantric Buddhism*. Wellcome Museum: Art Heritage Interviews, https://youtu.be/JTFyCskQ_Kk, accessed 22 September 2021.

Baker, I.A. (2019) *Tibetan Yoga: Principles and Practices*. London: Thames and Hudson.

Barnes, L.L. (2011) 'New Geographies of Religion and Healing: States of the Field', *Practical Matters*, 4: 1–82.

Bian, H. (2020) *Know Your Remedies: Pharmacy and Culture in Early Modern China*. Princeton, NJ: Princeton University Press.

Bourdieu, P. (1977) *Outline of a Theory of Practice*. Cambridge; New York: Cambridge University Press.

Bourdieu, P. (1986) 'The Forms of Capital', in J.G. Richardson (ed.) *Handbook of Theory and Research for the Sociology of Education*. New York, NY: Greenwood Press, pp. 241–60.

Bourdieu, P. (1990) *The Logic of Practice*. Stanford, CA: Stanford University Press.

Bourdieu, P. (1991) 'Genesis and Structure of the Religious Field', *Comparative Social Research*, 13: 1–44.

Bowker, G.C. (2005) *Memory Practices in the Sciences*. Cambridge, MA: MIT Press.

Brentjes, S. (2018) 'Visualization and Material Cultures of the Heavens in Eurasia and North Africa', in S. Schmidtke (ed.) *Near and Middle Eastern Studies at the Institute for Advanced Study, Princeton, 1935–2018*. Piscataway, NJ: Gorgias Press, pp. 134–53.

Buell, P. (2008) 'How did Persian and Other Western Medical Knowledge Move East, and Chinese West? A Look at the Role of Rashīd al-Dīn and Others', *Asian Medicine*, 3.2: 279–95.
Burchardt, M. and Wohlrab-Sahr, M. (2013) 'Multiple Secularities: Religion and Modernity in the Global Age', *International Sociology*, 28.6: 605–11.
Bynum, C.W. (1987) *Holy Feast and Holy Fast: The Religious Significance of Food to Medieval Women*. Berkeley, CA: University of California Press.
Cadden, J. (1993) *Meanings of Sex Difference in the Middle Ages: Medicine, Science, and Culture*. Cambridge; New York: Cambridge University Press.
Campany, R.F. (2003) 'On the Very Idea of Religions (in the Modern West and in Early Medieval China)', *History of Religions*, 42.4: 287–319.
Campany, R.F. (2005) 'The Meanings of Cuisines of Transcendence in Late Classical and Early Medieval China', *T'oung Pao*, 91: 1–57.
Campany, R.F. (2009) *Making Transcendents: Ascetics and Social Memory in Early Medieval China*. Honolulu, HI: University of Hawai'i Press.
Campany, R.F. (2010) 'Religious Repertoires and Contestation: A Case Study based on a Collection of Buddhist Miracle Tales, ca. 490 C.E', *Buddhism, Daoism, and Chinese Religion*, Princeton University, Oct. 8–10, 2010.
Campany, R.F. (2012) *Signs from the Unseen Realm: Buddhist Miracle Tales from Early Medieval China*. Honolulu, HI: University of Hawai'i Press.
Campany, R.F. (2018) '"Religious" as a Category: A Comparative Case Study', *Numen*, 65: 333–76.
Camus, A. (1946 [1942]) *The Stranger*, trans. S. Gilbert. New York, NY: Vintage Books.
Cerulli, A. (2014) 'Storytelling and Accountability for Illness in Sanskrit Medical Literature', in I.M. Vargas-O'Bryan and X. Zhou (eds) *Disease, Religion and Healing in Asia: Collaborations and Collisions*. Abingdon: Taylor & Francis, pp. 86–100.
Charon, R. (2008) *Narrative Medicine: Honoring the Stories of Illness*. New York, NY: Oxford University Press.
Chaudhary, A. and Singh, N. (2012) 'Intellectual Property Rights and Patents in Perspective of Āyurveda', *Ayu*, 33.1: 20–6.
Chen K.-H. (2010) *Asia as Method: Toward Deimperialization*. Durham, NC: Duke University Press.
Chen, K.-H. (2012) 'Takeuchi Yoshimi's 1960 'Asia as Method' Lecture', *Inter-Asia Cultural Studies*, 13.2: 317–24.
Chen, P.C.Y. (1976) 'Medical Systems in Malaysia: Cultural Bases and Differential Use', *Ekistics*, 41.245: 192–9.
Cohen, D. (2014) 'Ghost Exorcism, Memory, and Healing in Hinduism', in I.M. Vargas-O'Bryan and X. Zhou (eds) *Disease, Religion and Healing in Asia: Collaborations and Collisions*. Abingdon: Taylor & Francis, pp. 69–84.
Craig, S.R. (2012) *Healing Elements: Efficacy and the Social Ecologies of Tibetan Medicine*. Berkeley, CA: University of California Press.

Deeg, M., Freiberger, O. and Kleine, C. (eds) (2013) *Religion in Asien? Studien zur Anwendbarkeit des Religionsbegriffs*. Uppsala: Acta Universitatis Upsaliensis.

Despeux, C. (ed.) (2010) *Médecine, religion et société dans la Chine médiévale: étude de manuscrits chinois de Dunhuang et de Turfan*. Paris: Collège de France, Institut des hautes études chinoises.

Duden, B. (1991) *The Woman Beneath the Skin: A Doctor's Patients in Eighteenth-century Germany*. Cambridge, MA: Harvard University Press.

Editorial (2019) 'The World Health Organization's Decision about Traditional Chinese Medicine could backfire', *Nature*, 570.7759: 5. https://doi.org/10.1038/d41586–019–01726–1.

Elman, B.A. (2005) *On Their Own Terms: Science in China, 1550–1900*. Cambridge, MA: Harvard University Press.

Elman, B.A. and Pollock, S. (2018) *What China and India Once Were: The Pasts That May Shape the Global Future*. New York, NY: Columbia University Press.

Fabian, J. (2014) *Time and the Other: How Anthropology Makes Its Object*. New York, NY: Columbia University Press.

Fan Fa-ti (2012) 'The Global Turn in the History of Science', *East Asian Science, Technology and Society*, 6.1: 249–58.

Farquhar, J. (1994) *Knowing Practice: The Clinical Encounter of Chinese Medicine*. Studies in the Ethnographic Imagination. Boulder, CO: Westview Press.

Farquhar, J. (2020) *A Way of Life: Things, Thought, and Action in Chinese Medicine*. New Haven, CT: Yale University Press.

Farquhar, J. and Wang Jun (2011) 'Knowing the Why but Not the How: A Dilemma in Contemporary Chinese Medicine', *Asian Medicine*, 5.1: 57–79.

Feher, M., Naddaff, R. and Tazi, N. (1989) *Fragments for a History of the Human Body*. New York, NY; Cambridge, MA: Zone.

Feuerstein, G. (1998) *The Yoga Tradition: Its History, Literature, Philosophy and Practice*. Prescott, AZ: Hohm Press.

Fleck, Ludwik. (1927 [1986]), 'Some Specific Features of the Medical Way of Thinking', in R. S. Cohen and T. Schnelle (eds.) *Cognition and fact: materials on Ludwik Fleck*, Dordrecht: Boston, 39–46.

Foucault, M. (1978 [French edn. 1976]) *The History of Sexuality*. New York, NY: Pantheon Books.

Foucault, M. (2012) *The Birth of the Clinic*. Hoboken, NY: Taylor & Francis.

Franklin, J.J. (2012) 'Buddhism and Modern Existential Nihilism: Jean-paul Sartre Meets Nagarjuna', *Religion & Literature*, 44.1: 73–96. www.jstor.org/stable/23347059.

Fu Daiwie (2007) 'How Far Can East Asian STS Go?' *East Asian Science, Technology and Society*, 1.1: 1–14.

Gai Jianmin 盖建民 (2001) *Daojiao yixue* 道教医学 (Daoist Medicine). Beijing: Zongjiao wenhua chubanshe.

Garrett, F. (2008) *Religion, Medicine and the Human Embryo in Tibet.* London; New York: Routledge.
Gerke, B. (2021) *Taming the Poisonous: Mercury, Toxicity, and Safety in Tibetan Medical Practice.* Heidelberg: Heidelberg University Publishing.
Giles, B. and Finch, A. (2006) *The Science of Acupuncture*, BBC documentary, London.
Good, B. (1994) *Medicine, Rationality, and Experience: An Anthropological Perspective.* The Lewis Henry Morgan lectures. Cambridge: Cambridge University Press.
Grant, E. (2008) *A History of Natural Philosophy: From the Ancient World to the Nineteenth Century.* Cambridge: Cambridge University Press.
Greene, M. (2014) 'Wong Tai Sin: The divine and healing in Hong Kong', in I.M. Vargas-O'Bryan and X. Zhou (eds) *Disease, Religion and Healing in Asia: Collaborations and Collisions.* Abingdon: Taylor & Francis, pp. 54–68.
Gyatso, J. (2004 [2011]) 'The Authority of Empiricism and the Empiricism of Authority: Medicine and Buddhism in Tibet on the Eve of Modernity', *Comparative Studies of South Asia, Africa and the Middle East*, 24.2: 83–96.
Gyatso, J. (2015) *Being Human in a Buddhist World: An Intellectual History of Medicine in Early Modern Tibet.* New York, NY: Columbia University Press.
Gyatso, J. (2017) 'Review of C. Pierce Salguero, Translating Buddhist Medicine in Medieval China', *History of Religions*, 57.1: 96–9.
Hackett, E.J., Amsterdamska, O., Lynch, M. and Wacjman, J. (eds) *The Handbook of Science and Technology Studies.* 3 edn. Cambridge, MA: MIT Press.
Hansen, V. (2017) *The Silk Road: A New History with Documents.* New York, NY; Oxford: Oxford University Press.
Haraway, D. (1988) 'Situated Knowledges: The Science Question in Feminism and the Privilege of Partial Perspective', *Feminist Studies,* 14.3: 575–99.
Haraway, D. J. (2016) *Staying with the Trouble: Making Kin in the Chthulucene.* Durham, NC: Duke University Press.
Hofer, T. (ed.) (2014) *Bodies in Balance: The Art of Tibetan Medicine.* Seattle, WA: University of Washington Press.
Hsu, E. (1999) *The Transmission of Chinese Medical Knowledge.* Cambridge: Cambridge University Press.
Hulsewâe, A.F.P., Idema, W.L. and Zèurcher, E. (eds) (1990) *Thought and Law in Qin and Han China: Studies Dedicated to Anthony Hulsewâe on the Occasion of His Eightieth Birthday.* Leiden: Brill.
Ibrahim, N. and Shah, F.A. (2020) 'Prophetic Medicine in Malay Manuscripts: A Brief Study on the 19th Century Kitāb Ṭib Manuscript', *Hadis*, 10.19: 454–64.

Jiang Sheng 姜生 and Tang Weixia 汤伟侠 (2002) *Zhongguo daojiao kexue jishu shi: Han, Wei, Jin juan* 中国道教科学技术史: 汉魏两晋卷 (History of Daoist Science and Technology in China: Han, Wei and Jin Dynasties). Beijing: Kexue chubanshe.

Jiang Sheng 姜生 and Tang Weixia 汤伟侠 (2010) *Zhongguo daojiao kexue jishu shi: Nanbei chao, Sui, Tang, Wudai juan* 中国道教科学技术史: 南北朝隋唐五代卷 (History of Daoist Science and Technology in China: Northern and Southern Dynasties, Sui, Tang and Five Dynasties). Beijing: Kexue chubanshe.

Killinger, K., Kleine, C. and Triplett, K. (2019) 'Distinctions and Differentiations between Medicine and Religion', *Asian Medicine,* 14.2: 233–62.

King, R. (1999) *Orientalism and Religion: Post-Colonial Theory, India and 'The Mystic East'*. Abingdon: Routledge.

Kleine, C. (2013) 'Religion als begriffliches Konzept und soziales System im vormodernen Japan: Polythetische Klassen, semantische und funktionale Äquivalente und strukturelle Analogien', in M. Deeg, O. Freiberger and C. Kleine (eds) *Religion in Asien? Studien zur Anwendbarkeit des Religionsbegriffs*. Uppsala: Acta Universitatis Upsaliensis, pp. 225–92.

Kleine, C. and Wohlrab-Sahr, M. (2016) 'Research Programme of the HCAS: Multiple Secularities – Beyond the West, Beyond Modernities', *Working Paper Series of the HCAS*. Leipzig: Leipzig University.

Kleinman, A. (1980) *Patients and Healers in the Context of Culture: An Exploration of the Borderland between Anthropology, Medicine and Psychiatry*. Berkeley, CA: University of California.

Kleinman, A. and Benson, P. (2006) 'Anthropology in the Clinic: The Problem of Cultural Competency and How to Fix It', *PLOS Medicine,* 3.10: e294.

Kloos, S. (2014–2019) *RATIMED: Re-Assembling Tibetan Medicine: The Formation of a Transnational Sowa Rigpa Industry in Contemporary India, China, Mongolia and Bhutan*. Vienna: Österreichischen Akademie der Wissenschaften.

Krämer, H.M. (2013) 'How 'Religion' Came to Be Translated as 'Shūkyō': Shimaji Mokurai and the Appropriation of Religion in Early Meiji Japan', *Japan Review*, 25: 89–111.

Lackner, M., Tam, K.K., Gänssbauer, M., and Yip, T.S.H. (2020) *Fate and Prognostication in the Chinese Literary Imagination*. Leiden: Brill.

Lam, Wai Ching, Lyu, Aiping, and Bian, Zhaoxiang (2019) 'ICD-11: Impact on Traditional Chinese Medicine and World Healthcare Systems', *Pharmaceutical Medicine*, 33.5: 373–7. https://doi.org/10.1007/s40290–019–00295-y.

Lambert, H. (2014) 'The Management of Sickness in an Indian Medical Vernacular', in I.M. Vargas-O'Bryan and X. Zhou (eds) *Disease, Religion and Healing in Asia: Collaborations and Collisions*. Abingdon: Taylor & Francis, pp. 9–21.

Latour, B. (2007) 'A Textbook Case Revisited. Knowledge as Mode of Existence', in E.J. Hackett, O. Amsterdamska, M. Lynch and J. Wacjman (eds) *The Handbook of Science and Technology Studies*. 3 edn. Cambridge, MA: MIT Press, pp. 83–112.

Latour, B. and Woolgar, S. (1979) *Laboratory Life: The Construction of Scientific Facts*. Princeton, NJ: Princeton University Press.

Law, J. and Lin Wen-yuan (2010) 'Cultivating Disconcertment', *The Sociological Review*, 58.2: 135–53.

Lawson, D. (2022) 'Chinese Medicine has Blighted Billions', *Sunday Times*, London, 1 May, p. 28.

Leslie, C. (ed.) (1977) *Asian Medical Systems: A Comparative Study*. Berkeley, CA: University of California Press.

Lévi-Strauss, C. (1963) *Structural Anthropology*, trans. C. Jacobson and B.G. Schoepf. New York, NY: Basic Books.

Li Zhisui (1994) *The Private Life of Chairman Mao: The Memoirs of Mao's Personal Physician Dr. Li Zhisui*. New York, NY: Random House.

Libbrecht, U. (1990) 'Prāṇa = Pneuma = Ch'i?', in A.F.P. Hulsewâe, W.L. Idema and E. Zèurcher (eds) *Thought and Law in Qin and Han China: Studies Dedicated to Anthony Hulsewâe on the Occasion of His Eightieth Birthday*. Leiden: Brill, pp. 42–62.

Liu, Y. (2021) *Healing with Poisons: Potent Medicines in Medieval China*. Seattle, WA: University of Washington Press.

Lo, V. (ed.) (2018) *Imagining Chinese Medicine*. Leiden: Brill.

Lo, V. and Cullen, C. (eds) (2005) *Medieval Chinese Medicine*. London; New York: RoutledgeCurzon.

Lo, V. and Wang Yidan 王一丹 (2018) 'Chasing the Vermilion Bird: Late Medieval Alchemical Transformations in "The Treasure Book of Ilkhan on Chinese Science and Techniques"', in V. Lo (ed.) *Imagining Chinese Medicine*. Leiden: Brill, pp. 291–304.

Lo, V., Stanley-Baker, M. and Yang, D. (eds) (2022) *Routledge Handbook of Chinese Medicine*. Abingdon: Routledge.

Lomi, B. (2014) 'Dharanis, Medicines and Straw-dolls', *Japanese Journal of Religious Studies*, 41.2: 255–304.

Lomi, B. (2017) 'The Ox-Bezoar Consecration (Goo kaji) for Safe Childbirth', in P.C. Salguero (ed.) *Selected Readings from the Shingon Ritual Collections*. New York, NY: Columbia University, pp. 351–7.

Lomi, B. (2018) 'Ox Bezoars and the Materiality of Heian-period Therapeutics', *Japanese Journal of Religious Studies*, 45.2: 227–68.

Luhmann, N. (2013) *A Systems Theory of Religion*. Stanford, CA: Stanford University Press.

Mallinson, J. (2010) *Khecarividya of Adinatha: A Critical Edition and Annotated Translation of an Early Text of Hathayoga*. London: Routledge.

Mallinson, J. (2015–2020) *The Haṭha Yoga Project*. London: SOAS. http://hyp.soas.ac.uk/, accessed 22 September 2021.

Mandair, A.-P. S. (2009) *Religion and the Specter of the West: Sikhism, India, Postcoloniality, and the Politics of Translation*. New York, NY: Columbia University Press.

Masuzawa, T. (2005) *The Invention of World Religions, or, How European Universalism was Preserved in the Language of Pluralism*. Chicago, IL: University of Chicago Press.

McDonald, M. (2017) 'The Ontological Turn Meets the Certainty of Death', *Anthropology & Medicine*, 24.2: 205–20.

McGrath, W.A. (ed.) (2019) Knowledge and Context in Tibetan Medicine. Leiden: Brill.

Moerman, D.E. (2002) *Meaning, Medicine, and the 'Placebo Effect'*. Cambridge: Cambridge University Press.

Mol, A. (2002) *The Body Multiple: Ontology in Medical Practice*. Durham, NC: Duke University Press.

Mukharji, P. (2011) 'Lokman, Chholeman and Manik Pir: Multiple Frames of Institutionalising Islamic Medicine in Modern Bengal', *Social History of Medicine*, 24.3: 720–38.

Needham, J. and Wang, L. (1956) *Science and Civilisation in China, Vol. 2, History of Scientific Thought*. Cambridge: Cambridge University Press.

Netz, R. (2011) *The Shaping of Deduction in Greek Mathematics: A Study in Cognitive History*. Cambridge: Cambridge University Press.

Newcombe, S. (2019) *Yoga in Britain: Stretching Spirituality and Educating Yogis*. Sheffield: Equinox Publishing.

Newcombe, S. and O'Brien-Kop, K. (2021) *Routledge Handbook of Yoga and Meditation Studies*. Abingdon; New York, NY: Routledge.

Nicholson, A.J. (2010) *Unifying Hinduism: Philosophy and Identity in Indian Intellectual History*. New York, NY: Columbia University Press.

Onaga, L., Whyte, K.P., Nelson, M., Diaz, V.M. and Chivizhe, L.L.-. (2020) *Reclaiming Turtles All the Way Down (TAWD): Animal Cosmologies and Paths to Indigenous Sciences*. Berlin: Dept. III, Max Planck Institute for the History of Science, www.mpiwg-berlin.mpg.de/research/projects/reclaiming-turtles-all-way-down-tawd-animal-cosmologies-and-paths-indigenous, accessed: 22 September 2021.

Palmer, H. and Hunter, V. (2018) 'Worlding', *Newmaterialism: How Matter Comes to Matter*, https://newmaterialism.eu/almanac/w/worlding.html, accessed 29 May 2022.

Palmer, J. (2020) 'Chinese Media Is Selling Snake Oil to Fight the Wuhan Virus' *Foreign Policy*, February 3.

Parkin, D.J. (ed.) (1982) *Semantic Anthropology*. London: Academic Press.

Pollock, S. (ed.) (2011) *Forms of Knowledge in Early Modern Asia: Explorations in the Intellectual History of India and Tibet, 1500–1800*. Durham, NC: Duke University Press.

Pollock, S., Bronkhorst, J., Bronner, Y., Deshpande, M., Ganeri, J., Houben, J.E.M., McCrea, L., Minkowski, C., Nye, J.H., Preisendanz, K., Tubb, G. and Wujastyk, D. (2001–2005) *Sanskrit Knowledge Systems on the Eve of Colonialism*. New York, NY: Columbia University.

Poo Mu-chou (1998) *In Search of Personal Welfare: A View of Ancient Chinese Religion*. SUNY Series in Chinese Philosophy and Culture. Albany, NY: State University of New York Press.

Rankin, A. (2021) *The Poison Trials: Wonder Drugs, Experiment, and the Battle for Authority in Renaissance Science*. Chicago, IL: University of Chicago Press.

Richard, S.W. (2009) *Recipes for Immortality: Healing, Religion, and Community in South India*. New York, NY: Oxford University Press.

Richardson, J.G. (ed.) (1986) *Handbook of Theory and Research for the Sociology of Education*. New York, NY: Greenwood Press.

Richey, J.L. (ed.) (2015) *Daoism in Japan: Chinese Traditions and Their Influence on Japanese Religious Culture*. London: Routledge.

Salguero, C.P. (2014) *Translating Buddhist Medicine in Medieval China*. Philadelphia, PA: University of Pennsylvania Press.

Salguero, C.P. (2017) *Buddhism and Medicine: An Anthology of Premodern Sources*. New York, NY: Columbia University Press.

Salguero, C.P. (ed.) (2017) *Selected Readings from the Shingon Ritual Collections*. New York, NY: Columbia University Press.

Salguero, C.P. (ed.) (2020) *Buddhism and Medicine: An Anthology of Modern and Contemporary Sources*. New York, NY: Columbia University Press.

Salguero, C.P. (2022) *A Global History of Buddhism and Medicine*. New York, NY: Columbia University Press.

Salguero, C.P. and Macomber, A. (2020) *Buddhist Healing in Medieval China and Japan*. Honolulu, HI: University of Hawai'i Press.

Samuel, G. (2013) 'Subtle-body Processes: Towards a Non-reductionist Understanding', in G. Samuel and J. Johnson (eds) *Religion and the Subtle Body in Asia and the West: Between Mind and Body*. Abingdon: Routledge, pp. 249–66.

Samuel, G. and Johnston, J. (eds) (2013) *Religion and the Subtle Body in Asia and the West: Between Mind and Body*. Abingdon: Routledge.

Sartre, J.P. (1956) *Being and Nothingness: A Phenomenological Essay on Ontology*. New York, NY: Washington Square Press.

Schäfer, D. (2011) *The Crafting of the 10,000 Things: Knowledge and Technology in Seventeenth-century China*. Chicago, IL: University of Chicago Press.

Schäfer, D. and Yi, H. (2018) 'Great Plans: Song Dynastic (960–1279) Institutions for Human and Veterinary Healthcare', in D. Schäfer, M. Siebert and R. Sterckx (eds) *Animals through Chinese History: Earliest Times to 1911*. Cambridge: Cambridge University Press, pp. 160–80.

Schäfer, D., Siebert, M. and Sterckx, R. (eds) *Animals through Chinese History: Earliest Times to 1911*. Cambridge: Cambridge University Press.

Schmidtke, S. (ed.) *Near and Middle Eastern Studies at the Institute for Advanced Study, Princeton, 1935–2018*. Piscataway, NJ: Gorgias Press.

Selby, M.A. (2008) 'Between Medicine and Religion: Discursive Shifts in Early Ayurvedic Narratives of Conception and Gestation', in I.G. Županov and C. Guenzi (eds) *Divins remèdes: médecine et religion en Asie du sud*. Paris: Ecole des hautes études en sciences sociales, pp. 41–63.

Shapin, S. (2007) 'Science and the Modern World', in E.J. Hackett, O. Amsterdamska, M. Lynch, and J. Wacjman (eds) *The Handbook of Science and Technology Studies*. 3 edn. Cambridge, MA: MIT Press, pp. 433–48.

Shapin, S. (2010) *Never Pure: Historical Studies of Science as if it was Produced by People with Bodies, Situated in Time, Space, Culture, and Society, and Struggling for Credibility and Authority*. Baltimore, MD: Johns Hopkins University Press.

Shen, G. (2007) 'Murky Waters: Thoughts on Desire, Utility, and the "Sea of Modern Science"', *Isis*, 98.3: 584–96.

Sivin, N. (1995a) *Medicine, Philosophy and Religion in Ancient China: Researches and Reflections*. Aldershot: Variorum.

Sivin, N. (1995b) *Science in Ancient China: Researches and Reflections*. Aldershot: Variorum.

Staal, F. (1993) *Concepts of Science in Europe and Asia*. Leiden: International Institute for Asian Studies.

Stanley-Baker, M. (2009) 'Daoism and Medicine: A Review of Gai Jianmin's *Daojiao yixue* 道教醫學 (Daoist Medicine)', *Asian Medicine*, 4.1: 249–55.

Stanley-Baker, M. (2013) *Daoists and Doctors: The Role of Medicine in Six Dynasties Shangqing Daoism*, PhD thesis, University College London.

Stanley-Baker, M. (2018) *Drugs Across Asia: Tracing the Movement of Medicines across Space, Language and Time*, https://michaelstanley-baker.com/drugs-across-asia/, accessed 22 September 2021.

Stanley-Baker, M. (2019) '*Dao*ing Medicine: Practice Theory for Considering Religion and Medicine in Early Imperial China', *East Asian Science Technology and Medicine*, 50: 21–66.

Stanley-Baker, M. (2022) 'Qi 氣: A Means for Cohering Natural Knowledge', in V. Lo, M. Stanley-Baker and D. Yang (eds) *Routledge Handbook of Chinese Medicine*. Abingdon: Routledge, pp. 23–50.

Stanley-Baker, M. (unpublished MS) *Daoists, Doctors and Demons: Situating Religion and Medicine in Early Imperial China*.

Stanley-Baker, M., Chen Shih-pei 陳詩沛 and Tu Hsieh-chang 杜協昌 (2018) 'Daoist Buddhist and Medical Corpus for Six Dynasties [DaoBudMed6D]'. Taipei: National Taiwan University Press, https://doi.org/10.6681/NTURCDH.DB_DocuSkyDaoBudMed6D/Text, accessed 29 May 2022.

Stanley-Baker, M., Xu Duoduo 許多多. and Chong, W.E.K. (2020a) 'Bencaojing jizhu 本草經集注 in Three Layers' (Version 2). DR-NTU (Data), https://doi.org/10.21979/N9/K4WS29, accessed 29 May 2022.

Stanley-Baker, M., Xu Duoduo 許多多, Chen Shi-pei 陳詩沛, Zhang Duan 張端 and Tu Hsieh-chang 杜協昌 (2020b) *Bencao jing jizhu* 本草經集注 (Version 2) [*.xml]. Taipei: National Taiwan University Press, http://10.6681/NTURCDH.DB_DocuSkyBencaojing/Text, accessed 29 May 2022.

Stanley-Baker, M., Zakaria, F., Cacciafoco, F.P. and M.W. Goodman M.W. (2022) *Polyglot Medical Traditions in Southeast Asia*. Nanyang

Technological University, Singapore National Heritage Board, www.polyglotasianmedicine.com, accessed 22 September 2021.

Steavu, D. (2015) 'Delocalizing Illness: Healing and the State in Chinese Medicine', in W.S. Sax, and H. Basu (eds) *The Law of Possession: Ritual, Healing, and the Secular State*. New York, NY: Oxford University Press, pp. 82–116.

Stengers, I. (2010) *Cosmopolitics*, trans. R. Bononno, Vol. 1. Minneapolis, MN: University of Minnesota Press.

Subramaniam, B. (2000) 'Archaic Modernities: Science, Secularism, and Religion in Modern India', *Social Text*, 18: 67–86.

Takeda Kiyoko 武田 清子 (ed.) (1961) *Shisôshi no taishô to hôhô* 思想史の方法と大将 (Objects and Methods of Intellectual History). Tokyo: Sôbunsha.

Takeuchi Yoshimi (2005) 'Asia as Method', *What is Modernity? Writings of Takeuchi Yoshimi*. New York, NY: Columbia University Press, pp. 149–66.

Takeuchi Yoshimi 竹内 好 (1961) 'Hôhô to shite no Ajia', 方法としてのアジア (Asia as Method), in Takeda Kiyoko 武田 清子 (ed.) *Shisôshi no taishô to hôhô* 思想史の方法と大将 (Objects and Methods of Intellectual History). Tokyo: Sôbunsha.

Tambiah, S. J. (1990) *Magic, Science, Religion, and the scope of Rationality*. Cambridge: Cambridge University Press.

Taylor, K. (2005) *Chinese Medicine in Early Communist China, 1945–63: A Medicine of Revolution*. London: RoutledgeCurzon.

Triplett, K. (2019a) *Buddhism and Medicine in Japan: A Topical Survey (500–1600 CE) of a Complex Relationship*. Berlin; Boston: De Gruyter.

Triplett, K. (2019b) 'Pediatric Care and Buddhism in Premodern Japan: A Case of Applied "Demonology"?' *Asian Medicine*, 14.2: 313–41.

Triplett, K. (2021) 'Chinese-style Medicine in Japan', in V. Lo, M. Stanley-Baker and D. Yang (eds) *Routledge Handbook of Chinese Medicine*. London: Routledge, pp. 513–23.

Unschuld, P.U. (2003) *Huangdi neijing suwen: Nature, Knowledge, Imagery in an Ancient Chinese Medical Text*. Berkeley, CA: University of California Press.

Unschuld, P.U. (2009) *What Is Medicine? Western and Eastern approaches to healing*. Berkeley, CA: University of California Press.

Unschuld, P.U. (2010) 'When Health was Freed from Fate: Some Thoughts on the Liberating Potential of Early Chinese Medicine', *East Asian Science Technology and Medicine*, 31: 11–24.

Vargas-O'Bryan, I.M. (2014)'Balancing Tradition Alongside a Progressively Scientific Tibetan Medical System', in I.M. Vargas-O'Bryan and X. Zhou (eds) *Disease, Religion and Healing in Asia: Collaborations and Collisions*. Abingdon: Taylor & Francis, pp. 122–45.

Vargas-O'Bryan, I.M. and Zhou, X. (eds) (2014) *Disease, Religion and Healing in Asia: Collaborations and Collisions*. Abingdon: Taylor & Francis.

Verellen, F. (2019) *Imperiled Destinies: The Daoist Quest for Deliverance in Medieval China.* Cambridge, MA: Harvard University Press.

Verran, H. (2014) 'Working with Those who Think Otherwise', *Common Knowledge*, 20.3: 527–39.

von Richthofen, F. (1877) 'Über die zentralasiatischen Seidenstrassen bis zum 2. Jh. n. Chr (On the Central Asian Silk Roads until the 2nd century A.D.)', *Verhandlungen der Gesellschaft fu¨r Erdkunde zu Berlin,* 4: 96–122.

Wallace, V. (2014) 'The Method-and-Wisdom Model in the Theoretical Syncretism of Traditional Mongolian Medicine', in I.M. Vargas-O'Bryan and X. Zhou (eds) *Disease, Religion and Healing in Asia: Collaborations and Collisions.* Abingdon: Taylor & Francis, pp. 101–21.

Waugh, D. (2007) 'Richthofen's 'Silk Roads': Toward the Archaeology of a Concept', *The Silk Road*, 5.1: 1–10.

Weber, M. (1978) *Economy and Society: An Outline of Interpretative Sociology.* Berkeley, CA; London: University of California Press.

White, D.G. (1996) *The Alchemical Body: Siddha Traditions in Medieval India.* Chicago, IL; London: University of Chicago Press.

Wohlrab-Sahr, M. and Burchardt, M. (2012) 'Multiple Secularities: Toward a Cultural Sociology of Secular Modernities', *Comparative Sociology*, 11.6: 875–909.

Wohlrab-Sahr, M. and Kleine, C. (2021) 'Historicizing Secularity: A Proposal for Comparative Research from a Global Perspective', *Comparative Sociology*, 20.3: 287–316.

World Health Organization (2018) *ICD-11: International Classification of Diseases 11th Revision: The global standard for diagnostic health information.* Geneva: World Health Organization.

World Health Organization (2019) ICD-11: *International Classification of Diseases 11th Revision: The Global Standard for Diagnostic Health Information.* Geneva: World Health Organization.

World Health Organization (2022) *WHO International Standard Terminologies on Traditional Chinese Medicine.* Geneva: World Health Organization.

Wujastyk, D. (2015–2020) *AYURYOG: Entangled Histories of Yoga, Āyurveda and Alchemy in South Asia.* Vienna, Alberta: University of Vienna, University of Alberta.

Wujastyk, D., Plofker, K., Montelle, C., Speziale, F., Michio Yano, Bühnemann, G., Misra, A., Kolachana, A. and Wujastyk, D. (eds) (2013) *Journal of the History of Science in South Asia.* Edmonton: University of Alberta.

Xu Duoduo 許多多 and Stanley-Baker, M. (2021) '葛仙翁肘後備急方 Fulltext Database' (Version 1) [DocuXML]. DR-NTU (Data), https://doi.org/10.21979/N9/JUL0EO, accessed 29 May 2022.

Yahya, F. (2016) *Magic and Divination in Malay Illustrated Manuscripts.* Leiden: Brill.

Yamashita Shinji, Bosco, J. and Eades, J.S. (eds) (2004) *The Making of Anthropology in East and Southeast Asia*. New York, NY: Berghahn Books.
Yang, D. (2018) *Prescribing 'Guiding and Pulling': The Institutionalisation of Therapeutic Exercise in Sui China (581–618 CE)*, PhD thesis, University College London.
Yang, D. (2022) 'The Formalisation of Therapeutic Exercises in the Medical Practice of Sui China', in V. Lo, M. Stanley-Baker and D. Yang (eds) *Routledge Handbook of Chinese Medicine*. London: Routledge, pp. 109–119.
Yang, D. (2023) 'Knowledge Transfer of Bodily Practices between China and India in the Medieval World', *Journal of Yoga Studies* 4: 413–440.
Yoeli-Tlalim, R. (2021) *Reorienting Histories of Medicine: Encounters along the Silk Roads*. London; New York, NY: Bloomsbury Academic.
Zhan, M. (2009) *Other-worldly: Making Chinese Medicine through Transnational Frames*. Durham, NC: Duke University Press.
Ziegler, J. (1998) *Medicine and Religion, c. 1300: The Case of Arnau de Vilanova*. Oxford Historical Monographs. New York, NY: Variation.
Županov, I.G. and Guenzi, C. (eds) (2008) *Divins remèdes: médecine et religion en Asie du sud*. Paris: Ecole des hautes études en sciences sociales.

Part I

East Asia

1

Religion and health care in middle-period China

Nathan Sivin

Background

This study will explore religious curing from roughly 600 to 1400 CE. Before and after that interval, popular religion has been so little studied that a general exploration (which would necessarily include it) would be premature.[1]

The study of medical disorders and their treatment in the Chinese past has focused almost exclusively on the experience of physicians. Very few early sources are based on the patient's viewpoint. That makes for a remarkably biased approach.

Until modern times, in most of the world, including Western Europe, few people had access to doctors. There were not enough of them, and they were too expensive for most. A small minority of European and American doctors studied the state of their art at a university medical school. As late as the mid-nineteenth century in a few advanced Western European countries, and the 1920s in the United States, they were more likely to have learned medicine in an apprenticeship or a proprietary school of low standard, or – for that matter – might simply have done a little reading and, perfectly legally, hung up a shingle.

The earlier generations of medical historians, Chinese and foreign, were mostly educated as doctors or situated in medical schools. They saw their mission as chronicling the hard-won distinction of the scientific physician. From their viewpoint, legitimate healing was an endeavor to create and apply the modern state of the art. This was, in their eyes, an entirely rational and positivistic endeavour. Nothing else was worth studying.

But that tells us nothing about the public's health at a given time, and what people and governments did to improve it. Fantasying that the vast majority of Chinese – illiterate peasants in isolated villages and poor people in towns and cities – went to a doctor when they needed treatment will not do. It is merely sensible to ask whose help they could actually count on.

In the early twentieth century, it was still true that the sources of therapy available to ordinary people were almost entirely religious. There were popular priests in every village, Buddhist priests or monks in many, and Daoist priests or monks in a few. For that matter, over the last thousand years, local officials representing the imperial government were required to perform regular formal ceremonies of worship in popular and Buddhist temples and monasteries and Daoist abbeys that had passed the demanding requirements for government registration.[2]

Historians in China often noted that a good deal of therapy was done by people called 'wizards' (*wu* 巫), whose methods, seen from the viewpoint of modern medicine, seem highly irrational and dangerous.[3] Here is how the leading Chinese dictionary of the classical language defines *wu:*

> In antiquity, people who occupied themselves with praying, divination, and astrology, and who used medicines on behalf of others to pray for good luck, to dispel calamities, or to treat illness. In the Shang dynasty (fifteenth to eleventh century) their status was relatively high. In the Zhou period (eleventh to third century BCE) they were divided into male and female *wu,* with different responsibilities, all subordinate to the Director of Sorcery (*siwu* 司巫).[4] From the Spring and Autumn period (770–476) on, the medical art gradually differentiated itself from the techniques of wizards. Nevertheless, among the common people only wizards practiced their techniques, impersonating gods and ghosts to pray and cure disease on behalf of people for generation after generation (Luo Zhufeng 1988: 971).[5]

Early sources tend mysteriously to hint, as this modern quotation does, that physicians and wizards were originally one occupational group, and to think of the differentiation as a stage in the evolution of medicine, rather than involving human social action worth understanding.[6]

Scholars of religion now mostly understand *wu* as someone possessed by a god, temporarily having the power to exorcise spirits. But that is correct only for early China. From the beginning of the imperial period, in the late third century BCE, *wu* gradually came to be used, not as the name of a particular occupation, but as a negative epithet – a term used to characterise someone of whose religious activities the speaker disapproved, without finding it worthwhile to understand, describe or define them. The literate minority,[7] the only people who left written documents, used the word most often for popular priests, who mostly carried out their rituals while possessed by spirits, but as time went on conventional people routinely applied it to Daoist monks or priests and other religious operatives whom they did not see any need to distinguish from mediums.[8] But from the early days of Daoism, its operatives defined themselves by their attacks on popular religion.

From the eleventh century on, when the government began registering popular temples on a large scale, officials tended to apply it to priests of temples which had not met the stringent criteria for inclusion as an Orthodox Shrine (*zhengsi* 正祀) in the state's Register of Sacrifices (*sidian* 祀典), or clerics who had not bought the expensive government certificates of ordination (Sivin 2015: 96, 131).[9]

How do we know this? For most of Chinese history, only the literate minority could leave written records. Their idea of medical history was chronological accounts of the careers of eminent physicians. The celebrated *History of Medicine* (*Yi shi* 醫史, 1547), by Li Lian 李濂, is limited to precisely that. My concern here is not medicine in that narrow sense, but health care: everything, done no matter by whom, to restore health.[10]

We can hardly expect people in the stratum that studied classics for years in preparation for government service impartially to observe and systematically to record how their servants and tenant farmers cared for their health. On the other hand, in elite writings of various kinds are scattered a great many remarks on precisely that.

We can conclude from our knowledge of the scholar-official class and of aristocrats over many centuries that, far from being severely secular, they took the worship of spirits seriously (Johnson *et al.* 1985; Bell 1989; Chao 2011). Most emperors patronised at least one religion, and even high officials wrote prayers and other documents used in ceremonies.[11] The central government's registration of popular, Daoist and Buddhist temples over the last millennium depended mainly on the written testimony of the magistrate and the local gentry that each temple's gods were efficacious (*ling* 靈), that they responded to ritual and prayer (Sivin 2015: 163). Great numbers of prayers and other documents for curing rituals survive (still largely unread) in the collected writings of high officials and even emperors. A few literati, exceptionally curious about those around them, collected anecdotes of the remarkable, commonly giving space to miraculous cures.

Curing was the most-cited proof of the gods' efficacy. That is not surprising, for popular culture embodied its own perspectives on ailment and cure.

Most sickness in the popular milieu was the result of pollution of one kind or another, often due to violating a taboo or to the neglect of ritual. The popular priest (whom ordinary people called 'master of arts' [*fashi* 法師]), was usually part-time, often a neighbour or a fellow farmer, who had learned what he (or less commonly she) needed to serve as an intermediary with the otherworld. Some popular priests learned techniques such as thunder rites that let them actually exorcise the miscreant spirits.[12] Competing with them for a living were curers who had been trained as Daoists but were not ordained. There were also itinerant lay practitioners, who used a similar armamentarium without being possessed.

Buddhists and Daoists were much more powerful. The Buddhists were able to call upon their own divinities. Daoists, as members of the celestial bureaucracy, could take up such matters with divine colleagues. That let them identify guilty spirits directly and with exactitude, and ritually issue requests to bring them back into line. Even local government officials sometimes learned methods of exorcism that could augment their authority (Sivin 2015: 171–81).

The Celestial Masters, the first Daoist movement (second half of second century CE) about which we know the workings, lived in closed theocratic communities that believed illness was sin, whether from violating community rules or incorrectly carrying out ritual. The cure was a matter of identifying and ritually confessing the sin; the use of medicine or other secular therapy was expressly forbidden. But not long after the third century, the communities were transplanted to other parts of China, where they came in regular contact with non-members. They began using the full range of their neighbours' medical techniques alongside their spiritual cures.

From that time on, all three religions competed for clients, but that does not imply that patients simply chose. Most of the population of Imperial China did not have disposable income until quite late. Popular healers, who were not necessarily better off than their clients, could always accept gifts in kind from those who could not pay in cash. Buddhists were not as prevalent, but might also accept gifts in return for performing their rites. Daoists were a great deal thinner on the ground. According to what we have learned about the second millennium CE, there were about a twentieth as many of them as of Buddhist clerics. That ruled out serving everybody (Goosaert 2000, 2007).[13] They tended to concentrate on rituals for wealthy individuals, for communities, for periodic spiritual renewal, for health, or to prevent or stop epidemics; that is still the case. Their rituals were, to put it roughly, the most expensive.

It is natural to ask what the borders were between the methods of popular, Buddhist and Daoist priests, and between them and the therapies of physicians. That question, however, is based on two erroneous assumptions, namely that healers wanted to use only their own proprietary measures and to avoid those of their competitors, and that they could stop outsiders who adopted theirs.

Competition there certainly was. The case records of physicians survive from the eleventh century on. Their authors often specify, for a given case, what sort of healer had unsuccessfully preceded them – mostly other physicians, but fairly often religious healers. Clerics did not compile case records, but the ritual texts of Buddhists and Daoists make it clear that both were adapting therapeutic rites from popular priests, who in turn were freely adapting their methods. As lay popular therapists entered the picture, they used religious rituals, and their religious competitors used theirs.

Although this promiscuity is often explained by such concepts as 'influence' and 'borrowing', Stephen Bokenkamp has argued persuasively that when a therapy prominently associated with A shows up in the practice of B, this is not a case of influence but of appropriation. The motivation is not B's desire to resemble A, but to excel him (Orzech 2002; Bokenkamp 2004: 198).

We can also find medical methods being used by Buddhists and Daoists. For instance, the Daoist patriarch Tao Hongjing 陶弘景 (456–546) wrote the most important handbook of *materia medica* of his time. We also find Buddhist and Daoist methods in use by doctors. For example, the Daoist *Jin jing* 禁經 (Classic of Interdiction), is included in Sun Simiao's 孫思邈 (alive 673) *Qianjin yi fang* 千金翼方 (Revised Formulas Worth a Thousand in Gold), probably the most influential medical treatise of the seventh century.[14]

I will first summarise what sources are available for religious curing and its background.

Literature

The study of medical disorders and their treatment in the Chinese past has focused almost exclusively on the experience of physicians. Very few early sources are based on the patient's viewpoint. That makes for a remarkably biased approach.

The viewpoint of Sinologists has also been distorted by their unwillingness to look beyond the ingrained notion that there were three great religions (*sanjiao* 三教) – Confucianism, Daoism and Buddhism. The first of these labelled a kind of cultivation practised by some members of the elite, which did not directly affect even its majority, much less commoners. Literate adherents of all three were unwilling to acknowledge the importance of popular religion, the organised worship of the gods that had given rise to the elite religions.[15] Because their own liturgies were based on written scriptures, they considered the ceremonies of the illiterate majority nothing more than 'vulgar practices' (*su* 俗). Rather than acknowledging the ritualists as local healers and exorcists – that is, priests – they tended to look down upon them as 'wizards' (*wu* 巫).[16]

Religions

The scholarly literature on religious curing is astonishingly small, and mostly recent. Most pioneering specialists in premodern religious studies were uninterested in therapy, and the few historians of medicine who have looked into non-European matters have seldom challenged the prejudice that Chinese medicine is merely delusory and therefore irrelevant. Change has come about as anthropology and sociology have increasingly proven valuable in historical studies, shifting the focus away from political history and the careers of great men towards cultural and social analysis.

Buddhist studies have been canted towards philology and the explication of texts. One can occasionally find early generalist writings, but until the 1990s most Buddhological publications on medicine tended to be notes devoted to miniscule topics approached out of context.[17]

The study of Daoism was greatly deterred by the tendency of Sinologists to limit the word's scope to the *Laozi*, *Zhuangzi* and a few other classics written after 300 BCE. The only substantial studies undertaken before 1945 – but published later – that investigated the Daoist religious movements were, in Europe, those of Henri Maspero in Paris, and in Japan, those of Yoshioka Yoshitoyo and a few others who had observed Daoist monastic life in China (Maspero 1950; Yoshioka 1952: 1970–6). The Sino-Japanese War and then, from 1949 on, Chinese government pressure against the study of religion, minimised publication on both Buddhism and Daoism until the 1980s.

Until the late 1960s, a few scholars outside China in various fields delved in the Daoist Canon to investigate one or another topic that happened to interest them. What inspired a discipline that could be called Daoist studies was a series of three international conferences held between 1968 and 1979.[18] They brought together scholars who had studied some aspect of Daoism for discussions that related what understanding they had, revealing important questions likely to benefit from research. In the course of the three meetings, a first sense of the historical development of the Daoist religious movements began to emerge.[19]

The most striking outcome was the discovery at the second meeting that K. M. Schipper, who was trained in anthropology and Sinology in Paris, after a decade of apprenticeship in Tainan had been ordained as a Daoist priest. Scriptures centuries old that he had studied in the Daoist Canon, he discovered, were still being used in modern Taiwanese liturgy.[20]

The long-term result of the conferences was the emergence of Daoist studies as a distinct constituent of the history of religions. The surviving performance of Daoist liturgy meant that ethnology was feasible as well. Attendees began to teach; their students came to understand that the subject was worth deep study. International recognition led to a revival in China, and regular communication worldwide between specialists and students.[21] Daoist studies have grown quickly.[22]

Popular religion

Another outcome of the three conferences on Daoism was a first appreciation of popular religion as a related but distinct cultural entity. The consensus at that point was that popular religion was the historical backbone of religion in China, and that other religions evolved as elite adaptations of and reactions to it.[23] This view rejects the old mythology that claimed archaic rulers and their ministers invented all that was important in traditional culture.

Before 1985, only a handful of studies had examined popular religion and its relations with other religious phenomena. From the mid-1980s on, the Chinese Popular Culture Project at Berkeley and the theoretical analysis of Catherine Bell encouraged the growth of understanding in Western scholarship. Recovery from the Cultural Revolution led to valuable studies in China and elsewhere.[24] Peter Nickerson and Paul Katz have provided superior concise discussions of the relation of Daoism and popular religion.[25] But most scholarship on religion simply ignored popular religion, and still does so.

Curing

Scholars in China began publishing on the relations of Daoism with medicine as early as 1981.[26] Such studies often depended on extremely loose senses of both 'Daoism' and 'medicine', and quoted their sources out of context. Their analyses tended to be positivistic. This situation has improved as Chinese authors have had more contact with international networks of researchers. As a result, scholars elsewhere have also produced much valuable work.[27]

Japanese scholars of Buddhism have been taking up the role of curing since the work of Obinata Daijō 大日方大乘 in 1958. Obinata's scholarship was largely devoted to defining medical terms one by one. Fukunaga Katsumi's 福永勝美 studies of terminology (1972) were organised in biomedical categories, and concentrated on practices of Indian origin. Useful more recent publications include Geng Liutong 耿刘同 and Geng Yinxun 耿引循 (1993) and Birnbaum (1989). Particularly influential is Davis (2001), a study of thunder rites, Tantric in origin and widely used by Buddhists, Daoists, popular priests and local officials from about 1100 on. Salguero's *Translating Buddhist Medicine in Medieval China* (2014) is a detailed study of transmission from India and enrichment in China.[28]

Eventually there were a few studies of curing as an aspect of popular religion. Lin Fushi 林富士 (1999) and Liu Liming 劉黎明 (2004) looked at what they considered shamanistic healing, ignoring the social setting of these activities but revealing their character. Sivin (2015), on health care in the eleventh century, studied popular and other ritual therapies and their medical uses.

Sources

The view we find in medical books reflects the world view of the literati. The cosmos, the universal order, spontaneously tends towards internal harmony. Its dynamics were cyclical, and could be expressed in terms of *qi* and its divisions, *yin-yang* and the five phases. There were two microcosms, the state and the human body. In health they were part of the larger harmony, but humans could violate harmonious living, causing dysfunction. The physician, like the ruler and his high officials, could restore healthy functioning by correctly diagnosing what had gone wrong and counteracting it.[29] In a sense doctors were applied cosmologists.

Commoners lived in quite a different world. What organised it was not cosmic forces but human communities and the bureaucracy of the gods. Humans lived in close proximity to, and regularly came in contact with, the world of spirits. These (nature spirits aside) were remnant *qi* of the human dead, who survived in the otherworld[30] as gods, ghosts and ancestors. They became ancestors when their families ritually laid them to rest. If that did not happen, or if the rites were not correctly performed, their *qi*, as ghosts, could cause mischief for their progeny or other people. On the other hand, if the spirit of the deceased brought blessings to descendants, that made it a true ancestor. If the efficacy of its *qi* encouraged people from other families to pray to it and they too benefited, the spread of its worship might lead to its becoming a god (Sivin 2015: 100–4). Practically speaking, that meant an honored place in a shrine of its own, or eventually in the local temple.

Becoming a god was not just an increase in spiritual power. According to the Han people, the gods belonged to a bureaucracy parallel to that of the imperial government. Daoists too were gods.[31] The registers (*lu* 籙) that ordained Daoists received as proof of spiritual attainment specified the place in the pantheon's hierarchy to which they had been appointed, what gods were their colleagues, and what protective spirits they commanded. Buddhists, instead, had access to their own hierarchy of spirits, which remained exotic to worshippers even after they became familiar.

The main bodies of sources for religious curing are the Buddhist and Daoist Canons. The Daoist Canon also contains most of the surviving accounts of popular rituals. The latter were oral, performed in the vernacular, and were recorded only when transcribed – particularly when Daoist clergy performed or adapted them. Let me quote a most sensible note on method by Stephen F. Teiser (1994: 622):

> The overwhelming majority of sources for medieval society were authored by members of one elite or another. Scholar-officials sifted through records to construct edifying accounts of the past, while another elite, composed of the highest-ranking members of the Buddhist and Taoist churches, designed histories to provide to the state a justification of their respective institutions. All sources, of course, reflect the interests of their authors, and in our case that means that we gain knowledge of the past through the eyes of a very powerful but relatively tiny subset of medieval society.[32]

This is all the more evident when the subject of a given record is popular religion and its therapies.

A great many other primary sources are scattered through the general literature. For instance, the documents that high government officials often wrote for use in Daoist liturgy are regularly included in their collected works. Emperors who were devoted to Buddhism or Daoism also wrote ritual documents (Sivin 2015: 174–9). Comments on and descriptions of ceremonies and other activities occur in the collected jottings (*biji* 筆記) of many literati.[33] Poetry is a badly underused source.

In short, the sources reflect three main kinds of therapy. All elite writings accept the value of medicine, although none are attentive to the fact that its clientele was small and privileged. Writings of the office-holding class vary in their esteem for Buddhist and Daoist curing, depending on their status and experience. All of the written sources tend to disparage popular religion, and to see it as the practice of individual 'wizards' rather than as an enterprise rooted in communities.

Analysis

Three basic questions need to be clarified. The first is whether the efficacy of spiritual therapy can be taken seriously. The second is what we know about the varieties of religious curing. The third is about popular religion, the most neglected type: What was it? Who performed it? What was its relation with other religious traditions?

Efficacy

In studying efficacy in Chinese religious therapy, I have had to question the widespread assumption that its value is merely as a sort of folk psychotherapy (Sivin 2015: 9–30). This assumption is based on confidence that biomedical research offers the only way to determine what therapy is objectively valuable.

The Gold Standard of biomedical efficacy is double- or triple-blind testing on a large, statistically random sample of patients. Such tests compare the drug's effects with those of a biomedically inert substance, a placebo, that is given to part of the sample instead of the drug. The difference between positive results – a mere matter of subtraction – becomes a numerical measure of efficacy. This 'gold standard' is useless for studying medicine in, say, seventeenth-century China – or England – for which we have no statistics that satisfy biomedical criteria, and in which many therapies did not use medicines.

The anthropologist Daniel Moerman, based on his survey of the large literature of his field and his own field experience, has argued instead that efficacy in health care is of three distinct kinds (Moerman 2002: 16–21):

1. The **autonomous response** is the tendency of abnormal conditions of the body to regress to the normal mean; that is, the ability of the patient's body to recover spontaneously is probably responsible for most returns to health. Most doctors I have asked estimate the proportion of people who recover regardless of therapy at 65 to 80%. Most clinical problems are, after all, self-limiting.
2. The **specific response** to biological, chemical, or physical intervention. This is the response that biomedical therapy values, and is the only one that its practitioner is prepared to recognise and evaluate. Many physicians, particularly those with substantial experience in general practice, are aware of what they call the 'bedside manner', but most recent medical-school graduates are too rushed in the clinic to overcome a purely evidence-based or other reductive mindset that is useful in research but limiting in caring for patients.
3. The **meaning response** is the curative power of meaning – not only symbols, but 'meaningful events – involving relationship, discourse, form, belief, knowledge, commitment, history' (Moerman 2002: 56). Medical anthropologists and sociologists have examined ailment and its cure in many places and various periods. Their experience invalidates much of the conventional wisdom on efficacy. It shows that the responses of patients and healers to meaning vary greatly. Patients respond to therapists, whether cardiologists or mediums in trance, in ways that are part of their responses to other people in general, and in particular to people who can claim powerful knowledge or people whose status differs notably from theirs. Physicians are human beings interacting in complicated ways with other human beings who are suffering, and who have gone to them for help. For common ailments, doctors' prescriptions often matter less than their social, moral or spiritual influence. Spokesmen for medicine often argue that meaning can affect the patient's view of her experience (her 'illness') but cannot change the objective body states that constitute her 'disease'. But this dichotomy is fallacious.[34]

In Imperial China, as in the modern United States, the value of a technique depends on how it is used, how the therapist and patient understand it, and how the two (and other people present) interact.

In any culture, roles, attitudes, rituals and techniques combine through normal social processes to make available whatever provision of health care lies within the means of that people.[35]

Translating traditional accounts of disease directly into biomedical concepts leads to grossly inadequate understanding. We have seen that therapy depends as greatly on the body's tendency towards homeostasis, and on the patient's response to symbolic and personal interaction, as it does on technology – and often more so. In any system of health care, a practitioner who has learned how to facilitate more than the specific response is more likely to help patients than one who cannot. This implies that the present-day physician's personal cultivation, sensibility and empathy may play as large a role in the outcome as her mastery of pathology.

Popular religion

'Popular religion' is only one of a number of English terms that scholars use; 'folk religion', 'the common religion', 'local religion', 'folk Daoism', 'popular sects', 'local cults', 'shamanism' and others often appear, usually with no sign that all these terms designate the same thing. My preference for 'popular religion' is due to its breadth; unlike 'folk religion', which implies worship by the lower orders, everyone, high and low, experienced it.[36] Even literati who denounced it in official documents as wizardry had taken part in rituals as children; in their native places they supported their local temple and worshipped its gods (Sivin 2015: 93–5).[37]

Popular religion differed from Daoism and Buddhism in that its priesthood was usually part-time, poor and illiterate, so that its liturgy was performed in the local spoken dialect rather than the classical language. In South Chinese villages,[38] where *fashi* were mainly spirit mediums, they were chosen by the gods (often in childhood) because of their ability to enter trance and become possessed. In many cases these early experiences were involuntary, but novice mediums gradually learned to become possessed at will.

The gods that took over their bodies were those locally worshiped. Some of them were tutelary deities such as The Great Sage Equal of Heaven (Qitian Da Sheng 齊天大聖). He was a deified form of Sun Wukong 孫悟空, the mischievous monkey protagonist of *Journey to the West* (*Xi you ji* 西遊記), and his medium's movements resembled those of the monkey in the many operas based on the novel.

In the temple, the medium interacted with people who needed help because of illness and other personal difficulties – or who simply wanted to improve their luck. The god might speak through them, or (from the Ming period on) might leave a written message through the planchette. The local priest performed, in early times, the elite biennial *she* 社 ceremony at the rural altars of the Earth God and, from the eleventh century on, the urban *shehui* 社會, open to everyone, a celebration of the birthday of a tutelary deity (Davis 2001: 12–13).

The priest also conducted rituals at the homes of community members, spiritually purifying the building to interdict spirits, and performing life-cycle rites such as funerals. They also performed rites that spiritually purified people or buildings. That meant, among other things, diagnosing and treating illness. The form this diagnosis normally took was identifying the shade, the spirit, that had been offended, and was causing the trouble by harrassing or possessing the patient. The priest's therapy was analogous to the good offices that a well-connected neighbour could perform if a messenger from the local government headquarters was demanding a bribe you could not afford. The neighbour had no official power, but by asking around he could identify the greedy messenger and entreat his superiors to restrain him.

The local temple was a sort of club for various gods. It might well have been founded as a branch of a temple elsewhere,[39] but it often added gods that the community recognised. The popular pantheons were organised by Daoists, who imposed their empire-wide perspective on the scattered reverence of villages and neighbourhoods. The government's Register of Sacrifices was of course also empire-wide, but it included only temples and gods that had elicited the state's recognition (Sivin 2015: 95–8).

The temple was also a club for the people of the locality. In villages and small towns, it was likely to be the only public gathering-place. Group activities, not only religious but social, economic and military – anything involving too many people to fit in a private house – were centred there. Most of what Sinologists usually call Daoist temples are actually popular, in the sense that the community owned them. Daoists (who, for Imperial China's last millennium, had mostly monasteries and very few temples) simply used them along with popular priests.[40] In fact, many Daoists supplemented inadequate incomes by performing popular liturgies.

Varieties of popular curing

In Imperial China the range of religious therapies was enormous. In addition to those that originated in popular religion, many had been originally elaborated for Daoist and Buddhist use, and *fashi* then re-adapted them into their own vernacular liturgies. My concern here is not to catalogue all of the latter, but rather to give an idea of their range and of how they were adapted back and forth.

The most fundamental basis for most of them was sincere prayer. From at least the seventeenth century on, laymen normally tested themselves for sincerity before or after praying. Temples were provided with a set of two half-moon-shaped blocks (*gaozi* 筶子), one side rounded and one side flat, which the supplicant dropped onto the floor to see which sides faced upward. The pair's landing with one flat side and one rounded side up for three consecutive throws indicated that the god would accept the prayer. If not, the supplicant had to try for a more sincere state of mind or else give up.

The lay practitioner, who lacked the authority of both the Buddhist and Daoist priest, had to rely on the tools available to the popular priest and to him. One of these was knowledge of taboos. He often had to conceal from his patient the remedy that he was using for a particular ailment. In *The Penetrator Corrected* (*Chuan ya* 串雅) there is even a medicine guaranteed to enable pregnancy that carries a conventional taboo against letting dogs, chickens and women see the medicine being mixed. The practitioner was also constrained by special days on which to recite incantations and mix drugs, and special times of day to use drugs – the latter silently.[41]

It is impossible to clearly distinguish popular therapies from those of Buddhism and Daoism, or for that matter from those of physicians. The importance of curing to gaining public support led to a free-for-all of mutual appropriation.

Appropriation necessarily involved adaptation. Here is an example, from the most popular acupuncture treatise of late Imperial China, by Yang Jishi 楊濟時, a palace physician:[42]

> Men or women singing or laughing, weeping or groaning, talkative or silent for a long time, eyes staring wide open morning and evening, moving about wildly day and night, mouth and eyes both askew, going bareheaded or barefoot, exposing their bodies or naked, seeing[43] gods or ghosts, and things of this kind are the mischief of evil presences (*xie* 邪) that have invaded [i.e., possessed] them: flying worm-spirits, lingering *qi* of the dead (*jingling* 精靈), demons, and wild ghosts.
>
> When the time comes for therapy, what is essential in the first place is contentment. What I mean by this is that the patient must respect and trust the doctor, and the doctor must examine and treat the patient with a sincere heart, so that they are happy with each other. Only then can [the physician] expel the demons or ghosts. If the patient cannot stand the *bian* stone (*bian shi* 砭石), there is no point in discussing therapy.[44] If the physician is greedy, one cannot speak of his virtue.
>
> **Writing a talisman.** First use cinnabar [ink] to write Efficacious Talismans of the Supreme One.[45] Burn one of them to ashes, mix them in wine, and have the patient drink it. Paste up one in the patient's room. As you write the talismans, repeat the Small Incantation of the Big Dipper.[46]

The book then provides the words of the incantation and the pattern for the talisman. Its purpose is to drive out alien presences. Although this book recommends its procedure for physicians and other acupuncturists, it obviously originated in popular curing. Burning a talisman and drinking the ashes is still commonly a step in popular therapy.

Classical physicians, like everyone else except a few late intellectuals, did believe that spirits possessed people. They knew that clerics were specialists in curing possession. Some of them claimed that they too could control it. The passage above enumerates several conditions for successful therapy: a healthy relationship between the patient and the therapist, a patient who is prepared for the special kind of acupuncture required and a virtuous curer. Very few medical books spoke explicitly of the need for respect, trust and sincerity. Yang was maximising the effectiveness of what Moerman called the meaning response.

As for other popular therapies, there is no repertory of remedies before 1400. We are fortunate enough to have an eighteenth-century collection of an itinerant curer's remedies. Zhao Xuemin 趙學敏 (c. 1719–1805), a most eminent scholar of *materia medica* and other subjects, met his distant relation Zhao Boyun 趙柏雲, who practised itinerant therapy in North and South China. Zhao Xuemin compiled his methods, selected those 'able to benefit the world', and edited them into *Chuan ya* 串雅 (The Penetrator Corrected, 1759).[47] The book includes not only human disorders but those of animals, fish, insects (crickets kept as pets, silkworms raised for silk, etc.), plants (to prevent bamboos from dying the year after they bloom, etc.) and insects (actually on parasitic disorders in humans).

The author, Zhao Boyun, so far as we know, was not a cleric, but he freely used therapies of a religious nature. He earned his living by therapy. He used incantations, for example, this one for curing a baby that cried at night:[48]

> Take a poker and write[49] on it the words 'by command'. Silently repeat this incantation:
>
> Poker, poker, the Jade Emperor has made you Chancellor
> To grab the night-bawling ghost.
> Beat it to death, beat it to death, never let it go.
> I send thirty-six spirit generals, bearing iron rods and bronze flails
> To get rid of the evil and return it to the correct [way].
> I am carrying out the orders of the Supreme Old Lord;[50]
> Quickly, quickly, by lawful order!

This resembles Daoist incantations found in the late-seventh-century *Classic of Interdictions*. For instance, here is one for 'Violation by an Extrinsic Spirit' (*kewu qi* 客忤氣), a class of possession disorder that could indeed include children crying at night:[51]

> I am a Libationer of the Celestial Masters,
> Sent as an emissary of Heaven and Earth.
> On my body I wear mighty uranic (*qian* 乾) weapons.
> [Spirit soldiers] by the hundred, thousand, myriad, myriad myriad
> Before and behind me, arrayed to my left and right.
> What spirit dares stay? What ghost dares resist?
> Evil shades, quickly go!
> Quickly, quickly, by lawful order.

Zhao Boyun was a popular curer, not a priest, but he did not hesitate to use a therapy that wielded the authority of a Daoist master.

On the other hand, we can find eighth-century Buddhist clerics using popular rituals to cure illness. This story comes from an anthology of the early or mid-tenth century:[52]

> Zhou Xiang 周象 was fond of hunting. Later, when he was magistrate of Fenyang 汾陽 (in present Shanxi), he unexpectedly dreamt of being cornered by a tigress with cubs. Alarmed, he woke up. As a result [of the dream] he became ill.
>
> Afterward, the Buddhist monk Haining 海寧, as he was passing Zhou's house, remarked to an aged neighbor, 'That house has the *qi* of a demon in it; if that goes on much longer, it will be irredeemable'. The old neighbor reported this to Zhou. Zhou summoned the monk, and ordered him to investigate. The monk announced, 'I will exorcise it on your behalf'. He chose a suitable day and set up an altar [outside the house]. Carrying a sword, he did the Pace of Yu and chanted an incantation. He then entered the front gate and proceeded to Zhou's bedroom. He circumambulated the ailing man several times and then shouted in the direction of Zhou. Suddenly from under the bed there came the growl of a tiger. The members of Zhou's family, terrified, scattered. Zhou himself, without waking up, threw himself out of bed, landing unconscious on the floor. The monk sprayed him with water,[53] and in a few moments he recovered (Harper 1998: 159–60, 167–9).[54]

In the Northern Song period (960–1127), as Asaf Goldschmidt has shown, there were important changes in every aspect of medicine. This was due to the activity of the state, which sought to control practice. The same was true of local religion. The state, which had been registering Daoist and Buddhist monasteries and temples for some time, began doing the same for popular temples on a large scale for the first time. What qualified them was the efficacy (*ling* 靈) of their deities, a matter of which ability to cure serious illness was a major sign (Goldschmidt 2009; Sivin 2015: 95–6, 102–3). This registration was extremely selective. Temples that were not chosen were often persecuted by local officials (Hinrichs 2003).

Another significant change in the eleventh and twelfth centuries was the proliferation of new Daoist movements. One of these, the Heart of Heaven movement, plays a part in an anecdote below. A third change was the extraordinary popularity of thunder rites (*leifa* 雷法), which originated much earlier but became a major activity of Daoist priests in the Song period. These two changes were due in part to imperial patronage of thunder rites. They quickly spread to Daoists who could not qualify for ordination by the government, and then to practitioners of popular religion, and even to officials, as in this example:[55]

> Yu Ronggu 余榮古 of Leping 樂平 (Jiangxi), in 1165/1173, because of a famine, left his home and sailed along the Huai river. He had an unanticipated opportunity to learn the rites of the Five Thunder Gods; he studied and practised them to some extent.
>
> At the time, the water buffalo that did the ploughing in the villages often suffered from an epidemic. He went to treat them, and regularly succeeded. He received enough rewards to keep his stomach filled, so he decided to settle down there.
>
> In 1185 he made his way back to his old home. The parents of his cousin Zhiquan's 知權 wife, née Zhan 詹, had just gone to the Huai river area, and Zhiquan and his wife had accompanied them [part way] to see them off. The wife, after returning home, got an ailment that made her talk wildly as if she were crazy or demented; she was no longer conscious of what went on around her (*buxing ren shi* 不省人事). [Her husband] summoned Yu to examine her. When he began carrying out the rites of Investigating and Summoning (*kaozhao* 考召), he found that [the responsible shade] was that of her dead ancestor.
>
> Yu looked at [the wife] and said, 'She can be tied up'. At the time, the patient was lying down in the bedroom. She immediately thrust her hands forward, and meekly allowed herself to be bound. He next had her whipped and interrogated until she cried out and confessed her guilt. He unhurriedly spoke to her, 'You are an ancestor of the Zhan family who has attached herself[56] to this house so that incense will be burnt for you. How dare you arbitrarily enter the domicile of living people and cause such calamity? I am aware that you are a relative by marriage, and do not want to bring the law to bear on you, but you had better leave quickly!' She apologized for her misconduct and asked to be released, and he assented. In just a moment the patient returned to normal.

This is a typical example of 'investigating and summoning', a major component of thunder rites, as Davis has analysed them (Davis 2001: 107–8). The term *kaozhao* often stands for the entire procedure.[57] The curer forces the shade to confess – in this case by whipping the body of the possessed woman, and then persuades it to transform from a harmful presence to a benevolent one, or at least (as here) to leave.

Finally, an intriguing example of lay use of Daoist authority:[58]

A wizard of Huaijin township in Wuyuan 婺源懷金鄉 (present Zhejiang) named Zhang (*wuzhe* Zhang sheng 巫者張生) was skilled in the arts of sorcery; he was able to visit calamities on people. He often visited the houses of the rich to demand money or food. If what he received was less than he wanted, he would begin jumping and hopping about; [people] called it 'turning somersaults'.[59] Such a family would become ill with sores and rashes, or some of them would die. Because of this, everyone feared him.

A gentleman, Wang Tingrui 汪廷瑞, admired Zhang's ability to come by money dishonestly, so he became his follower, helping him with this and that. He wrote a signboard in large characters that said, 'Those who go to audience in heaven *(chao tian men* 朝天門)' and hung it on [Zhang's] house.

The wizard wore a high hat, a dark red gown with broad sleeves and a wide yellow belt. Every day he climbed into a high chair and spoke freely about good and bad fortune. He had thirty [disciples] who respectfully served him.

A district headquarters underling, Wang Zao *(Xian shouli Wang Zao* 縣手力汪早), had occasion to stop by [Zhang's] house, and became angry because he did not burn incense.[60] He sent people to catch him and bring him back [to headquarters] for interrogation. [When he arrived,] Wang said, 'permit me to wash my hands and pay my respects' (*rong xi shou zhijing* 容洗手致敬). When he had [done so and] burnt incense, he had Zhang tied up, and said, '[Your conduct] will not do. If you have a way of using talismans, you might as well have *yin* soldiers suspend me in mid-air and beat me with rods. If you can't, I will go and tell the district magistrate about you'. He then had him unbound. [Since the wizard could not stop him,] Wang went to prepare charges, and proceeded to the magistrate to report them.

The magistrate, Hong Bangzhi 洪邦直,[61] had him brought in to the hall, where he pressed him for a confession, interrogating him about his sorcery. Zhang replied, 'What I practise is the Rectifying Rites of the Heart of Heaven,[62] which is best for curing people's ailments. When I began, I was not doing sorcery'. His words and his expression

> were haughty. The magistrate said, 'You are able to turn somersaults. If you can do one higher than the drum tower, I'll let you go!' At that, Zhang became visibly frightened. He begged for pity, but was ordered put in jail.
>
> The next day, [the magistrate] himself conducted the trial. He also carried in his hand a Celestial Masters register with a demon-subjugating seal, and he said to the wizard, 'You always say that you are in touch with spirits, and know things that have not yet happened. Now tell me what I am holding in my hand'. [Zhang] was stupefied; he had no answer. [The magistrate] without further ado had him flogged twenty strokes and then ejected from his district. ...

This is a typically conventional Song dynasty account of the villainy of a local *fashi*, and his comeuppance at the hands of a representative of the imperial government. TJ Hinrichs has discussed the political significance of this type of story, common in historical writing as well as in jottings based on hearsay (Hinrichs 2003: 9–14, 39–47, 93–6). It has religious repercussions as well. Such stories document the widespread persecution of popular priests who practised in temples that, because they were unregistered, government officials did not recognise (they were required to worship in registered temples). This story is typical in another sense; those who approved and proposed this persecution tended, like Hong Yingxian, to be southerners (Sivin 2015: 96–7).

But this anecdote is exceptional in a different sense. It is about the judgement of an official on a commoner. In addition to the power wielded *ex officio* by the magistrate, the magistrate also had religious power at his disposal. Two Daoist movements encounter each other in the persons of two people who are apparently not ordained Daoists. One is the wizard who claims to be practising the exorcistic Rectifying Rites of the Heart of Heaven. The second is the magistrate who exerts superior religious authority because he carries in his hand an orthodox Daoist register along with a seal typical of someone initiated into the Rites of the Five Thunder Gods. How he got them is not mentioned.

As the challenge by Wang Zao reveals, magical cures often formed a locus of contestation wherein folk practice, official powers, and elite Celestial Master authority were negotiated and defined. The *wu*, despite what are described as his calamitous rites, does not actually control the talismans of dreadful gods that are the chief weapons of Heart of Heaven liturgy – perhaps because he is illiterate.[63] But the imperial official does not have to use his Daoist powers; he finds his conventional tools, flogging and exile, quite adequate.[64]

Conclusions

Physicians played a very small role in Chinese health care. For most people the only therapy available was religious, and that offered by priests of popular religion was most accessible.

The Chinese elite, like everyone else in China, believed that gods, ghosts and ancestors affected their lives. For the last three centuries of Imperial China, many educated men rejected this understanding, but it was practically universal between 600 and 1400.

The understanding of Chinese religion has been greatly distorted because students of that topic have generally accepted the biases of the late imperial elite and their successors. This attitude has encouraged Sinologists to disregard popular religion, or to treat its priests as mere 'wizards'.

Sacred cures in use at a given time cannot be sorted into such neat categories as popular, Buddhist and Daoist. The cutting edge of religious organisation in China was curing. For that reason, every religious movement nurtured its own methods of health care, and its initiates adapted those of other religions. The outcome was a free-for-all of appropriation.

Notes

1 A study of 'shamanism' in the third to sixth centuries (Lin Fu-shih 1999), although out of date in its scholarship, gives the impression that, before the wide impact of Buddhism and Daoism, popular religion differed greatly from the forms it took from the seventh century on. The spread of education and wealth beyond the old elite in the Ming period also made a great difference.

2 I have documented all the assertions in this paragraph in Sivin (2015).

3 On the efficacy of religious ritual see Sivin (2015: 31–52).

4 The standard reference work for official titles, Hucker (1985, #5814), describes the civil service post this way: 'Director of Sorcery: … members of the Ministry of Rites (*Chunguan* 春官) responsible for

all sorcery at court including appeals for rain in times of drought and various activities in response to other sorts of calamities; participated in all court ceremonies and funerals'.

5 The description of *wu* in the Zhou period is based on the *Zhou li* 周禮 (The Rites of Zhou), 6: 39b, a late, unreliable depiction of the dynasty's civil service. Note that I speak of 'curing' instead of 'healing'. Primary sources unambiguously claim to cure disease.

6 For a digest of the exceedingly varied data on pre-Han curing, see Cook (2013).

7 A tiny minority in the first millennium CE, and not a large one until well after 1949. See two essays on *wu* in Li Ling (2000).

8 J.J.M. de Groot, who studied in Imperial China from 1886 to 1890, wrote about *wu* at considerable length under the heading 'The Priesthood of Animism'. He considered Daoists a kind of *wu*. See Groot (1892–1910: 1187–341).

9 Robert Hymes (2015: 531–2) has shown that in the Southern Song period, these certificates were widely sold and resold as a speculative investment.

10 Health care decidedly includes self-therapy and care by family members. See Sivin (2015: 4). Preserving health was in Chinese eyes a separate but intimately related matter (*yangsheng* 養生, 'nurturing life'), largely concerned with longevity. I do not take up these topics here.

11 For examples from Northern Song, see Sivin (2015: 172–79).

12 In the Song period, when unordained Daoists and Buddhists joined their ranks, this became more prevalent than before. See Davis (2001).

13 For the Northern Song, when government censuses included only officially ordained clerics. See Sivin (2015: 163).

14 Tao's handbook was *Bencao jing jizhu* 本草經集注. On his career see Espesset (2008). The manual of interdictions is j. 29–30 of *Qianjin yi fang*. 'Interdiction' (*jin* 禁) is a term for methods that both keep spiritual impurities from entering the body and drive them out if they are present. It is thus wider in scope than 'exorcism'.

15 Buddhism was already formed when it entered China, but most of the ways in which it adapted to its new milieu were shaped by popular religious customs.

16 Sinologists also translate this term as 'sorcerer' or 'shaman'. Puett (2002: 36–40, 117) argues strongly that shamanism is a misleading term. See Davis (2001: 7–11) for a more defensible and cogent trio.

17 The best-known exception is Paul Demiéville (1937). See also Birnbaum (1989).

18 They were held in Europe and Japan, but the main source of funding was the American Council of Learned Societies. The end of the

Cultural Revolution enabled two Chinese scholars to attend the third conference.

19 The papers and discussions are summarised and evaluated in Sivin (1979).

20 His many important contributions include both analytic studies (Schipper 1982, 1995) and reference tools (Schipper 1975; Schipper and Verellen 2004). For an account of his career and contributions see Zurndorfer's foreword to Meyer and Engelfriet (2000).

21 The early publications of Liu Zhiwan 劉枝萬 (1967, 1972) were mainly based on the observation of large-scale Daoist ceremonies in Taiwan.

22 A few of the most important contributions to Daoist studies are Kohn (2000), Kohn and Roth (2002), Goossaert (2000 and 2007), Lagerwey (2004), Pregadio (2008) and Chao (2011). For the relations of popular religion and Daoism, see Little and Eichman (2000: 255–73) and Matsumoto Koichi 松本浩一 (2006). For recent reference works, see Sivin (2010).

23 The forms that Buddhism took in China differed considerably from those in India. Daoism developed mainly in opposition to popular religion, whose animal sacrifices and worship of humans who had died unnatural deaths it condemned as diabolic. This relationship also had its complementary aspects. See Schipper (1994: 7). At another point (1994: 19) he remarks 'in modern China, in local society, the strength and scope of popular beliefs and practices surpass Taoism'.

24 Johnson *et al.* (1985) and Johnson (2009). See Bell (1989). Feuchtwang (2001) is a pioneering attempt at synthesis; see also Ma Xisha 马西沙 and Han Bingfang 韩秉方 (2004). Among other important early publications were Teiser (1993), Anonymous (1994), Li Fengmao 李豐楙 (1994), Zheng Tuyou 郑土有 and Wang Xiansen 王贤森 (1994), Orzech (2002), Zong Li 宗力 and Liu Qun 刘群 (1987), Dean (1993), Katz (1995 and 2009), Li Zhitian 黎志添 (1999), Wang Jianchuan 王見川 (1999) and Zhang Zehong 张泽洪 (1999).

25 Nickerson (2008a, 2008b), Katz (2008). The topic is essentially the same, but the approaches are different.

26 Wei Qipeng 魏启鹏 (1981). See the extensive list of publications in Gai Jianmin 蓋建民 and He Zhenzhong 何振中 (2014: 4–6).

27 Exceptional are Strickmann (1985, 1987, 2002), Nickerson (1994, 2002), Lin Fushi 林富士 (1999, 2001), Sakade (2007), Kleeman (2005, 2009), Lai (2010), Despeux (2010), and Stanley-Baker (2013).

28 See also Salguero (2015).

29 Lloyd and Sivin (2002: 214–26) discuss the relationship between macrocosms and microcosms. It supersedes the discussion in Sivin (1995).

30 Because in China gods were part of the natural order, many scholars use this or similar terms rather than the misleading 'supernatural'.

31 The form and import of registers varied to some extent between Daoist movements; see Miller (2008). The relation between liturgical ordination within Daoism and ordination by the state, confirmed by issuing a certificate, is entirely unclear. Most specialists in Daoism ignore the latter.

32 Teiser also recommends 'adopting a suspicious attitude towards all sources'.

33 The richest and most often studied is *Yijian zhi* 夷堅志 (completed 1202). See especially Davis (2001: 5) which notes that *Yijian zhi* contains nearly two hundred instances of spirit possession.

34 On the fallacy of the illness–disease dichotomy, see Sivin (2015: 24–5).

35 A complicating factor is the variation over space and time in definitions not only of disease but also of symptoms. In other words, the nosology of biomedicine is likely to be misleading unless one first understands the kind of therapy being studied. On this topic, see Sivin (2015: 41–7).

36 On the other hand, my preference for 'popular religion' over 'common religion' is arbitrary.

37 The remainder of this subsection is largely based on Schipper unpublished. It gives an account of late-twentieth-century practices in Taiwan. Although much of it is in line with fragmentary early sources, there is still no even-handed and general description of popular religion in Imperial China.

38 The situations in North and Southwest China have still to be closely studied. This is even true of Daoism. 'Fieldwork for rural North China by Daoist scholars is even more seriously flawed in that, basically, there is none' (Jones 2013: 3009).

39 See Dean (1993: 99–130), on the 'division of incense'.

40 See Steinhardt (2000) on the fuzziness of the distinction.

41 *Chuan ya, wai bian* 串雅外遍, 1.33b, 1.18b, 1.20b, and 1.30a; *Chuan ya quan shu, wai bian*, 1.186–87, 1.175, 1.176, and 1.183.

42 *Zhenjiu dacheng* 針灸大成 (1601) 9.33b–34b. The modern critical edition excludes this section as 'superstitious and absurd'. Heilongjiang Zuguo Yiyao Yanjiusuo 黑龙江祖国医药研究所 (1984).

43 The text reads *sangjian* 桑見, clearly a copyist's error.

44 On this stone surgical tool, see Lo (2002).

45 The text says 'write one Efficacious Talisman of the Supreme One' (*shu Taiyi ling fu yidao* 書太乙靈符一道) but at least two are required.

46 *Tiangang* 天罡 is a star in the handle of the Big dipper, here synecdoche for the Dipper.

47 Preface to *Chuan ya*. *Chuan* 串 was itinerant doctors' slang for drugs of downward-tending function (laxatives, etc.).

48 *Chuan ya, wai bian* 外遍, 1.15b–16a (printed ed., pp. 131–2), part of a whole chapter on incantations and related methods (1. 9a–19b; printed ed., pp. 126–35).

49 The text reads '*yi jian jue shou shu* 以劍訣手書'; the meaning of the first three characters is something like 'using the instructions for [writing on] swords'.

50 Laozi as one of the three divine emanations of the Way. Since the Way itself is ineffable, the three are the primary objects of Daoist rites.

51 *Qianjin yifang*, 29.14a. 347b.

52 *Kaiyuan Tianbao yi shi* 開元天寶遺事, 1.14.

53 In a fine spray from his mouth, as Chinese still do to moisten clothes while ironing, and as a stage of ritual.

54 Harper cites or translates occurrences in manuscripts of the third and second centuries BC. The Pace of Yu in Daoist ritual was a kind of dance performed to clear away in advance the hazards of a cosmic journey. 'Common to magic in the north and south during the third century BC', it originated in popular rites of at least the third century BC. Its meaning and function that early are not clear.

55 *Yijian zhi, zhi yi* 支乙, 3.815. Ordination required either passing a demanding examination or buying an expensive certificate.

56 There is no clue about whether the ghost is male or female.

57 The term is often translated 'summoning and investigating' but that ignores the order of the words. The therapist first determines which shade is responsible for the medical disorder, and then summons it to possess the body of the afflicted person. If the patient is too weak to handle the stress, the ritualist may cause the shade to possess a spirit medium or a child.

58 *Yijian zhi* 夷堅志, *zhi ding*支丁, 4.995.

59 This may very well have been a strongly unsympathetic way of describing the Pace of Yu or a similar ritual dance at an early stage in certain ceremonies.

60 I suspect this implies that the wizard did not give him a tip.

61 Hong was a member of the clan of Hong Mai, the compiler of the Yijian zhi, and appears often in his collection. Sometimes Hong refers to him by name, and sometimes (as here) by his courtesy name, Yingxian 應賢. See *Yijian zhi, jiazhi* 甲志, 13.112 and *yizhi* 乙志, 15.309.

62 *Tianxin zheng fa* 天心政法 (Rectifying Rites of the Heart of Heaven), an important new Daoist movement of the tenth century. It was widely known that it used talismans and seals.

63 On Heart of Heaven talismans see Andersen (1996).
64 For an anecdote from the same source in which an official does use thunder rites effectively, see Sivin (2015: 135).

Bibliography

Andersen, P. (1996) 'Taoist Talismans and the History of the Tianxin Tradition', *Acta Orientalia*, 57: 141–52.

Anonymous (1994) *Minjian Xinyang yu Zhongguo Wenhua Guoji Yantao Lunwenji* 民間信仰與中國文化國際研討會論文集 (Proceedings of International Conference on Popular Beliefs and Chinese Culture). Center for Chinese Studies Research Series, 4. 2 vols. Taipei: Hanxue yanjiu zhongxin.

Bell, C. (1989) 'Religion and Chinese Culture: Toward an Assessment of "Popular Religion"', *History of Religions*, 29: 35–57.

Bencao jing jizhu 本草經集注 (The [Heavenly Farmer's] Canon of *Materia Medica*, with Collected Annotations). Tao Hongjing 陶弘景 (456–536 CE) (1955). Shanghai: Qunlian chubanshe.

Birnbaum, R. (1989) 'Chinese Buddhist Traditions of Healing and the Life Cycle', in L.E. Sullivan (ed.) *Healing and Restoring: Health and Medicine in the World's Religious Traditions*. New York: Macmillan, pp. 33–57.

Bokenkamp, S.R. (2004) 'The Silkworm and the Bodhi Tree: The Lingbao Attempt to Replace Buddhism in China and Our Attempt to Place Lingbao Daoism', in J. Lagerwey (ed.) *Religion and Chinese Society. A Centennial Conference of the École française d'Extrême-Orient.* Volume 1. *Ancient and Medieval China*. Hong Kong: The Chinese University Press, pp. 317–39.

Chao, Shin-yi (2011) *Daoist Ritual, State Religion, and Popular Practices: Zhenwu Worship from Song to Ming (960–1644)*. Routledge Studies in Daoism. New York: Routledge.

Chuan ya 串雅 (The Penetrator Improved). Zhao Boyun 趙柏雲 and Zhao Xuemin 趙學敏 (eds.) (1759). Japanese MS copy of 1836 in library of Jimbun Kagaku Kenkyujõ. Kyoto. An early study is Unschuld (1978).

Chuan ya quan shu 串雅全书 (The Complete Penetrator Improved), includes the original *Chuan ya* and *Chuan ya bu* 串雅補 (Supplement to *The Penetrator Improved*, 1875) (1998). Beijing: Zhongguo zhongyiyao chubanshe.

Cook, C.A. (2013) 'The Pre-Han Period', in TJ Hinrichs and L.L. Barnes (eds) *Chinese Medicine and Healing: An Illustrated History*. Cambridge, MA: The Belknap Press of Harvard University Press, pp. 5–30.

Davis, E.L. (2001) *Society and the Supernatural in Song China*. Honolulu: University of Hawai'i Press.

Dean, K. (1993) *Taoist Ritual and Popular Cults of Southeast China*. Princeton: Princeton University Press.
Demiéville, P. (1937) 'Byô', in S. Levi, J. Takakusu and P. Demiéville (eds) *Hōbōgirin. Dictionnaire Encyclopedique de Bouddhisme d'apres les Sources Chinoises et Japonaises*. Tokyo: Maison Franco-Japonaise, 3, pp. 224–70.
Despeux, C. (ed.) (2010) *Médecine, Religion et Société dans la Chine Médiévale. Étude de Manuscripts Chinois de Dunhuang et de Turfan*. 3 vols. Paris: Institut des Hautes Études Chinoises.
Espesset, G. (2008) 'Tao Hongjing', in F. Pregadio (ed.) *The Encyclopedia of Taoism*. London: Routledge, pp. 968–71.
Feuchtwang, S. (2001) *Popular Religion in China: The Imperial Metaphor*. Richmond, Surrey: Curzon.
Fukunaga Katsumi 福永勝美 (1972) *Bukkyō igaku shōsetsu* 仏教医学詳説 (Detailed explications of Buddhist medicine). Tokyo: Yūzankaku.
Gai Jianmin 蓋建民 and He Zhenzhong 何振中 (2014) *Daojiao yixue jingyi* 道教医学精义 (Essential Meanings of Daoist Medicine). Beijing: Zongjiao wenhua chubanshe.
Geng Liutong 耿刘同 and Geng Yinxun 耿引循 (1993) *Foxue yu Zhongyixue* 佛学与中医学 (Buddhism and Chinese Medicine). Fuzhou: Fuzhou kexue jishu chubanshe.
Goldschmidt, A. (2009) *The Evolution of Chinese Medicine. Northern Song Dynasty (960–1127)*. Needham Research Institute Series, 8. London: Routledge.
Goossaert, V. (2000) 'Counting the Monks: The 1736–1739 Census of the Chinese Clergy', *Late Imperial China*, 21.2: 40–85.
Goossaert, V. (2007) *The Taoists of Peking, 1800–1949: A Social History of Urban Clerics*. Harvard University Center for Asian Studies.
Groot, J.J.M. de (1892–1910) *The Religious System of China, its Ancient Forms, Evolution, History and Present Aspect, Manners, Customs and Social Institutions Connected Therewith*. Leiden: Brill.
Harper, D. (1998) *Early Chinese Medical Literature: The Mawangdui Medical Manuscripts*. London: Royal Asiatic Society.
Heilongjiang Zuguo Yiyao Yanjiusuo 黑龙江祖国医药研究所 (1984) *Zhenjiu dacheng jiaoshi* 針灸大成校释 (Acupuncture Omnibus, Critical Edition). Beijing: Renmin weisheng chubanshe. Expurgated.
Hinrichs, TJ (2003) *The Medical Transforming of Governance and Southern Customs in Song Dynasty China (960–1279 C.E.)*. PhD thesis, East Asian Languages, Harvard University.
Hucker, C.O. (1985) *A Dictionary of Official Titles in Imperial China*. Stanford University Press.
Hymes, R. (2015) 'Sung Society and Social Change', in J.W. Chaffee and D. Twitchett (eds) *The Cambridge History of China*, vol. 5, part 2. Cambridge: Cambridge University Press, pp. 526–664.
Jin jing 禁經 (Canon of Interdiction). In *Qianjin yifang*, j. 29–30.

Johnson, D.G. (2009) *Spectacle and Sacrifice: The Ritual Foundations of Village Life in North China*. Cambridge: Harvard University Press.

Johnson, D.G., Nathan, A.J., Rawski, E.S. and Berling, J.A. (eds) (1985) *Popular Culture in Late Imperial China*. Berkeley, CA: University of California Press.

Jones, S. (2013) 'Temple and Household Daoists: Notes from North China', in Liu Xun and V. Goossaert (eds) *Quanzhen Daoists in Chinese Society and Culture, 1500–2010*. Berkeley: Institute of East Asian Studies, University of California, pp. 308–33.

Kaiyuan Tianbao yi shi 開元天寶遺事 (Accounts that Survived from the Early Eighth Century). Wang Renyu 王仁裕 (mid tenth-century), in *Tang Song shiliao biji congkan* 唐宋史料筆記叢刊 (1981). Beijing: Zhonghua shuju.

Katz, P.R. (1995) *Demon Hordes and Burning Boats. The Cult of Marshal Wen in Late Imperial Chekiang*. Albany: State University of New York press.

Katz, P.R. (2008) 'Taoism and Local Cults', in F. Pregadio (ed.) *The Encyclopedia of* Taoism. London: Routledge, pp. 152–6.

Katz, P.R. (2009) *Cong diyu dao xian jing: Hanren minjian xinyang de duoyuan mianmao* 從地獄到仙境. 漢人民間信仰的多元面貌 (From Hell to the Realm of the Immortals: the Many Facets of Han Popular Belief). Taipei: Boyang wenhua shiye gongsi.

Kleeman, T. (2005) 'The Evolution of Daoist Cosmology and the Construction of the Common Sacred Realm', *Taiwan Journal of East Asian Studies*, 2.1: 89–110.

Kleeman, T. (2009) 'The Ritualized Treatment of Stroke in Early Medieval Daoism and the Secret Incantation of the Northern Thearch', in F. Reiter (ed.) *Foundations of Daoist Ritual, A Berlin Symposium*. Wiesbaden: Harrassowitz, pp. 227–38.

Kohn, L. (ed.) (2000) *Daoism Handbook*. Leiden: Brill.

Kohn, L. and Roth, H.D. (eds) (2002) *Daoist Identity. History, Lineage and Ritual*. Honolulu: University of Hawai'i Press.

Lagerwey, J. (ed.) (2004) *Religion and Chinese Society. A Centennial Conference of the École française d'Extrême-Orient*. Volume 1. Ancient and Medieval China. Hong Kong: The Chinese University Press.

Lai Chi-tim [Li Zhitian 黎志添] (2010) 'The Ideas of Illness, Healing, and Morality in Early Heavenly Masters Daoism', in A.K.L. Chan and Yuet-Keung Lo (eds) *Philosophy and Religion in Early Medieval* China. Albany: SUNY Press, pp. 173–202.

Li Feng-mao 李豐楙 (1994) 'Xing wen yu song wen. Daojiao yu minzhong wenyiguan de jiaoliu yu fenji' 行瘟與送瘟. 道教與民衆瘟疫觀的交流與分歧 (Parading the Epidemic Gods and Sending Them Off. The Interaction and Divergence of Daoist and Popular Views of Epidemics), in Anonymous (ed.) *Minjian Xinyang yu Zhongguo Wenhua Guoji Yantao Lunwenji* 民間信仰與中國文化國際研討會論文集 (Proceedings of International Conference on Popular Beliefs and Chinese Culture). Center for Chinese Studies Research Series, 4. 2 vols. Taipei: Hanxue yanjiu zhongxin, pp. 373–422.

Li Ling 李零 (2000) *Zhongguo fangshu xu kao* 中国方术续考 (Further Studies of Chinese Technical Arts). Beijing: Dongfang chubanshe.

Li Zhitian 黎志添 [Lai Chi-tim] (ed.) (1999) *Daojiao yu minjian zongjiao yanjiu lunji* 道教与民间宗教论集 (Collected Researches on Daoism and Popular Religion). Hong Kong: Xuefeng wenhua shiye gongsi.

Lin Fushi 林富士 (1999) 'Zhongguo liuchao shiqi de wushi yu yiliao 中國六朝時期的巫覡與醫療' (Wizards and Healing in China during the Six Dynasties Period). *Bulletin of the Institute of History and Philology, Academia Sinica*, 70.1: 1–48.

Lin Fushi 林富士 (2001) *Jibing zhongjiezhe – Zhongguo zaoqi de daojiao yixue* 疾病終結者 – 中國早期的道教醫學 (Terminators of Illness: Daoist Medicine in Early China). Taipei: Sanmin shuju.

Little, S. and Eichmann, S. (2000) *Taoism and the Arts of China*. Art Institute of Chicago. Catalogue of Exhibition, Nov 2000–Jan 2001. Chicago: Art Institute of Chicago; Berkeley, CA: University of California Press.

Liu Liming 劉黎明 (2004) *Songdai minjian wushu yanjiu* 宋代民間巫術研究 (Studies of wizardry in the Song period). Chengdu: Bashu shushe.

Liu Xun and Goossaert, V. (eds) (2013) *Quanzhen Daoists in Chinese Society and Culture, 1500–2010*. Berkeley, CA: Institute of East Asian Studies, University of California.

Liu Zhiwan 劉枝萬 (1967) *Taibei shi Songshan Qi'an Jianjiao jidian: Taiwan qi'an jiao xisu yanjiu zhiyi* 臺北市松山祈安建醮祭典: 臺灣祈安醮祭習俗研究之一 (Great Propitiatory Rites of Petition for Benificence at Sungshan, Taipei, Taiwan). Nangang: Institute of Ethnology, Academia Sinica.

Liu Zhiwan (1974) *Zhongguo minjian xinyang lunji* 中國民間信仰論集 (Essays on Chinese Folk Belief and Folk Cults). Nangang: Institute of Ethnology, Academia Sinica.

Lloyd, G.E.R. and Sivin, N. (2002) *The Way and the Word. Science and Medicine in Early China and Greece*. New Haven: Yale University Press.

Lo, V. (2002) 'Spirit of Stone: Technical Considerations in the Treatment of the Jade Body', *Bulletin of the School of Oriental and African Studies*, 65.1: 99–128.

Luo Zhufeng 羅竹風 (ed.) (1997–1985) *Hanyu Dacidian* 漢語大辭典 (Unabridged Chinese Dictionary). Hong Kong: Joint Publishing Co.

Ma Xisha 马西沙 and Han Bingfang 韩秉方 (2004) *Zhongguo minjian zongjiao shi* 中国民间宗教史 (History of Chinese Popular Religion). Corrected ed., 2 vols. Beijing: Shehui kexue chubanshe.

Maspero, H. (1950) *Le Taoïsme et les Religions Chinoises*. Paris: Gallimard. 1971; trans. F.A. Kierman, Jr. (1981) *Taoism and Chinese Religion*. Amherst: University of Massachusetts Press.

Matsumoto Koichi 松本浩一 (2006) *Sōdai no dōkyō to minkan shinko* 宋代の道教と民間信仰 (Daoism and Popular Belief in the Song Dynasty), Tokyo: Kyuko shoin 汲古書院.

Meyer, J.A.M. de and Engelfriet P.M. (eds) (2000) *Linked Faiths: Essays on Chinese Religions and Traditional Culture in Honour of Kristofer Schipper*. Leiden: Brill.

Miller, A.L. (2008) 'Register', in F. Pregadio (ed.) *The Encyclopedia of Taoism*. London: Routledge, pp. 39–42.

Moerman, D. (2002) *Meaning, Medicine and the Placebo Effect*. Cambridge: Cambridge University Press.

Nickerson, P. (1994) 'Shamans, Demons, Diviners, and Taoists: Conflict and Assimilation in Medieval Chinese Ritual Practice (c. A.D. 100–1000)', *Taoist Resources*, 5.1: 41–66.

Nickerson, P. (2002) '"Opening the Way": Exorcism, Travel, and Soteriology in Early Daoist Mortuary Practice and Its Antecedents', in L. Kohn and H. Roth (eds) *Daoist Identity: History, Lineage, and Ritual*. Honolulu: University of Hawai'i Press, pp. 58–77.

Nickerson, P. (2008a) 'Taoism and Popular Religion', in F. Pregadio (ed.) *The Encyclopedia of Taoism*. London: Routledge, pp. 145–50.

Nickerson, P. (2008b) 'Taoism and Medium Cults', F. Pregadio (ed.) *The Encyclopedia of Taoism*. London: Routledge, pp. 156–9.

Obinata Daijō 仏日方大乗 (1958) *Bukkyō igaku* 佛教医学 (Buddhist Medicine), Tokyo: Sanko Shuppan.

Orzech, C.D. (2002) '*Fang Yankou* 放炎口 and *Pudu* 普度: Translation, Metaphor, and Religious Identity', in L. Kohn and H. Roth (eds) *Daoist Identity: History, Lineage, and Ritual*. Honolulu: University of Hawai'i Press, pp. 213–34.

Qianjin yifang 千金翼方 (Revised Formulas Worth a Thousand in Gold). Sun Simiao 孫思邈 (late seventh century) (1955). Beijing: Renmin weisheng chubanshe. Qianjin

Pregadio, F. (ed.) (2008) *The Encyclopedia of Taoism*. 2 vols., London: Routledge.

Puett, M. (2002) *To Become a God. Cosmology, Sacrifice, and Self-divinization in Early China*. Harvard-Yenching Monograph Series, 57. Cambridge, MA: Harvard University Asia Center.

Sakade Y. (2007) *Taoism, Medicine and Qi in China and Japan*. Osaka: Kansai University Press.

Salguero, C.P. (2014) *Translating Buddhist Medicine in Medieval China*. Philadelphia: University of Pennsylvania Press.

Salguero, C.P. (2015) 'Reexamining the Categories and Canons of Chinese Buddhist Healing', *Journal of Chinese Buddhist Studies*, 28: 35–66.

Schipper, K.M. (1975) *Concordance du Tao-tsang. Titres et ouvrages*. Paris: École Française d'Extrême-orient.

Schipper, K. (1982) *The Taoist Body*, trans. Karen C. Duval (1993). Berkeley, CA: University of California Press.

Schipper, K. (1994) 'Sources of Modern Popular Worship in the Taoist Canon: A Critical Appraisal', in Anonymous (ed.) *Minjian Xinyang yu Zhongguo Wenhua Guoji Yantao Lunwenji* 民間信仰與中國文化國際研討會論文集 (Proceedings of International Conference on Popular

Beliefs and Chinese Culture). Center for Chinese Studies Research Series, 4. 2 vols. Taipei: Hanxue yanjiu zhongxin, pp. 1–21.

Schipper, K. (1995) 'The Inner World of the *Lao-tzu chung ching*', in Chun-chieh Huang and E. Zürcher (eds) *Time and Space in Chinese Culture*. Leiden: Brill, pp. 114–31.

Schipper, K. (unpublished) 'On Chinese Folk Religion', distributed at the Second International Conference on Daoism, Tateshina, Japan, 1972.

Schipper, K. and Verellen F. (eds) (2004) *The Taoist Canon. A Historical Companion to the* Daozang. 3 vols, Chicago: University of Chicago Press.

Sivin, N. (1978) 'On the Word Taoism as a Source of Perplexity. With Special Reference to the Relations of Science and Religion in Traditional China', *History of Religions*, 17: 303–30.

Sivin, N. (1979) 'Report on the Third International Conference on Taoist Studies', *Society for the Study of Chinese Religions Bulletin*, 7: 1–23.

Sivin, N. (1995) 'State, Cosmos, and Body in the Last Three Centuries B.C.', *Harvard Journal of Asiatic Studies*, 55.1: 5–37. Superseded by Lloyd and Sivin 2002.

Sivin, N. (2010) 'Old and New Daoisms', *Religious Studies Review*, 36.1: 31–50.

Sivin, N. (2015) *Health Care in Eleventh Century China*. Cham, Switzerland: Springer.

Stanley-Baker, M. (2013) *Daoists and Doctors: The Role of Medicine in Six Dynasties Shangqing Daoism*, PhD thesis, University of London.

Steinhardt, N.S. (2000) 'Taoist Architecture', in S. Little and S. Eichman (eds) *Taoism and the Arts of China*. Chicago: Art Institute of Chicago; Berkeley and Los Angeles, CA: University of California Press, pp. 57–75.

Strickmann, M. (1985) 'Therapeutische Rituale und das Problem des Bösen im fruhen Taoismus', in G. Naundorf, K.-H. Pohl and H.-H. Schmidt (eds) *Religion und Philosophie in Ostasien: Festschrift fur Hans Steininger zum 65. Geburtstag*. Wurzburg: Verlag Dr. Johannes Konigshausen and Dr. Thomas Neumann, pp. 185–200.

Strickmann, M. (1987) 'Dreamwork of Psycho-Sinologists: Doctors, Taoists, Monks', in C.T. Brown (ed.) *Psycho-Sinology: The Universe of Dreams in Chinese Culture*. Washington: Asia Program, Woodrow Wilson International Center for Scholars, pp. 25–46.

Strickmann, M. (2002) *Chinese Magical Medicine*, ed. Bernard Faure. Stanford University Press.

Teiser, S.F. (1993) 'The Growth of Purgatory', in P.B. Ebrey and P.N. Gregory (eds) *Religion and Society in T'ang and Sung China*. Honolulu: University of Hawai'i Press, pp. 115–46.

Teiser, S.F. (1994) 'The Ten Kings of Purgatory in Popular Belief', in Anonymous (ed.) *Minjian Xinyang yu Zhongguo Wenhua Guoji Yantao Lunwenji* 民間信仰與中國文化國際研討會論文集 (Proceedings of International Conference on Popular Beliefs and Chinese Culture). Center for Chinese Studies Research Series, 4. 2 vols. Taipei: Hanxue yanjiu zhongxin, pp. 621–53.

Unschuld, P.U. (1978) Das *Ch'uan-ya* und die Praxis chinesischer Landärtzte im 18. Jahrhundert', *Sudhoffs Archiv*, 62.4: 378–407.

Wang Jianchuan 王見川 (1999) *Ming Qing minjian zongjiao jing juan wenxian* 明清民間宗教經卷文獻 (Manuscript Scriptures of Popular Religion in the Ming and Qing Periods), 12 vols. Taipei: Xinwenfeng chuban gongsi.

Wei Qipeng 魏启鹏 (1981) 'Taiping jing *yu Dong Han yixue*' 太平经与东汉医学 (The *Scripture of Great Peace* and Eastern Han Medicine), *Shijie zongjiao yanjiu* 世界宗教研究, 1: 101–9.

Xi you ji 西遊記 (Journey to the West). Attributed to Wu Cheng'en 吳承恩 (1506–1582) (2006). Beijing: Zuojia chubanshe.

Yijian zhi 夷堅志 (Records of the Listener). Hong Mai 洪邁 (parts completed from 1161 to 1198 or later). 4 vols. (2006). Beijing: Zhonghua Shuju.

Yi shi 醫史 (History of Medicine). Li Lian 李濂 (1547) (1992). Xiamen: Xiamen University Press.

Yoshioka Yoshitoyo 吉剛義豐 (1952) *Dōkyō no kenkyū* 道教の研究 (Studies in Daoism). Kyoto: Hōzōkan.

Yoshioka Yoshitoyo 吉剛義豐 (1970–1976) *Dōkyō to Bukkyō* 道教と仏教 (Daoism and Buddhism), 3 vols. Tokyo: Kokusho kankōkai.

Zhang Zehong 张泽洪 (1999) *Daojiao zhaijiao keyi yanjiu* 道教斋醮科仪研究 (Studies of Major Taoist Rituals). Chengdu: Bashu shushe.

Zhenjiu dacheng 針灸大成 (Acupuncture Omnibus). Yang Jishi 楊濟時 (or Jizhou 繼洲). 1601 (1993). Changsha: Yue Lu shushe. See also Heilongjiang Zuguo Yiyao Yanjiusuo (1984).

Zheng Tuyou 郑土有 and Wang Xiansen 王贤森 (1994) *Zhongguo chenghuang xinyang* 中国城隍信仰 (Chinese Belief in the City Wall God). Shanghai: Sanlian shudian.

Zhou li 周禮 (Rites of the Zhou dynasty). End of first century. Some scholars defend an earlier date, e.g., W. G. Boltz in Loewe 1993, 25–9. in *Shisanjing chushu* 十三經註疏 1815 (1997). Shanghai: Shanghai guji chubanshe.

Zong Li 宗力 and Liu Qun 刘群 (1987) *Zhongguo minjian zhu shen* 中国民間诸神 (Popular Gods of China). Shijiazhuang: Hebei renmin chubanshe.

2

Religion and medicine in premodern Japan

Katja Triplett

Background

Religion and medicine, with their individual ideas and practices concerned with healing, have long been connected in Japan. As the modern categories of religion and medicine did not exist in premodern Japan, scholars investigating the relationship between the two fields must instead focus on the forces by which they were constructed in the period under investigation. One could ask whether the sources contain certain features or traits that are characteristic of what would later be referred to as, and even in some way pre-structured as, these two distinct categories. To enable me to provide some background information, in this section I will use the categories of religion and medicine as they are employed in everyday speech.[1] In the Literature Review, I will then explore how modern Japanese scholars have dealt with the categories of religion and medicine in their work.

Looking at the history of religion and medicine in ancient and medieval Japan, the distinction between what is regarded as foreign and what is regarded as native seems to have been an important factor guiding the incorporation of new forms of religion and medicine into Japanese society and the interpretation of those new forms in historiographical works. Japan's geography may have encouraged such a native/foreign paradigm. Japan is an archipelago of four large and numerous smaller islands that forms an arc in the Pacific Ocean close to the eastern coast of continental East Asia and Russia. The northernmost island of the archipelago, Hokkaidō, is in the Sea of Okhotsk, while the southern coast of the main island of Kyūshū is located in the East China Sea. The western part of Honshū, the largest of the four main islands, is separated from the Korean Peninsula by just a short expanse of the Japanese Sea. Ancient seafarers used some smaller islands in the Japanese Sea to travel back and forth between Yamato, as Japan was known in ancient times, and the kingdoms of Korea. The waters between Japan and the Asian continent were frequently traversed, resulting in intense cultural exchange; the spread of technological skills, including medicine, to Yamato, and occasional warfare. Nagasaki and other harbour towns on Kyūshū, which were important areas of cultural exchange, traded in goods, tools and skills, first with other parts of Asia, and, from the sixteenth century CE, also with Europe. Trade with Europe was often via the European nations' colonies in India, China and maritime Southeast Asia.

From the sixth century onward, Buddhist texts, statues and other expressions of material culture, as well as Chinese medicine, entered Japan from Korea and later directly from China. Different actors in various social fields circulated, reproduced and further developed the new knowledge, tools and materials. State-sponsored educational institutions, the imperial court, religious sanctuaries and hospitals are some of the establishments important for the present study. Ancient Japanese medicine before the establishment of state institutions for training *ishi* 醫師 (medical doctors) and *kusushi* 藥師 (masters of medicines), and before the creation of a Buddhist ordination platform (*kaidan* 戒壇) in the then capital of Nara, appears to have been dominated by the idea of diseases caused by divine wrath (*tatari* 祟), curses and divine punishment for moral misdeeds. One important written source for the understanding of the worldviews prevalent at the time is the *Nihon shoki* 日本書紀 (Record of Japan, 720), which describes how a particular clan managed to gain political hegemony in wide areas of the Japanese archipelago[2] by chronicling events from a distant Age of the Gods. The compiler(s) of the chronicle was interested in legitimising the victorious clan's military conquests by referring to the actions of illustrious divine ancestors and protectors of the land. The chronicle also mentions two deities responsible for creating the available methods for healing both humans and animals in the land: Ōnamuchi no mikoto 大汝命 and Sukunabikona no mikoto 少彦名命.[3] These two gods of healing also gave people the means to protect the land from calamities caused by pests. For most of Japanese history, however, the Chinese founding figure of pharmacology, Shennong (Japanese: Shinnō) 神農, was the medical healers' central focus of reverence, although Ōnamuchi no mikoto also enjoyed some popularity. Other early texts such as the local gazetteers (*fudoki* 風土記) mention the use of exorcisms (*majinai* 呪い), prayer and apotropaic methods, as well as bathing in natural hot springs. While there were no Daoist institutions in Japan as such, exorcisms from the Daoist tradition, imported from China, appear to have been frequently practised. During the phase of state-building in the eighth century, Daoist ritual forms became popular at court and within court institutions. The inclusion of certain Daoist ritual forms and techniques contributed not only to the plurality of religious practices but also to the plurality of curative techniques, including some that used talismans.[4]

The Chinese tradition of presenting and preserving medical and religious knowledge, and other imported cultural techniques were adapted, applied and reworked, often to serve new purposes on the Japanese archipelago. A short note on textual tradition, language, speech and translation is in order here because of the intricate challenges this poses for research. Written treatises used in the context of healing the physical body often, if not always, appeared in sizable compilations. As in other parts of the world where writing was a means of recording knowledge, compilers of medical compilations in East Asia usually included selections from as many earlier texts as were available to them. Some compilations were made up of sources by a single author, while others were drawn from collections of traditional knowledge ascribed to a famous sage or divinity. In some cases, both types of sources were used. As a result, the compilations generally included multiple voices. Texts that circulated for a longer period of time started to serve different purposes within their respective historical contexts, not least due to the practice of adding commentaries to the texts. Colophons provide valuable insights into the possible political and social circumstances in which the commentaries were written. The same applies to new editions and, in the case of Buddhist texts, also to translations from Sanskrit into Chinese.

In addition to the heterogeneous nature of compilations, a further challenge faced by modern (and not only modern) scholars is the complex writing system of texts circulating in Japan. Writers of scholarly texts and some genres of literature in East Asia used Classical Chinese script. In this script, the shape of the logographic characters conveys meaning, though the phonetic value – i.e. how the character is pronounced or read – can change. While the shape of the characters has broadly remained stable over centuries, if not millennia, the meanings associated with the characters have altered with the result that commentaries on an authoritative text can differ, even to the extent of saying the complete opposite of the 'original' text. Commentators used the 'original' texts to serve their own agendas, reinterpreting the original characters. In Japan, texts continued to be written in Classical Chinese and many Chinese classics and Buddhist texts remained 'untranslated' until the seventeenth to eighteenth centuries. This is curious given that there has been a Japanese writing system since at least the eighth century and that the Japanese language bears no resemblance to Chinese. Rather than translating the Chinese texts, the Japanese developed a complex system of annotation, which elaborated on the meaning of the Chinese text and allowed them to read it in Japanese. To study textual sources, therefore, we need to deal with the intricate complexities of the various writing styles involving several scripts, as well as signs and glosses used for indicating pronunciation or transposing Chinese into Japanese grammar, the so-called *kundoku* 訓読 system. In addition, manuscripts appear in calligraphic styles meaning the study of such source materials must take into consideration the intended presentation of aesthetic qualities. The calligraphic presentation of a text enhances the enjoyment of reading. Where the calligrapher demonstrates extraordinary skill, their art also gives the text greater authority. While most texts were copied by hand, some appeared in woodblock prints. There were large print runs of some texts, particularly certain Buddhist scriptures. Scholarly treatises and Buddhist scriptures were written and printed in regular characters for representative purposes, giving them an official appearance, while more literary texts and personal commentaries appeared in cursive styles. Buddhist texts in the esoteric tradition contain passages in an Indic script, *Siddhaṃ*, in addition to Sinitic scripts. Sacred sounds, such as root syllables, mantras or *dhāraṇī*, appear in this Indic script. Many texts include images and thus communicate meaning in both writing and pictures. Since calligraphic writing of Chinese characters has a pictorial quality as well, the products often transcend boundaries between what is regarded as script and as picture in the European tradition.

While textual production was limited to a learned elite, this group did comprise both men and women, as well as members of monastic orders. Given that Buddhist clerics trained as medical doctors, who administered care to everyone, the textual production of medical and pharmaceutical texts was firmly in the hands of Buddhist monastics. This only changed in the seventeenth century when the new military government started to curb Buddhist temples' monopoly on medical training.

Family genealogies as well as Buddhist monastic lineages passed on the coveted medical knowledge. Secular and religious medical practitioners were in competition in ancient and medieval times, and well into the early modern period when doctors were increasingly trained outside monastic circles in Neo-Confucian academies. Knowledge about Chinese *materia medica* (*honzō* 本草), formulae and therapies (*hō* 方), including needling and moxibustion (*shinkyū* 鍼灸) and Indian-style eye surgery and other treatments, were available only to individuals initiated formally into the familial or monastic lineage. However, the knowledge appears to have been shared despite initiatory vows to keep it secret, not least because members of both groups of doctors sometimes shared family ties. In the early modern period, orally transmitted medical lore was increasingly written down and previously secret records (*hiden* 秘伝, *kuden* 口伝) became available to a wider circle of practitioners and, last but not least, to modern researchers.[5]

When traders and Catholic missionaries from Europe started introducing new knowledge to Japan in the late sixteenth century, doctors and scholars in Japan adopted early modern and modern European medical ideas, further adding to an already hybrid and highly dynamic medical culture. European medical knowledge continued to reach Japan even during a period of close control and censorship of foreign books, primarily via the Dutch trading post near Nagasaki. These developments, among others, marked the beginning of the early modern period. Civil laws officially separated religion and medicine in 1874, with the result that formerly Buddhist doctors either changed to a secular status and obtained a state medical licence or gave up medicine altogether. In the latter case, they devoted themselves to 'religious' Buddhist practice only, providing pastoral care and facilitating fundraising for the former temple hospitals. Today, longstanding cults of Buddhas and bodhisattvas with curative powers, especially Yakushi Nyorai 薬師如来 (Sanskrit: Bhaiṣajyaguru), the 'Medicine Buddha', and the bodhisattva Kannon (Sanskrit: Avalokiteśvara), remain popular. While such cults engage in the 'core activity' of the system of religion, that is, in prayer and rituals, religious organisations such as pilgrimage sanctuaries also provide medicinal substances, a core activity of the system of medicine.[6] The close tie between religion and medicine continues to be discernible today, despite the conceptual distinction between the two emphasised by the civil legal framework.

Much of the Chinese-style medicine popularly referred to today as 'Kampo' (from *kanpō* 漢方, literally 'Han [Chinese] methods') is a continuation of earlier forms of medicine in Japan. The term 'Kampo' came into use at the end of the nineteenth century when the Japanese government increasingly supported and finally adopted European-style medicine, not quite to the joy of everyone involved. After relative neglect of Chinese medicine around the end of the nineteenth century and the beginning of the twentieth century, efforts to revive Kampo came to fruition in the 1970s. Although Kampo is often practised alongside biomedicine today, and both are taught at educational institutions recognised by the state, some argue that Kampo is not part of the secular sphere as its cosmological foundation suggests otherwise. Discourses about whether Kampo constitutes religion or medicine have been influenced by the continued struggle to achieve recognition and legitimation of complementary and alternative medicine. As we will see, the developments in Japan following the rather abrupt adoption of European medicine at the end of the nineteenth century, and the initial prohibition on practising Chinese-style medicine without approbation from a Western-style medical facility, had a significant impact on intellectual writing about the history of medicine in Japan.

Literature

The first historiographies of medicine in Japan began to appear after the 'modernisation' of Japan's medical system had taken root. Some of the authors of these historiographies wanted to provide an overview of a tradition that was being lost or changed radically. In the following section, the oeuvres of some of those early authors will be briefly introduced and assessed to explore how 'religion' and 'medicine' as intellectual categories shaped their narratives and frameworks, whether tacitly or explicitly. I will also introduce selected authors from various academic fields,[7] as well as editors of text-critical editions of primary sources from more recent decades, and elucidate how 'religion' and 'medicine' are presented in these publications.

Fujikawa Yū (1865–1940) is well known for his now classic volumes on the history of medicine in Japan. This towering figure in the field collected and preserved medical sources from the Japanese traditions in a period of profound changes with the shift to European medicine. He was trained in modern European medicine and worked initially as a journalist of medicine and author. Fujikawa's oeuvre includes the 1934 (revised edition 1978) outline of Japanese medical history in English based on a translation from German (1911). As such, his work has been known outside Japan for over a century. Fujikawa, who studied medicine in Jena, Germany,[8] from 1889 to 1890, also wrote extensively on Buddhist thought, as well as education and social matters. In his writings on *shūkyō* 宗教, the modern term coined for the European term *religion*, Fujikawa confidently presents the 'essence' of the influential medieval Buddhist thinker Shinran's (1173–1262) thought. To Fujikawa, religion – true religion – is in fact Shinran's teaching of *naikan* 内観, 'internal observation' and *jinen hōni* 自然法爾,[9] 'naturally occurring as it is'. While these teachings have a long and complex history, it is important to note here that Fujikawa equates Shinran's teaching to European concepts of *religion*, rather than philosophy. He also employs contemporary modes of thought he encountered through publications and during his studies in Germany.

Fujikawa, for example, argues in an essay published in the widely read general interest magazine *Chūō kōron* (Central Review) in 1915 that the idea of the 'other power [of Buddha Amitābha]', another of Shinran's central ideas, is equivalent to German zoologist Ernst Haeckel's (1834–1919)[10] idea of Monism.[11] Haeckel's Monism went through different stages of development and it can be assumed that Fujikawa is referring to the latest stage when Haeckel postulated a 'new religion, rooted in scientific knowledge as well as emotional attachment'.[12] This corresponds well with what Fujikawa outlines in a later essay, published in 1937, in which he presents a fundamental critique of modern medicine. To Fujikawa, the modern achievements of humankind in science, philosophy and art are admirable but, in fact, too mechanical and materialistic. He argues that only (true) religion can provide human beings with warmth and emotional strength. The experience of unity and freedom transcends ethics and morality. He sees both ethics and morality as merely leading to affectation and finger-pointing.[13] This in turn creates a feeling of incompetence and ineptitude. To come to an honest and devout subjective attitude one needs, according to Shinran, to practise 'internal observation' (*naikan*). To practise medicine and medical care, Fujikawa continues, one also needs to approach the patient with a compassionate attitude arrived at by having insight into 'naturally occurring as it is' (*jinen hōni*).[14]

Fujikawa not only disseminated his religious thought in various publications but also founded a missionary association to propagate Shinran's teachings.[15] Between 1936 and 1941 he published fourteen volumes on exemplary devotees of the True Land Buddhist School (*Jōdo shinshū*) for the association.[16] In these volumes he provided psychograms of each of the devotees to guide members of the religious community. However, Fujikawa's writings on the history of medicine and his religiously motivated writings present two different worlds, i.e. we do not find any religious teachings in his historiographies, while his essays and books on religion and *Jōdo shinshū* doctrine represent his personal and normative views on the attitude of a doctor or nurse.

More recent works by authors who are both doctors and Buddhist teachers writing on Japanese Buddhism and medicine reveal, as do Fujikawa's religious writings, apologetic propensities.[17] They emphasise compassion for suffering beings and the social dimension of medical practice in their strand of Buddhism from a normative standpoint.

A contrasting stance can be seen in the work of the doctor and historian of medicine Hattori Toshirō 服部敏良 (also: Tōrō, Toshiyoshi, 1906–1992), who wrote extensively on the history of medicine in Japan. He held both a doctorate in medicine, awarded in 1936 from Nagoya Medical University, and one in literature, awarded in 1973 from Komazawa University, a private Buddhist university in Tokyo. His history of medicine appeared in several volumes from 1945 to 1978 covering the Nara to the Edo periods, i.e. from the era of early state-building in the eighth century to the end of the early modern period in the late nineteenth century. In Hattori's first book, the volume on the history of medicine in Nara-period (710–794) Japan, which he penned during his time as a medical officer during the Asia-Pacific War, he explains in his foreword that he wants to focus not only on the main themes of the historical period but also to highlight 'the connections (*kanren* 関連) between medicine (*igaku* 医学) and both the culture of the period and the intellectual environment (*shichō* 思潮)' (Hattori 1945: iii). Hattori outlines the influence of 'Buddhist medicine' (*bukkyō no igaku* 仏教の医学), including Indian medicine, and the activities of 'care-giving monks' (*kanbyō-sō* 看病僧) and 'monastic doctors' (*sōi* 僧医). He also mentions influences from foreign cultures (*gairai bunka* 外来文化) by which he means the teachings of the Confucian tradition (*jukyō* 儒教) and Christianity (*kirishitankyō* 基督教) (Triplett 2019a: 61–2). Because of the political climate at the time his book was published, Hattori needed to explain that these foreign influences, especially religion from abroad and in particular Buddhism, did not completely replace the 'national religion' (*kokufū shūkyō* 国風宗教); and that the impact of Chinese-style medicine was beneficial to the nation because it represented a step towards scientific medicine (Hattori 1945: 1–3). He regards religion as a part of, or expression of, culture and argues that religion as culture significantly shaped medicine.

In a book published over two decades later, in 1968, Hattori revisits the topic of Buddhism as a cultural force in the development of medicine, and explores early Indian Buddhist sources to describe what he calls 'Shakyamuni's medicine' (*Shaka no igaku* 釈迦の医学). Interestingly, he starts his narrative with a personal anecdote about his 1945 volume on medicine in the Nara period. In it Hattori openly expresses his admiration for Buddhist culture. In the fall of 1943, when the situation in Japan had worsened during the war, Hattori took a study tour and happened to visit the ancient Murōji temple near Nara. The beauty of the temple and its statuary inspired him to learn more about the history of Buddhist art. He started conversations with an authority on art history and their conversations led to Hattori's interest in Nara-period medicine and eventually to the 1945 volume. Hattori continues his narrative by addressing his dissatisfaction with that volume: At first, he felt painfully ignorant about the intrinsic connection between medical history and Buddhist history in the Nara period but when he actually looked closely at Buddhist texts (*butten* 仏典) that he had always considered to be 'those incomprehensible sutras (*o-kyō* お教) full of complicated Buddhist philosophy', he was surprised to find that they carefully explained ancient Indian medicine. To him, the Buddhist texts suddenly turned into medical texts. After that, he continued to extract passages relating to medicine from Buddhist texts, adding his own comments, but then he realised that 'the wealth of medical matters in the Buddhist texts are all related to the greatness of the founder of Buddhism, Shakyamuni himself' (Hattori 1968: 1), so he came to admire Shakyamuni's wisdom and kindness. To him, a professed amateur when it comes to Buddhism, 'ancient Indian medicine reveals something about Shakyamuni. Of course, Shakyamuni was not actually a physician (*ishi*). [...] The aim of the book is not to describe a scientific systematisation of medicine in the Buddhist texts but to introduce Shakyamuni as a great religious figure (*shūkyōjin* 宗教人) to a general audience. Shakyamuni was not only a philosopher but he also showed a deep interest in natural science in regard to medicine' (Hattori 1968: 2). Hattori assumes that, although Shakyamuni, the founder of Buddhism, was not actually a doctor, he knew about medicine because he must have studied it as a required subject during his youth when he was raised as a princely ruler (Hattori 1968: 240). Hattori's book also draws parallels with other systems of medicine in other regions of the world, for example Egypt, Greece and China, during Shakyamuni's time.

Unlike Fujikawa's writing on Shinran, Hattori's discussion remains outside the system of religion, and clearly treats the Buddhist texts as historical and not as 'sacred' sources. Instead of treating the Buddhist texts as medical texts, as he did in his early work, Hattori explores what the texts reveal about ancient India's culture, education, intellectual environment and various knowledge systems that indirectly form part of Japan's cultural heritage.

Publications on 'Buddhist medicine' (*bukkyō igaku* 仏教医学), a modern term, also refer to medical ideas and practices from India as contained in Buddhist texts known in East Asia. An example is the encyclopedia compiled by Fukunaga Katsumi.[18] In a similar vein to Hattori's book on Nara-period medicine, Buddhist texts in the encyclopedia are 'medicalised', and the medical lore explored in them is grouped into modernised categories while ancient categories are ignored. Another example of such a modern classification of concepts and terms is the twentieth-century indices to the Taishō-period (1912–1924) edition of Buddhist texts in Chinese and, to a lesser extent, Japanese, that also includes volumes on matters of iconography. The indices, the *Taishō shinshū daizōkyō sakuin* 大正新脩大藏經索引 (1926–1985), uses modern or material-medical categories such as *eisei* 衛生, 'hygiene', and *sōyaku* 草藥, 'medical herbs', but ignores commonly used practices like treatments with talismans, meditation and karmic treatments. This may be because these methods were deemed 'irrational', 'occult' or otherwise not in line with modern scientific medicine. Christoph Kleine notes how the modernised categories in the otherwise Chinese-style encyclopedia *Koji ruien* 古事類苑 (Garden of Categories of Old Matters, 1896–1913) include 'monk healers' under 'occult arts' (*hōgi* 方技部) and not under 'religion' (*shūkyōbu* 宗教部), while 'Confucian healers' (*jui* 儒醫), interestingly, constitute an entirely separate category (Jingū shichō 1914; Killinger *et al.* 2019, n. 58, 250–1). This last example does not see 'monk healers' as belonging to 'religion' (*shūkyō*), let alone 'medicine', but to a third category akin to 'magic'.

While Fujikawa and Hattori are representative of modern scholars who viewed the role of religion, here Buddhism, as positive – albeit from rather different perspectives – other scholars regarded Buddhism and religion as irrelevant, or even as hindrances, to the development of medicine in Japan. We can discern two different, sometimes overlapping trends: some scholars saw Buddhism as irrelevant or as an obstacle to the development of traditional Japanese medicine, while others considered religion in general to be hindering the emergence of scientific medicine, here Western medicine.

The pioneer of Western ophthalmology and scholar Ogawa Kenzaburō 小川劍三郎 (1870–1933) deems the theory of the Five Buddhas as guardians of the Five Viscera linked to the five parts of the human eye – as found in many premodern texts – meaningless to the medical healing of sight-related diseases (Ogawa 1971:

57–8; Triplett 2019a: 189). Ishihara Akira 石原明 (1924–1980), who sympathised with the cause of the Kampo restoration movement and penned a seminal book on the history of medicine in Japan (1959), even spoke of a 'suppression' of empirical medical knowledge by the restrictions of Buddhist theory (quoted in Mura'i *et al.* 1994: 466; Triplett 2019a: 190). Examples also include other proponents of traditional Japanese medicine who were active in the period of its decline and the ensuing struggle for official recognition. Ōtsuka Keisetsu 大塚敬節 (1900–1980) was, along with Yakazu Dōmei 矢数道明 (1905–2002) and others, a main player in the field of creating a system of Kampo compatible with the Western system of medicine, for instance by matching historical clinical symptoms from the classical Chinese medical texts to the symptoms of diseases as described by modern biomedicine. Typically, they do not deny the impact of religion but simply ignore it. In a seminal article in English (1976), Ōtsuka Keisetsu's son Yasuo 大塚恭男 (1930–2009), who also engaged in the practice of Kampo, mentions medieval-period physicians whose works are generally regarded as significant in the history of traditional medicine. He does not mention that these physicians were learned Buddhist monks, instead referring to them only as medical doctors. Ōtsuka's chapter focuses on medical practices for healing the physical body and he describes physicians who follow particular textual and practical traditions within the Chinese–Japanese medical system. Religion and the role of Buddhist institutions do not feature at all. Here, religion is arguably excluded from traditional medicine.

Some scholars classify religious beliefs, ritual practices and taboos as 'superstition', and present them as misguided and even harmful. This scholarly attitude can be seen, for example, in some of the comments in the critical text edition and translation into modern Japanese of the thirty-volume tenth-century compilation of medical texts from Sui and Tang-period China, the *Essentials of Medicine* 医心方 (*Ishinpō*). The editor, Maki Sachiko 槇佐知子, a historian and literary author, provides short introductions throughout the edited volumes. Her introductions sometimes present premodern medicine as primitive and proto-scientific. For instance, she declares food taboos for pregnant women to be 'superstitious' (*meishinteki* 迷信的) (Maki 1995: 22 iii–iv; Triplett 2019a: 124).

This evolutionist way of relating the history of medicine as the story of a continuous progression is shared by other authors in the field.

Another scholarly attitude considers ritual healing practices in the context of both religion (Buddhism) and medicine. In his works on the use of ritual substances in the Japanese Buddhist tradition, historian Nihonyanagi Kenji (1994, 1997) shows that the complex rituals of esoteric Buddhism engage the practitioner in action towards supramundane transformation while also involving the use of substances with medicinal qualities. As such, he argues, the ritualists consciously and contentiously combine both religion and medicine. The subjects of healing and medicine in Japanese Buddhism are also explored in Buddhist folklore studies (*bukkyō minzokugaku* 仏教民俗学). Historian Gorai Shigeru 五来重 (1908–1993), a pioneer in the field, edited a volume (1986) on devotional practices to Yakushi Nyorai. Gorai's work challenged more narrowly nativist, and often anti-Buddhist movements in the study of folk practices in Japan (Triplett 2019a: 64–5). He focused on everyday religious life and medical-material activities related to coping with illness and impairment.

Similarly, historian Shinmura Taku writes of an 'interplay between healing by prayer and healing by medical means' (Shinmura 2013: 47–63). His volume on the history of medical therapeutics (*iryō* 医療) in Japanese Buddhism (2013)[19] is aimed at a general (Japanese) readership. It contains chapters on theories of the origin of disease and therapies, as well as discussions of terminal care and birth in the Pure Land; care provided to the ruler and his family; epidemics; popular cults of itinerant ascetics; and images of illness in illustrated scrolls. Shinmura also writes about views on sickness held by influential monks of the Kamakura period (1185–1333) and describes the activities of monastics engaged in pharmaceutics and medicine. His book is organised chronologically and provides an overview of pertinent events in the evolution of medicine within the framework of Buddhism in Japan. It briefly touches on developments in early modern Japan.

These scholars, who draw on a great variety of sources to explore religion and medicine as cultural and social forces, highlight historical developments and situate various topics in the wider context of Buddhist Asia. However, the notion of there being an 'interplay' between the two fields is rather vague, and several questions remain regarding the exact relationship between the two fields in premodern Japan.

The section below provides a brief overview of some of the sources that can be analysed with the aim of exploring conceptual distinctions between religion and medicine, as well as practices of social differentiation. It also explores problems that these sources present when it comes to distinguishing and differentiating more precisely between religion and medicine.

Sources

The selection of sources is usually guided by the specific requirements of a given academic discipline, with the result that the outcome of the selection is somewhat predetermined. As the topic at hand – the conceptual distinctions between religion and medicine, and practices of social differentiation – is very general, all types of sources could theoretically be employed. As a minimum, the source, whatever its nature or medium, has to fulfil two basic requirements: that the topic has a connection to the physical and mental healing of a human or animal and that there is a link to premodern Japan. Since there are rich collections of textual as well as material sources in Japan, some of them as yet unstudied, the scope of such a study is practically without limit. This should not deter the modern researcher from investigating the topic. Instead, the increased wealth of possible materials should liberate the scholar from the confines of certain ideological biases. The near limitlessness of the sources that can be included should result in a fundamental rethinking of the 'canon' of the history of religion in conjunction with the history of medicine. This will lead to concrete suggestions for the study of religion and medicine in premodern Japan, which will be addressed in the concluding part of the chapter along with issues for future research.

The standard texts that the ancient government in Japan prescribed for students of medicine are fairly well-known. Legal and penal codes issued by the newly formed centralised government in the eighth century set out a list of texts for medical students. The government wanted them to have access to cutting-edge knowledge in order to ensure the best care was available for both elite members of society and the population as a whole. Extended copies of such codes list Chinese medical classics in the section on medicine (*ishitsu-ryō* 醫疾令).[20] The government also ordered the establishment of a medical council (*ten'yakuryō* 典薬寮) in the capital to oversee the training and appointment of doctors, acupuncturists, exorcists and pharmacologists both in the capital and in the provinces. The codes introduced a quota for (male and female) medical students but expressly made allowances for the children of the families that had trained doctors in the past (Rosner 1989: 16; Michel-Zaitsu 2017: 29). The tradition of passing on knowledge within a family or clan was therefore maintained during this phase of incorporation of Chinese-style structures into Japanese society and culture. The challenge posed by this genre of texts is to discover which parts of the legal codes were actually followed.

At the same time as court medicine flourished, eighth-century chronicles compiled by imperial order, such as the *Nihon shoki*, tell of charismatic monastics who conducted ceremonies and rituals for the healing and welfare of members of the imperial family and other nobility. Monks and nuns were ordained according to governmental guidelines and were thus subject not only to monastic but also to secular law. The secular codes forbade them the use of Daoist techniques and non-Buddhist curative spells (Triplett 2019a: 67). We can assume that the government wanted to keep the expertise and actual practices of the two groups of religious specialists – the exorcists and the Buddhist monastics – apart.[21] We can also understand from the sources that these practices must have been popular; in fact, the codes did not have a lasting impact on society for various reasons, and a dynamic religious pluralism entailing both Daoistic and Buddhist ritual techniques continued to evolve during the medieval period. Still, the codes and chronicles are valuable sources for assessing which medical texts were officially seen as authoritative and prescribed for training doctors and what was regarded as proper Buddhist curative care. The Chinese texts imported from Korea and China provided knowledge for the doctors in Japan. Following Chinese precedent, doctors on Japanese soil, many of whom were of foreign descent, started commenting on the texts. One such doctor was the court physician Tanba Yasuyori 丹波康頼 (912–995). All standard introductions to the history of medicine in Japan mention the thirty-volume *Essentials of Medicine*

(*Ishinpō* 醫心方, 984) put together by him and regarded as the first medical work extant that was compiled in Japan. It is, in fact, a compilation of citations from numerous works produced and circulated in China which Tanba Yasuyori selected and added his comments to. *Essentials of Medicine* is a good example of the way medical knowledge was coveted in Japan: Only very few copies of the work ever existed and the Tanba clan and one of its branches, the Taki 多紀, apparently managed to keep the work from the prying eyes of competing medical clans for centuries. It was only in the nineteenth century that the *Essentials of Medicine*, a reconstruction made from the then only existing copy and available fragments, was printed and circulated more widely.

New Chinese works on medicine and extensive *materia medica* collections kept being imported and continued to exert an influence on developments in Japan. Medicine in Japan also developed autonomously, as Rosner has emphasised, although the establishment of medical schools closely followed Chinese models, often as a result of the involvement of doctors from the kingdoms on the Korean peninsula. Buddhist traditions and schools also formed in Japan in an autonomous manner. While major steps towards both Japanese medicine and religious traditions involved charismatic individuals, other less prominent figures and groups also contributed to shaping what we can term medicine and religion in premodern Japan. Charismatic individuals who are often considered founders or reformers of principal lineages, whether medical or Buddhist or both, receive considerable attention in academic research because of their central role in the circulation of knowledge. While Japanese-language introductions to the life and work of famous doctors and monks abound, such research is less available in European languages. Biographical studies of historical figures in Japan provide valuable insights into the combined fields of religion and medicine. Examples include publications on the Buddhist priest and physician Kajiwara Shōzen 梶原性全 (1265–1337) and his two influential medical works, the *Book of the Simple Doctor* (*Ton'ishō* 頓医抄, 1303) and the *Myriad Relief Formulas* (*Man'anpō* 万安方, 1315) (e.g. Goble 2009, 2011). The charismatic monk and Buddhist reformer Eison (or Eizon 叡尊, 1201–1290) famously established bathhouses and other facilities to provide relief for outcasts, including those afflicted by leprosy (Quinter 2015: 105).

His disciple Ninshō 忍性 (also Ryōkan-bō 良観房, 1217–1303) is known to have engaged in welfare activities, such as building care facilities for both humans and animals, namely horses and oxen (Yoshida 1983; Hidaka 2009; Triplett 2019a: 183–4). The monk Myōan Eisai (or Yōsai 明菴栄西, 1141–1215), revered as the founder of Rinzai Zen Buddhism, compiled the noteworthy work *Nurturing Life by Drinking Tea* (*Kissa yōjōki* 喫茶養生記, 1211).[22] He modelled the work on Chinese sources he encountered during his stays in monasteries in China. Among physicians in late medieval Japan, Manase Dōsan 曲直瀬道三 (1507–1594) stands out as having had a significant impact on medical culture. The Neo-Confucian physician Kaibara Ekiken 貝原益軒 (or Ekken, 1630–1714) and his ideas on medicine and other related fields have also been studied widely (e.g. Asuka 2003).

Social actors on the margins of society must also be considered. As the textual production of these social actors was less prolific, their activities and roles have to be gleaned from written evidence, such as court diaries or other narrative genres including fiction. As briefly mentioned above, modern scholars include various genres of literature in the archive on religion and medicine in premodern Japan. These include narratives in the form of picture scrolls (*emakimono* 絵巻物). Some picture scrolls include images of the sick, and medical treatments, providing insights into the medical culture of the past (e.g. Shinmura 2013: 151–74). The best known of these picture scrolls relating to the history of religion and medicine are the twelfth-century *Stories of Diseases* (*Yamai no sōshi* 病草紙) and *Stories of the Hungry Ghosts* (*Gaki zōshi* 餓鬼草紙).

Buddhist legends (*setsuwa* 説話) often report miracle healings, as does Heian (794–1185) court literature. Myths and legends relating to *jindō* 神道, a tradition centred on the reverence of local deities (*kami*), and Buddhist traditions also describe physical disorders and their treatment in the context of religious ideas and rituals. These narratives are valuable sources in the field of healing, medical and religious culture in premodern Japan.

The archive also includes early bibliographies of available books in Japan, such as the *Catalogue of Extant Texts in the Country of Japan* (*Nihonkoku genzai shomokuroku* 日本國現在書目録, 891) by Fujiwara no Sukeyo 藤原佐世 (847–897). These bibliographies give us valuable insights into the materials for knowledge production available at court. Encyclopedias modelled on Chinese works sought to explain the use and etymology of words, terms and names of both Chinese and Japanese origin. We can glean from these encyclopedias the current state of medical and other knowledge. The intense interest in gathering knowledge about all things Japanese is evident in efforts to identify indigenous plants, animals, minerals and other *materia medica* for use in healing illnesses and for the correct diet to ensure longevity. The Japanese faced, and continue to face, significant difficulties in obtaining rare and costly substances for medical use despite considerable efforts to identify useful *materia medica* in Japan from as early as the tenth century with the publication of the *Japanese Names for the Materia Medica* (*Honzō wamyō* 本草和名, 901–923) by the court physician Fukane Sukehito 深根輔仁 (dates unknown).[23] A unique source of *materia medica* imported into the ancient capital of Nara from China and other parts of Asia is a collection of drugs that was kept in the Tōdaiji temple repository, the famous Shōsōin, for over a thousand years.[24]

A wide range of writings linked to Buddhism in the broadest sense comprise a further important part of the archive. Among these texts are sutras, treatises, commentaries, practice and iconographic manuals and collections of hagiographic material. Most of the sutras and treatises arrived from China, bringing the practice of 'Buddhist medicine', i.e. Indian-style medicine in Chinese garb, to the Japanese archipelago. Influential texts such as the sixth-century Chinese Buddhist treatise on meditation, the *Treatise on Stopping and Contemplating* (*Mohe zhiguan* 摩訶止観) based on the teachings of master Zhiyi 智顗 (538–597), played a significant role in shaping views on the causes of sickness and physical and mental diseases.[25] In Japan, unlike in China, esoteric Buddhism, which included the practice of uttering *dhāraṇī* for curing patients and prolonging life, remained a dominant cultural force. The art of dying and various forms of spiritual and palliative care also feature prominently in Japanese Buddhist writings. Court diaries and other records attest to the popularity of death ceremonies that aimed at being born in the Pure Land.

In addition to all of these prescriptive and descriptive texts, there are also the materials and documentation found in the Shōsōin temple repository and other archaeological evidence. The basic challenge is not dealing with the immensity of the archive but enlarging it further by unearthing unstudied or neglected sources. The more extensive the archive, the more opportunities there are for discovering conceptual distinctions between religion and medicine and practices of social differentiation.

Analysis

Addressing the challenges outlined above and avoiding the pitfalls of studying premodern medical systems in connection with religion requires new approaches in methodology and theoretical considerations. Micro-historical studies employing philological methods are necessary in order to scan the vast number of textual sources in search of words and terms relating to the categories of religion and medicine. There are a number of possible avenues for determining the relationship between these two categories. We could follow the trend set by Fujikawa Yū in his religious writings and guide the readers to improve their personal lives as a response to the modernising processes. He advocated the scientific changes but felt the urge to share traditional teachings, 'true religion', on how to be a compassionate person.

Or we could follow in Hattori Toshirō's footsteps by 'medicalising' religious writings and extracting medical information from them, as well as using the ancient sources to bring Shakyamuni to life, in a similar vein to studies that seek to resurrect Jesus of Nazareth as an historical person. We may also decide to ignore the role religion played as a cultural or even intellectual source as Ōtuska Yasuo did in his history of traditional medicine in Japan. To advance our search for conceptual distinctions and social differentiations I, however, would suggest that we distance ourselves from more apologetic, rationalist or traditionalist approaches, instead pursuing Shinmura's approach, and seeking to specify further what he called the 'interplay' of religion and medicine.

For several years now, scholars at Leipzig University have been exploring the notion of *secularity*, a concept which describes how conceptual distinctions and social differentiations are made between religious and non-religious spheres.[26] Some of the scholars have been working to identify specific modes of distinguishing conceptually between religion and medicine, as well as practices of social differentiation between these two fields in premodern Asian societies. A working group on Religion and Medicine, of which I am a member, has proposed certain analytical tools for distinguishing between 'religious' and 'secular' healing practices, and applied them in various contexts including premodern Japan.

Inspired by Niklas Luhmann's systems theory, the working group on Religion and Medicine looked at binary oppositions, which Luhmann sees within communication in religion and medicine. In the system of religion, there is the transcendent/immanent binary; in the system of medicine, there is the health/illness binary. In ancient and early medieval Japanese society, Buddhism came to provide important epistemes,[27] which allow an interpretation that healing from sickness is a transcendent goal. One episteme is that the Buddha is seen as the King of Doctors or the Supreme Healer and the eradication of sickness considered the ultimate, irreversible liberation from suffering, a transcendent goal. The Buddha taught Four Noble Truths that are often related in the language of medicine: he identified the symptoms of suffering (diagnosis), revealed the causes of suffering (aetiology), stated that there is a way to heal the disease (recovery), and finally prescribed a treatment to end the suffering (therapy) and heal the beings from the 'three poisons' (Jp. *sandoku* 三毒) of craving, aggression and ignorance.

While such epistemes permit an interpretation that healing is a *transcendent* goal, the strands of Mahāyāna Buddhism dominant in Japan also provide the concept of the bodhisattva, a future Buddha who vows to engage in helping the suffering beings in the world, which is an *immanent* goal. The authoritative texts not only encouraged monks and nuns to act as bodhisattvas and train in medicine but also stated that this training was a requirement to fulfil the monastics' duty of compassionate action (Salguero 2018). Here, medical healing appears to be *both* transcendent – aimed at liberation from 'sickness' (Jp. *byō* 病), i.e. from all suffering and future birth in the six realms – and immanent – relieving the suffering beings by treating their concrete physical and mental ailments and illnesses. This explains why Buddhism and medicine were deeply intertwined from the incorporation of Buddhism into Japanese culture in the sixth and following centuries CE, until Buddhist and medical practice were officially separated in the late nineteenth century during a phase of profound social and political change and, as detailed above, continue to be intertwined even today.

While Buddhism is concerned with healing as salvation as an ultimate goal, medicine is focused on healing the physical bodies of humans and animals by alleviating pain, ensuring wellbeing and protecting medical knowledge. Let us look more closely at the *means and methods* employed in the field of healing in premodern Japan in order to discover conceptual distinctions. We will see that the approach to finding distinctions between religion and medicine in the means and methods that the social actors used, results here more in a proof of the close correspondence and not a clear distinction between the two. Buddhist rituals that pertain to healing are traditionally referred to as *kaji* 加持 (Sanskrit: *adhiṣṭhāna*, 'assistance') rituals. *Kaji* has remained the dominant paradigm of Esoteric Buddhist healing since the Heian period when Esoteric Buddhist culture became firmly established in Japan. Temples of various denominations also offered panaceas.[28] Pure Land Buddhist references to medicine directly link it to the attainment of a transcendent goal. The practice of saying Buddha Amitābha's name (*nenbutsu* 念佛) and directing one's thoughts to being born in Amitābha's Pure Land, which is a realm free from sickness.

The knowledge system available to practitioners in the social field of healing included records of *materia medica*, medical formulae and therapies including manuals for making amulets and talismans. In Japan, where Buddhist monastics cared for people's physical wellbeing, religious and medical practice overlapped for centuries. Not all monastics were doctors and there were also doctors outside Buddhist institutions. Both medically trained Buddhist monastics,[29] called 'monastic doctors' (*sōi*) in modern literature, and secular court doctors, who usually belonged to medical families and were trained either in state institutions or within their families, treated members of Japan's ruling elite. Other members of society were treated by the monastics as well as by healers from the religious tradition of Shugendō 修験道. Practitioners of the ascetic tradition of Shugendō attempted to obtain superhuman powers by conducting austerities in the mountainous wilderness in order to benefit the community. The mountain ascetics also administered medicinal herbs and other remedies to the sick.[30] These religious healers conducted rituals and cured by eradicating 'transcendent forces', such as demons, evil spirits, goblins and other disease-causing agents.[31] Because they involved intermediary beings, their methods could be rather easily distinguished from those of the physicians who treated the patient's body directly with acupuncture or poultices. However, 'secular' physicians also had knowledge of amulets and other methods that were supposed to activate unseen forces. And monastic physicians and other 'religious' healers also had knowledge of acupuncture and other Chinese-style medical therapies.

The Religion and Medicine working group at Leipzig University also explored other approaches to distinguishing conceptually between religion and medicine, such as looking through the source material for signs of distinctions being made through individuals being ascribed *charisma* on the basis of their particular training and authority. Charisma could also be earned on the basis of the *competencies* individuals gained during training or through authority and processes of legitimisation. Other forms of distinction that the working group discussed involved identifying the *functions and services* of the social systems, religion and medicine.

The Leipzig working group determined that, while religious experts in premodern Japan were ascribed the power of guiding suffering beings to salvation, which included liberation from sickness, they had in addition the means and methods to provide medicines for healing. As Christoph Kleine has also pointed out, 'the interpretation of the causal relationships between means and purposes' (Killinger *et al.* 2019: 59), i.e. that religious healers heal by proxy in order to eradicate evil influences and thereby heal the patient, on the *epistemic* level excludes religious healers from the modern category of medicine and firmly places them in the realm of religion.

While epistemes shape social structures, social structures shape the social activities of groups as well as individuals, which in turn can bring about change in those very structures. So, in addition to searching for conceptual distinctions, we should also focus on practices of social differentiation conceptualised on a semantic level. The boundaries are, however, as I discovered through my topical survey of various sources in early and medieval Japan, 'difficult to discern and to cast the findings into a simple binary is even less feasible' (Triplett 2019a: 196).

This should not keep us from re-reading the textual materials as a step towards assessing semantics and meaning-making in the social fields of religion and medicine. Additionally, we should continue to search for neglected or newly discovered textual and material sources.

Historian Anna Andreeva, for example, surveys several rediscovered manuscripts of the modern Kanagawa Bunko in Yokohama. This institution holds part of the outstanding collection of the former library of the Hōjō family who ruled Japan for nearly one and a half centuries (1185–1333) from their residence in Kamakura. The Hōjō family's library was once housed and administered by the family's temple. Andreeva, in her study on women, Buddhism and medicine, analyses the origin of the numerous sources quoted in the Kanagawa Bunko *Encyclopedia of Childbirth* (*Sanshō ruijūshō* 産生類聚抄, ca. 1318) (2017, 2018: 55).

Studies that are based entirely on written texts do not allow researchers to gain a comprehensive perspective on either medicine or religion. Recent research has thus increasingly paid more attention to material culture beyond the content of written texts and picture scrolls. Such research includes academic studies of talismans and effigies, and how these objects were used. East Asian Buddhist art historian Benedetta Lomi, for example, highlights the production of a talismanic medicine in relation to the Heian-period 'Ritual of the Six-syllable Sūtra' (*rokujikyōhō* 六字経法) (2014). In this ritual, three effigies of initially dangerous 'foxes' are burned during a fire ceremony to transform their destructive power into curative power. The ash from the burnt effigies was used to make a medicine to be taken orally (Lomi 2014: 291).[32] This exorcism ritual makes use of Daoist techniques, indicating that the religious tradition of Daoism survived in ritual technology. Studies such as this highlight the religious and medical plurality in premodern Japan. In modern terminology, such cures are designated 'magic' cures.

I would like to point out briefly several topics in the field of religion and medicine in premodern Japan where there is still a lack of research. I highlighted some of these in previous publications (Triplett 2019a, 2019b).

The history of medicine and science has focused on contributions made by men and neglected those made by women.[33] Similarly, there has been insufficient research on the role of women in religions. The same is true of studies in the field of medicine and religion in Japan. The early Japanese legal code explicitly provided for the selection and training of female doctors (*nyoi* 女醫), but it is currently unclear who these doctors were and how established they were in court circles. There has been insufficient research on the contribution of the women in medical clans, and on monastic women who trained as physicians. We do know that pious Buddhist lay women are reported to have contributed significantly to charity and welfare.[34]

Scholars of the history of medicine have not paid much attention to veterinary medicine and the healing of animals. As animal studies has developed as a field within the study of religions in Japan,[35] veterinary medicine and religion should also receive more attention as an area of study.[36] General encyclopedias, often compiled by Buddhist monks, are important sources for this topic because they are founts of contemporary knowledge and ideas about the ordering of the 'natural' world including animals and plants.

Conclusion

To address adequately the multi-disciplinary field of religion and medicine in premodern Japan, research from various disciplines in current academia needs to be integrated. Micro-historical approaches are helpful in the first instance to assess processes of shifting boundaries between religion and medicine, whether by applying basic philological methods to a text or investigating the work and lives of individual charismatic monks. The compartmentalisation of research cannot be overcome by merely accumulating available knowledge on texts and authors; we need to look at the correlations between social actors, institutions and wider cultural exchange processes in ancient and medieval Asia in order to understand better the historical conditions under which both religion and medicine developed in premodern Japan. It is evident that all social actors – from the empress to the low-ranking officer, from the military hegemon's personal doctor to the itinerant blind shamaness – were affected by the paradigm of esoteric Buddhism with its notions of secrecy, initiation and ultimate benefit for the world. When this esoteric Buddhist paradigm is seen as 'magic' from a modern perspective, it either means it is regarded as an obstacle to progress or deemed a way of life that has regrettably been lost. In order to move beyond embracing rationalism or nostalgic traditionalism, a different approach is suggested here, namely considering esoteric Buddhism as the dominant paradigm that remained despite some individuals distancing themselves from it and expressing ideas that represented a break from tradition.

It should be recognised moreover that Japan is not the only place where the fields of religion and medicine have been shaped by esoteric Buddhism. This is also true for Tibet. Although Japan and Tibet do not have a history of direct cultural exchange, they form part of an entangled Asian history created and fostered by a similar repertoire of Vajrayāna Buddhist ideas and practices. A comparative study of religion and medicine in regard to these Buddhist cultures may yield new insights into the relationship between state sponsorship, temple economies and non-monastic actors and other salient topics.

Notes

1 For general overviews on the topic, see also my contributions for academic handbooks in both fields of religion and medicine (Triplett 2021a, 2021b, 2022).
2 See Kidder (1993: 48).
3 The relevant passage is in *Nihon shoki*, book 1, *Kamiyo* (Age of the Gods), trans. Aston (1896: 141).
4 For works in English about the history of Daoist deities and rituals in Japan, see Como (2015) and Ooms (2009), esp. Chap. 6 on Daoism; Ooms (2015).
5 For examples from the field of ophthalmology, see Okuzawa (1997). For bone-setting, see Chang (2019).
6 For medical discourses and practices in contemporary Japanese religions including Buddhism, see Schrimpf (2018).
7 My focus is on Japanese language material; for an assessment of the seminal article on 'sickness' (*byō* 病) in French by Paul Demiéville (1937; English trans. 1985), see Triplett (2019a: 13–14, 41–43).
8 During the Japanese Meiji period (1868–1912), medical science and practice taught by German scholars was especially influential in the formation of modern biomedicine in Japan.

9 The focus of Shinran's teachings is the abandonment of 'self-power'; 'self-power' involving resorting to calculation. As Dessì explains, quoting Dennis Hirota: '[T]he abandonment of self-power does not mean that no positive action can be performed. Rather, compassionate acts can then arise 'naturally and inevitably' (*jinen*), and the discovery of a dimension where one is not possessed by blind passions any more [...] becomes possible'. (Dessì 2007: 90; Hirota 2000: 180). *Hōni*, the natural arising of all things in reality, further qualifies the arising of 'naturalness' (*jinen*). In Pure Land Buddhism, *hōni* means occurring through the power of the vow of Amitābha Buddha, the 'other-power'.

10 Haeckel was at the University of Jena, but Fujikawa and Haeckel seem to have never met in person.

11 Fujikawa, H. (1990: 243), quoted in Tsuchiya and and Horiguchi (2012: 178).

12 Holt (1971: 268), quoting from a speech held by Haeckel's private secretary Heinrich Schmidt (1914: 21).

13 On the problem of Jōdo shinshū ethics in contemporary Japan, see Dessì (2007).

14 For a detailed study on the *jinen hōni* thought in Fujikawa's work, see Yoshida (1986).

15 *Shinran shōnin sangyō-kai* 親鸞上人讃行会, later renamed *Shōshin kyōkai* 正信協会.

16 The fourteenth volume came out posthumously. A second, two-volume edition came out in 1954–1956, reprinted in 1971.

17 See e.g. Kawada (1976, 2013) and Obinata (e.g. 1965).

18 For a critique, see Salguero (2015: 50–1).

19 Shinmura has published several books on the history of medicine and medical culture in Japan (e.g. 2006).

20 For a translation of the pertinent sections (into German) of the eighth century *Yōrō Code*, see Dettmer (2010: 438–42).

21 See the study of Miyata (2012).

22 On the religious and cultural history of drinking tea in China (and in Japan), see Benn (2015). On the reception of Eisai's work in Japan and the notion of longevity, see Drott (2010).

23 For the reception of Chinese compilations of *materia medica* in Japan, see the works by historian Mayanagi Makoto, for example Mayanagi (1993).

24 For some details on the collection, see e.g. Triplett (2019a: 80, 129, 142–5).

25 For an English translation and contextualisation of the chapter on treating illness from the *Treatise*, see Salguero (2015).

26 Centre for Advanced Studies in the Humanities and Social Sciences 'Multiple Secularities – Beyond the West, Beyond Modernities' at Leipzig University 'investigates forms and arrangements of differentiation between religious and other social spheres, practices, interpretive frameworks, institutions and discourses in different eras and regions' referring 'to such arrangements, which are often contentious, with the heuristic term "secularities"'. This chapter results in part from research conducted at the Centre. The Centre is funded by the German Research Foundation (DFG). For further information, please consult www.multiple-secularities.de.
27 These are defined as epistemic structures that are culturally transmitted patterns of perception and interpretation, see Killinger *et al.* (2019: 239).
28 For a discussion of the tradition of offering such medicines in Zen Buddhist temples, see Williams (2005: 86–116).
29 For monks as healers in early and medieval Japan, see Kleine (2012).
30 On mountain ascetics' healing services and trade in pharmaceuticals, see Nei (1976, 1980).
31 For a discussion of male and female 'demons' that were thought to cause children's diseases, see Triplett (2019b).
32 See also her study on the use of an ox bezoar in rituals for fertility and safe childbirth, Lomi (2017).
33 For a revisionist European history of e.g. botany, see Schiebinger (2004).
34 A key example of such women is Kōmyō kōgō (光明皇后, 701–760).
35 See the study by Ambros (2012).
36 On equine medicine and Buddhism, see Triplett (2019a: 163–88).

Bibliography

Premodern sources

Book of the Simple Doctor, see *Ton'ishō*.
Catalogue of Extant Texts in the Country of Japan, see *Nihonkoku genzai shomokuroku*.
Encyclopedia of Childbirth, see *Sanshō ruijūshō*.
Essentials of Medicine, see *Ishinpō*.
Gaki zōshi 餓鬼草紙 (Stories of the Hungry Ghosts), late twelfth century, Kyoto National Museum (sign. AK 229).
Honzō wamyō 本草和名 (Japanese Names for the *Materia Medica*), 901–923, Fukane Sukehito 深根輔仁 (dates unknown), NKZ 27, 35 (1926).

Ishinpō 醫心方 (Essentials of Medical Treatment), 984, compiled by Tanba (no) Yasuyori 丹波康頼 (912–995), NKZ 186, 187, 189, 191, 192, 196, 197 (1935) and Maki (1993).
Japanese Names for the Materia Medica, see *Honzō wamyō*.
Kissa yōjōki 喫茶養生記 (Nurturing Life by Drinking Tea), 1211, Myōan Eisai (or Yōsai 明菴栄西, 1141–1215).
Koji ruien 古事類苑 (Garden of Categories of Old Matters), 1896–1913. Jingū shichō ed. (1914).
Man'anpō 万安方 (Myriad Relief Formulas), 1315, Kajiwara Shōzen 梶原性全 (1265–1337).
Mohe zhiguan 摩訶止観 (Treatise on Stopping and Contemplating), 594, T 1911, teachings of master Zhiyi 智顗 (538–597), compiled by Guanding 灌頂 (561–632). Trans. Salguero (2012).
Myriad Relief Formulas, see *Man'anpō*.
Nihon shoki 日本書紀 (Record of Japan), 720, NKBT 67, 68 (1965–1967). Trans. Aston 1896.
Nihonkoku genzai shomokuroku 日本國現在書目録 (Catalogue of Extant Texts in the Country of Japan), 891, compiled by Fujiwara no Sukeyo 藤原佐世 (847–897).
Nurturing Life by Drinking Tea, see *Kissa yōjōki*.
Record of Japan, see *Nihon shoki*; Sakamoto ed. (1965–1967).
Sanshō ruijūshō 産生類聚抄 (Encyclopedia of Childbirth), c. 1318, Kanazawa Bunko (sign. MS 5–3–1).
Stories of Diseases, see *Yamai no sōshi*.
Stories of the Hungry Ghosts, see *Gaki zōshi*.
Ton'ishō 頓医抄 (Book of the Simple Doctor), 1303, Kajiwara Shōzen 梶原性全 (1265–1337).
Treatise on Stopping and Contemplating, see *Mohe zhiguan*.
Yamai no sōshi 病草紙 (Stories of Diseases), 1193, edition Akiyama *et al.* (1977).
Yōrō Code (*Yōrō-ryō* 養老令), ca. 718–722, analysis and trans. Dettmer (2009–2015).

Modern Sources

Akiyama Ken 秋山虔 *et al.* (1997) Yamai no sōshi 病草紙 (Stories of Diseases), in S. Komatsu 小松茂美 (ed.) *Nihon emaki taisei* 日本絵巻大成 (Complete Japanese Picture Scrolls), vol. 7. Tokyo: Chūō Kōron.
Ambros, B. (2012) *Bones of Contention: Animals and Religion in Contemporary Japan*. Honolulu: University of Hawai'i Press.
Andreeva, A. (2017) 'Explaining Conception to Women? Buddhist Embryological Knowledge in the Sanshō ruijūshō 産生類聚抄 (Encyclopedia of Childbirth, ca. 1318)', *Asian Medicine*, 12, 170–202.

Andreeva, A. (2018) 'Devising the Esoteric Rituals for Women: Fertility and the Demon Mother in the *Gushi nintai sanshō himitsu hōshū*', in K.M. Gerhart (ed.) *Women, Rites, and Ritual Objects in Premodern Japan*. Leiden; Boston: Brill, pp. 53–88.

Aston, W.G. (1896) *Nihongi: Chronicles of Japan from the Earliest Times to A.D. 697*. Transactions and Proceedings of The Japan Society, London. Supplement I. Vols. I, II. London: Kegan Paul, Trench, Trübner & Co.

Asuka, R. (2003) *La médecine traditionnelle japonaise*. Paris: L'Harmattan.

Benn, J.A. (2015) *Tea in China: A Religious and Cultural History*. Honolulu: University of Hawai'i Press.

Chang, C. (2019) 'A Wooden Skeleton Emerges in the Knowledge Hub of Edo Japan', in P.H. Smith (ed.) *Entangled Itineraries: Materials, Practices, and Knowledges Across Eurasia*. Pittsburgh, PA: University of Pittsburgh Press, pp. 258–82.

Como, M. (2015) 'Daoist Deities in Ancient Japan: Household Deities, Jade Women and Popular Religious Practice', in J.L. Richey (ed.) *Daoism in Japan: Chinese Traditions and Their Influence on Japanese Religious Culture*. London; New York: Routledge, pp. 24–36.

Demiéville, P. (1937) 'Byō' in P. Demiéville (ed.) *Hōbōgirin; Dictionnaire encyclopédique du bouddhisme d'après les sources chinoises et japonaises (reprint in Siary & Benhamou 1994: 349–412)*. Tokyo: Maison franco-japonaise, pp. 224–65.

Demiéville, P. (1985) *Buddhism and Healing (=Hōbōgirin entry on 'Byō', trans. by Mark Tatz)*. Lanham, MD: University Press of America.

Dessì, U. (2007) *Ethics and Society in Contemporary Shin Buddhism*. Studies in modern Asian religions / Religiöse Gegenwart Asiens; 5. Berlin (*et al.*): Lit.

Dettmer, H.A. (2010) *Der Yōrō-Kodex: Die Gebote; Übersetzung des Ryō no gige, Teil 2 Bücher 2–10,* Veröffentlichungen des Ostasien-Instituts der Ruhr-Universität Bochum; 55. Wiesbaden: Harrassowitz.

Drott, E.R. (2010) 'Gods, Buddhas, and Organs: Buddhist Physicians and Theories of Longevity in Early Medieval Japan', *Japanese Journal of Religious Studies*, 37.2: 247–273.

Fujikawa Hideo 富士川英郎 (1990) *Fujikawa Yū* 富士川游. Tokyo: Ozawa Shoten.

Fujikawa, Y. (1911) *Geschichte der Medizin in Japan. Kurzgefaßte Darstellung der Entwicklung der japanischen Medizin mit besonderer Berücksichtigung der europäischen Heilkunde in Japan*. Tokyo: Kaiserlich Japanisches Unterrichtsministerium.

Fujikawa Yū 富士川游 (1915) 'Shinran Shōnin dan'yo 親鸞聖人談餘' (Saint Shinran Conversations), *Chūō kōron* 中央公論 November, 37–42.

Fujikawa, Y. (1934) *Japanese Medicine*, trans. J. Ruhräh. New York: P.B. Hoeber.

Fujikawa Yū 富士川游 ([1937] 2010) *Ijutsu to shūkyō* 医術と宗教 (Medicine and Religion). Tokyo: Orig. Daiichi shobō, Repr. Shoshi Shinsui.

Fujikawa Yū 富士川游 ([1954–1956] 1971) Shinsen myōkō-nin den 新選妙好人伝 (New Selection of Reports about Exemplary Devotees). *Daizō sensho* 大蔵選書, 8. Tokyo: Daizō Shuppan.

Fujikawa Yū 富士川游 and Shōshin kyōkai 正信協会 (eds) (1936–1941) *Shinsen myōkō-nin den* 新選妙好人伝 (New Selection of Reports about Exemplary Devotees). 14 vols. Tokyo: Kōtoku Shoin.

Fujikawa, Y. (1978) *Japanese Medicine*. New York: AMS Press.

Fukunaga Katsumi (1990) *Bukkyō igaku jiten: ho, Yōga* 仏教医学事典: 補・ヨーガ (Dictionary of Buddhist Medicine: Supplement, Yoga). Tōkyō: Yuzankaku Shuppan.

Goble, A.E. (2009) 'Kajiwara Shōzen (1265–1337) and the Medical Silk Road: Chinese and Arabic Influences on Medieval Japanese Medicine', in A.E. Goble, K.R. Robinson and H. Wakabayashi (eds) *Tools of Culture – Japan's Cultural, Intellectual, Medical and Technological Contacts in East Asia, 1000–1500s*. Ann Arbor, Michigan: Association for Asian Studies, pp. 231–57.

Goble, A.E. (2011) *Confluences of Medicine in Medieval Japan: Buddhist Healing, Chinese Knowledge, Islamic Formulas, and Wounds of War*. Honolulu: University of Hawai'i Press.

Gorai, Shigeru 五来重 (ed.) (1986) *Yakushi shinkō* 薬師信仰 (The Yakushi Cult), Minshū shūkyo-shi sōsho, 12 vols. Tokyo: Yūzankaku Shuppan.

Hattori Toshiyoshi [Toshirō] 服部敏良 (1945) *Nara jidai igaku no kenkyū* 奈良時代醫學の研究 (Studies in Nara-period Medicine). Tōkyō: Tōkyōdō.

Hattori Toshiyoshi [Toshirō] 服部敏良 (1968) *Bukkyō kyōten o chūshin toshita Shaka no igaku* 仏教経典を中心とした釈迦の医学 (Shakyamuni's Medicine According to Buddhist Classical Texts). Nagoya: Reimei Shobō.

Hidaka Yōko 日高洋子 (2009) 'Ninshō to fukushi no ryōiki ni kan suru ikkōsatsu' 忍性と福祉の領域に関する一考察 (Ninshō and Thought Relating to the Field of Welfare), *Saitama gakuen daigaku kiyō* (*ningen gakubuhen*) 埼玉学園大学紀要(人間学部篇), 9: 145–58.

Hirota, D. (2000) 'Dialogic Engagement and Truth', in D. Hirota (ed.) *Toward a Contemporary Understanding of Pure Land Buddhism: Creating a Shin Buddhist Theology in a Religiously Plural World*. Albany, NY: State University of New York Press, pp. 163–98.

Holt, N.R. (1971) 'Ernst Haeckel's Monistic Religion', *Journal of the History of Ideas*, 32.2: 265–80.

Ishihara Akira 石原明 (1959) *Nihon no igaku: sono nagare to hatten* 日本の医学: その流れと発展 (Japanese Medicine: Traditions and Developments). Tokyo: Shibundō.

Jingū shichō 神宮司庁 (ed.) (1914) *Koji rui'en* 古事類苑. Sōmokuroku 総目録 1. Tokyo: Jingū Shichō Koji Rui'en Shuppan Jimusho.

Kawada Yōichi 川田洋一 (ed.) (1976) *Bukkyō shisō to igaku* 仏教思想と医学 (Buddhist Thought and Medicine). Tokyo: Tōyo Tetsugaku Kenkyūsho.

Kawada, Yōichi 川田洋一 (ed.) (2013) *Bukkyō kango to kanwa kea* 仏教看護と緩和ケア (Buddhist Health Care and Palliative Care), Seimei tetsugaku nyūmon 生命哲学入門; 3. Tōkyō: Daisan Bunmeisha.

Kidder, J.E., Jr. (1993) 'The Earliest Societies in Japan', in D.M. Brown (ed.) *Ancient Japan*, The Cambridge History of Japan 1. Cambridge; New York: Cambridge University Press, pp. 48–107.

Killinger, K., Kleine, C. and Triplett, K. (2019) 'Introduction: Distinctions and Differentiations between Medicine and Religion', *Asian Medicine* (Special Issue 'Religion and Medicine' ed. by K. Killinger, C. Kleine and K. Triplett), 14.2: 275–304.

Kleine, C. (2012) 'Buddhist Monks as Healers in Early and Medieval Japan', *Japanese Religions* (Special Issue: Religion and Healing in Japan, ed. by C. Kleine and K. Triplett), 37.1&2: 13–38.

Lomi B. (2014) 'Dharanis, Talismans, and Straw-Dolls Ritual Choreographies and Healing: Strategies of the *Rokujikyōhō* in Medieval Japan', *Japanese Journal of Religious Studies*, 41: 255–304.

Lomi, B. (2017) 'The Ox-Bezoar Empowerment for Fertility and Safe Childbirth: Selected Readings from the Shingon Ritual Collection', in C.P. Salguero (ed.) *Buddhism and Medicine: An Anthology of Premodern Sources*. New York: Columbia University Press, pp. 351–7.

Maki Sachiko 槇佐知子 (ed.) (1993–2012) *Ishinpō: Maki Sachiko zenshaku seikai* 医心方: 槇佐知子全訳精解 (Ishinpō: Maki Sachiko's Complete Translation and Commentary). Tōkyō: Chikuma Shobō.

Maki Sachiko 槇佐知子 (ed.) (1995) 'Taikyō shussan hen' 胎教出産篇 (Volume on Prenatal Care and Childbirth), in Maki Sachiko 槇佐知子 (Hg.) *Ishinpō: Maki Sachiko zenshaku seikai* 医心方: 槇佐知子全訳精解. Tokyo: Chikuma Shobō.

Mayanagi Makoto 真柳誠 (1993) 'Chūgoku honzō to Nihon no juyō' 中国本草と日本の受容 (Chinese *Materia Medica* and Their Reception in Japan), in Xiao Peigen 蕭培根 and Mayanagi Makoto 真柳誠 (trans.) (eds) *Chūgoku honzō zuroku* 中国本草図録, 9. Tōkyō: Chūō Kōronsha, pp. 218–29.

Michel-Zaitsu, W. (2017) *Traditionelle Medizin in Japan von der Frühzeit bis zur Gegenwart*. München: Kiener Verlag.

Miyata, N. (2012) *Die Übernahme der chinesischen Kultur in Japans Altertum. Kultureller Wandel im innen- und außenpolitischen Kontext*. Berlin: Lit.

Mura'i Hideo 村井秀夫, Matsuo Shin'ichi 松尾信一 and Shira'i Tsunesaburō 白井恒三郎 ([1961] 1994) 'Ba'i makimono (Bunroku yonnen) ni tsuite 馬医巻物（文禄四年）について' (On the Scroll of Equine Medicine [Bunroku Era Year 4]), in Matsuo Shin'ichi 松尾信一 (ed.) *Bagaku: Uma o bungaku suru* 馬学: 馬を科学する. Uma no bunka sōsho 馬の文化叢書 7. Yokohama: Baji bunka zaidan, pp. 537–8.

Nei Kiyoshi 根井浄 (1976) 'Shugendō no iryō ni tsuite' 修験者の医療について (Medical Therapeutics in Shugendō), *Journal of Indian and*

Buddhist Studies/Indogaku Bukkyōgaku kenkyū 印度學佛教學研究, 24.2: 893–6.

Nei Kiyoshi 根井浄 (1980) 'Toyama baiyaku to shugenja ni tsuite' 富山売薬と修験者について (On the Pharmaceutical Trade and Mountain Ascetics in Toyama), *Journal of Indian and Buddhist Studies/Indogaku Bukkyōgaku kenkyū* 印度學佛教學研究, 28.2: 624–5.

Nihonyanagi Kenji 二本柳賢司 (1994) *Bukkyō igaku gaiyō* 佛教医学概要 (Outline of Buddhist Medicine). Kyōto: Hōzōkan.

Nihonyanagi Kenji 二本柳賢司 (1997) 'Nihon mikkyō igaku to yakubutsugaku' 日本密教医学と薬物学 (Japanese Esoteric Buddhist Medicine and Pharmaceutics), in K. Yamada and S. Kuriyama (eds) *Rekishi no naka no yamai to igaku* 歴史の中の病と医学. Kyōto: Kokusai Nihon Bunka Kenkyū Sentā; Shibundō, pp. 545–66.

NKBT *Nihon koten bungaku taikei* 日本古典文學大系 (Complete Works of Japanese Classical Literature) (1957–1969) Kurano K. 倉野憲司 ed. Tokyo: Iwanami shoten 岩波書店.

NKZ *Nihon koten zenshū* 日本古典全集 (Complete Works of Japanese Classic Texts) (1925–1944) Yosano Hiroshi 与謝野寛 *et al.* and Masamune, Atsuo 正宗敦夫 eds, Tōkyō: Nihon koten zenshū kankōkai 日本古典全集刊行會.

Obinata Daijō 大日方大乗 (1965) *Bukkyō igaku no kenkyū* 仏教医学の研究 (Buddhist Medical Studies). Tōkyō: Kasama Shobō.

Ogawa Kenzaburō 小川剣三郎 ([1904] 1971) *Nihon gankashi, kōhon* 日本眼科学史: 稿本 (The History of Japanese Ophthalmology: Manuscripts). Kyoto: Shibunkaku.

Okuzawa Yasumasa 奥沢康正 (1997) 'Me'ishi-tachi no hidensho to ryūha' 目医師達の秘伝書と流派 (The Secret Records and Schools and Branches of the Ophthalmologist Doctors), in K. Yamada and S. Kuriyama (eds) *Rekishi no naka no yamai to igaku* 歴史の中の病と医学. Kyōto: Kokusai Nihon Bunka Kenkyū Sentā, pp. 195–228.

Ooms H. (2009) *Imperial Politics and Symbolics in Ancient Japan: The Tenmu Dynasty, 650–800*. Honolulu: University of Hawai'i Press.

Ooms H. (2015) 'Framing Daoist fragments, 670–750', in J.L. Richey (ed.) *Daoism in Japan: Chinese Traditions and Their Influence on Japanese Religious Culture*. London; New York: Routledge, pp. 37–59.

Otsuka, Y. (1976) 'Chinese Traditional Medicine in Japan', in C. Leslie (ed.) *Asian Medical Systems*. Berkeley, CA: University of California Press, pp. 322–40.

Quinter, D. (2015) *From Outcasts to Emperors: Shingon Ritsu and the Mañjuśrī Cult in Medieval Japan*. Brill's Japanese studies library 50. Leiden; Boston: Brill.

Rosner E. (1989) *Medizingeschichte Japans,* Handbuch der Orientalistik Abt. 5: Japan Bd 3 Abschnitt 5. Leiden: E.J. Brill.

Sakamoto Tarō 坂本太郎 *et al.* (eds) (1965–1967) *Nihon shoki* 日本書紀 (Record of Japan). Nihon koten bungaku taikei 日本古典文學大系; 67, 68. Tōkyō: Iwanami Shoten.

Salguero, C.P. (2012) '"Treating Illness": Translation of a Chapter from a Medieval Chinese Buddhist Meditation Manual by Zhiyi (538–597)', *Asian Medicine*, 7.2: 461–73.

Salguero, C.P. (2015) 'Reexamining the Categories and Canons of Chinese Buddhist Healing', *Journal of Chinese Buddhist Studies*, 28: 35–66.

Salguero, P. (2018) 'Healing and/or Salvation? The Relationship Between Religion and Medicine in Medieval Chinese Buddhism', Working Paper 4, *Working Paper of the HCAS Multiple Secularities – Beyond the West, Beyond Modernities*. Leipzig.

Schiebinger, L.L. (2004) *Plants and Empire: Colonial Bioprospecting in the Atlantic World*. Cambridge, MA: Harvard University Press.

Schmidt, H. (1914) *Ernst Haeckel Rede, gehalten am 16. Februar 1914 im großen Volkshaussaal zu Jena zur Feier von Haeckels 80. Geburtstag*. Leipzig: Alfred Kröner.

Schrimpf, M. (2018) 'Medical Discourses and Practices in Contemporary Japanese Religions', in D. Lüddeckens and M. Schrimpf (eds) *Medicine – Religion – Spirituality: Global Perspectives on Traditional, Complementary, and Alternative Healing*. Bielefeld: Transcript, pp. 57–90.

Shinmura Taku 新村拓 (2006) *Nihon iryō shi* 日本医療史 (History of Medical Therapeutics in Japan). Tōkyō: Yoshikawa Kōbunkan.

Shinmura Taku 新村拓 (2013) *Nihon bukkyō no iryōshi* 日本仏教の医療史 (History of Japanese Buddhist Medical Therapeutics). Tōkyō: Hōsei Daigaku Shuppankyoku.

Taishō Shinshū Daizōkyō Kankōkai (ed.) (1926–1985) Taishō shinshū dai zōkyō sakuin 大正新脩大藏經索引. Reprinted Tokyo: Taishō Shinshū Daizō kyō Kankōkai (1964–). Tokyo: Daizō Shuppan.

Triplett, K. (2019a) *Buddhism and Medicine in Japan: A Topical Survey (500–1600 CE) of a Complex Relationship*. Religion and Society 81. Berlin: De Gruyter.

Triplett, K. (2019b) 'Pediatric Care and Buddhism in Premodern Japan: A Case of Applied 'Demonology'?' *Asian Medicine* (Special Issue 'Religion and Medicine' ed. by K. Killinger, C. Kleine and K. Triplett), 14.2: 355–82.

Triplett, K. (2021a) 'Medicine', in E. Baffelli and F. Rambelli (eds) *Bloomsbury Handbook of Japanese Religions*. London: Bloomsbury, pp. 151–6.

Triplett, K. (2021b) 'Medicine in Japanese Buddhism', in *The Oxford Research Encyclopedia of Religion*. Oxford: Oxford University Press. https://doi.org/10.1093/acrefore/9780199340378.013.614, accessed 25 May 2022.

Triplett, K. (2022) 'Chinese-style Medicine in Japan', in V. Lo and M. Stanley-Baker (eds) *Routledge Handbook of Chinese Medicine*. London: Routledge, pp. 513–23.

Tsuchiya Hisashi 土屋久 and Horiguchi Kyūgorō 堀口久五郎 (2012) 'Fujikawa Yū no shūkyō shisō: 'naikan' kara 'myōkō-nin' e 富士川游の宗教思想: 「内観」から「妙好人」へ' (Fujikawa Yū's Religious Thought:

From 'Naikan' to 'Exemplary Devotees'). *Seikatsu kagaku kenkyū* 生活科学研究 (Bulletin of Living Science) 34, 177–86.

Williams, D.R. (2005) *The Other Side of Zen: A Social History of Sōtō Zen: Buddhism in Tokugawa Japan*. Princeton, NJ: Princeton University Press.

Winfield, P.D. (2005) 'Curing with *kaji*: Healing and Esoteric Empowerment in Japan', *Japanese Journal of Religious Studies*, 32.1: 107–30.

Yoshida Fumio 吉田文夫 (1983) 'Ninshō no shakai jigyō ni tsuite' 忍性の社会事業について, (Ninshō's Social Engagement), in Nakao Takashi 中尾堯 and Imai Masaharu 今井雅晴 (eds) *Chōgen, Eison, Ninshō* 重源・叡尊・忍性. Tōkyō: Yoshikawa Kōbunkan, pp. 392–433.

Yoshida Kyūichi 吉田久一 (1986) '"Jinen hōni" ni tsuite – fukushi jissen no kontei: Shinran to Fujikawa Yū 「自然法爾」について- 福祉実践の根底: 親鸞と富士川游' (About 'Jinen hōni' – Foundation of Welfare Practice: Shinran and Fujikawa Yū), *Tōyō daigaku jidō sōdan kenkyū* 東洋大学児童相談研究, 5: 72–82.

3

Female alchemy in late imperial and modern China

Elena Valussi

Background

Inner alchemy

Female alchemy is part of the earlier tradition of Daoist inner alchemy (*neidan*). *Neidan* employs a series of physiological and mental practices like breathing, gymnastics, concentration and meditation intended to prolong one's life and to attain transcendence from this world. This set of internal practices developed fully in the Song dynasty (960–1279) through the modification of techniques and terminology from the earlier *waidan* 外丹 (external alchemy) tradition. The *waidan* tradition has a long history; starting in the early part of Western Han dynasty (202 BCE–9 CE), it flourished through the Tang dynasty (618–907), and declined in the Song and Ming dynasties. While in early sources this tradition was mostly concerned with performing rituals to connect with gods and spirits, practitioners during the Tang worked in a laboratory (*danshi* 丹室, Chamber of the Elixir) to transform mineral, metal and other natural substances, melting them inside a crucible (*ding* 鼎) on top of a furnace (*lü* 爐), and producing an elixir (cinnabar, or *dan* 丹). The elixir was then ingested, and was thought to cure diseases, extend one's life-span, and eventually lead to immortality (Pregadio 2008: 1002–4). In the Song and later times, as *waidan* declined, we see the soteriological import of alchemy being transferred to *neidan*. For *neidan* practitioners, the body became the crucible, and internal bodily essences became the primary materials to be melted, refined and sublimated (*xiulian* 修煉). The body became the centre of this transformation, and the goal was still long life and immortality.

With the focus of the practitioner squarely on the transformation of the body, an important element that influenced *neidan* was earlier Daoist, *yangsheng* 養生 or nurturing life practices, which developed even earlier than *waidan*. *Yangsheng* is a general term that can involve a variety of physiological practices, from breathing, to moving and stretching, to sexual hygiene. The first reference to *yangsheng* appears in the *Zhuangzi*, but it was in the former Han dynasty that it flourished. *Yangsheng* practices are described in the *Mawangdui* corpus of scriptures, dating to about 200 BCE, where dietary regimens, breathing and sexual practices are described in detail. While *yangsheng* is later extensively used in and transmitted through Daoist sources, its aims were initially mainly prophylactic and therapeutic, not soteriological, and it continued to be present in medical literature as well (Despeux 2008).

Traditional ideas of the interdependence of body and cosmos, the five agents, and the *yin-yang* theory also deeply inform *neidan*. Specifically, cosmological understanding derived from *Yijing* 易經 theory is central to the development of *neidan* theory and practice. The *Yijing* is a divination manual dated mostly to the Zhou period (1046–256 BCE). It is based on the interpretations of eight trigrams and sixty-four hexagrams (*gua* 卦), which variedly combine broken (*yin*) and unbroken (*yang*) lines, stacked on top of each other in groups of three (trigrams) or six (hexagrams). When received through a divination process, each trigram and hexagram has a specific meaning that is interpreted and applied to different life circumstances. In *neidan*, trigrams and hexagrams are used differently: they can be used as cosmic reference points for the ordering of the universe and, at the same time, they are a cosmological representation of the physical body and its processes, therefore they connect the universe to the body of the practitioner. Trigrams and hexagrams can also symbolise the alchemical ingredients to be transformed in the *neidan* process (Robinet 2008). Finally, influences from Chan Buddhism and from Confucianism also appear in *neidan* texts.

As for the aims of *neidan*, they are defined differently throughout its long history, but generally speaking they are described as achieving immortality (*chengxian* 成仙), forming an immortal embryo (*xiantai* 仙胎) or obtaining 'release from the corpse' (*shijie* 屍解).[1] The process of transformation is not only a process of refinement, but it is an inversion of the life-course (*diandao* 顛倒; *niliu* 逆流). Life energies are understood as being finite, and they are gradually lost as we age; *neidan* reverses that course, and redirects those energies towards the formation of an immortal embryo.[2] The process of reversal is codified in steps, and the practitioner is instructed to go through them in a sequence of refinement through which their own bodily essences become more ethereal and contribute to the formation of the immortal embryo. For standard *neidan* theory, the steps are as follows: *lianjing huaqi* 煉精化氣 (refining the essence into *qi*), *lianqi hua shen* 連氣化神 (refining the *qi* into spirit), and *lianshen hua xuwu* 煉神化虛無 (refining the spirit into emptiness). *Jing* 精 (essence), *qi* 氣 and *shen* 神 (spirit), also called *sanbao* 三寶 (the three Jewels), are essential elements of the *neidan* process.

Here is a typical description of the process of refinement:

> 'The Dao generates the One, the One generates the Two, the Two generate the Three, the Three generate the ten thousand things' (*Daodejing*, ch. 42). Emptiness transmutes itself into Spirit, Spirit transmutes itself into Breath, Breath transmutes itself into Essence, and Essence transmutes itself into form. The above is called 'following the course' (*shun* 順). The ten thousand things hold the Three, the Three return to the Two, the Two return to the One. Having refined [the form] into the perfect Essence, Essence transmutes itself into Breath, and Breath transmutes itself into Spirit. The above is called 'inverting the course'(*ni* 逆). The books on the Elixir say that 'following the course' forms the human being, while 'inverting the course' forms the elixir.[3]

More specifically, the process goes from 'building the foundations' (*zhuji* 築基), to refining the self (*lianji* 煉己), to gathering the ingredients for the elixir (*caiyao* 採藥), forming and nourishing the immortal embryo (*yangtai* 養胎) and eventually letting it go (*tuotai* 脫胎). On the physiological level, *jing* is refined by a repeated and continuous circular motion (*zhoutian* 周天) that makes it ascend through the back of the body through the three passes (*weilü* 尾閭, *jiaji* 夾脊, *yuzhen* 玉枕), arriving at the top of the head (*niwan* 泥丸) and descending through the front; *qi* is refined through meditation and breathing exercises, also connected to the circular motion described above.[4] *Shen* is refined by calming the mind (*xin*) and the emotions (*qing*). The process is described on the physiological plane, but this transformation also happens simultaneously on a cosmological level. On the physical level, grosser essences are refined into more ethereal ones; on the cosmological level, what transforms are the above-mentioned trigrams of the *Yijing*. The trigrams *Qian* ☰ and Kun ☷, formed by three unbroken *yang* lines and three broken *yin* lines respectively, symbolise the mother and father of the universe; when they unite, they create the cosmos. Their union forms eight children, the eight trigrams combining broken and unbroken lines. Of these trigrams, *Kan* ☵ symbolises water and female, *Li* ☲ symbolises fire and male. The final outcome of the self-cultivation process is the elimination of all *yin* elements, therefore all the broken lines, and the recreation of the *yang* trigram, *Qian* ☰, equivalent to the pure *yang* body.

Female alchemy

In the Qing dynasty (1644–1911) we see the emergence of a full-fledged tradition of female alchemy, born within the religious practice of spirit writing and aided by the expansion of cheap printing and the wide dissemination of textual corpuses. While there are previous references to female practices in Daoist texts prior to this time, for the first time we have whole manuals dedicated just to female practice. These manuals bring together longer texts, divided in different chapters, discussing the female practice step by step. They contain large sections on proper female behaviour, warnings against improper physical practices, hagiographies of female immortals, and a mostly female lineage of transmission. The understanding of the female body and its processes exemplified in these manuals is an expansion and a systematisation of earlier materials. Both *neidan* and *nüdan* share attention to the body, and to its relations to the structure of the cosmos; they also share much terminology and many techniques. The maturity and coherence of *nüdan* texts and collections thus owe much to *neidan*, in terms of textual origins and structure, cosmological discourse, techniques and terminology, processes and goals. *Nüdan* is, however, specifically directed at women, and thus also defines itself as different, first and foremost in the gendering of the language. The exchange of the word *nei* (内 internal) with the word *nü* (女 female) does not change the location of the work, as was the case with the shift from *waidan* to *neidan*, but it genders the term. *Nüdan* uses the same *neidan* process but applies it to the female body.

This shift from a genderless to a gendered term immediately lends itself to a gender analysis. The distinction is important because, before the appearance of *nüdan*, *neidan* was considered a path open to both men and women (social realities notwithstanding). From this moment onwards, however, *nüdan* would become the only viable practice for women, and *neidan*, by contrast, clearly became the purview of male practitioners.

In terms of physiology, prior to the emergence of *nüdan*, Daoist self-cultivation texts display some knowledge of female processes, but little evidence of gender-specific techniques (see the examples in the Daoist Canon below). From the seventeenth century onwards, on the other hand, the texts insist on the different physiological structures of men and women as the basis for a complex, and markedly different process, both at the physiological and at the cosmological level. In more than one preface to female alchemy texts, we see the emergence of the term *nandan* (男丹),[5] male alchemy, as a counterpart to female alchemy, forming a pair (*nüdan* – *nandan*) that did not exist before. In one case, we have a whole collection (the *Jinhua zhizhi* 金華直指) describing two specific and different processes for males and for females, presented side by side, with cosmological and physiological processes. Therefore, we can definitely say that the emergence of *nüdan* genders *neidan*.

The path to transcendence, in *neidan*, always involves forming an embryo of immortality inside the body of the practitioner. This embryo will exit the body from the top of the head when the process of refinement is complete, and the practitioner thus attains immortality. Even when talking about material, physiological processes of the standard *neidan*, however, discourse remains highly symbolic, and does not really mirror the physical body in detail. In female alchemy, on the other hand, the cosmological changes *are* changes in the female body. While from the discursive point of view, therefore, *nüdan* borrows extensively from *neidan*, the ideas about the female body that we find in *nüdan* texts are in large part within the domain of Chinese medical ideas. There is a specific attention to the female body and the female reproductive system, and especially the role of the breasts, of the uterus, and of blood. Blood, the central element of female physiology, is understood to have various manifestations throughout the female body, as a basic energy source, as menstrual blood and placenta, as breast milk. Thus, it also manifests itself in different parts of the female body: the heart (*xin* 心) where it is produced, the point between the breast (*ruxi* 乳溪) where it is gathered, the breasts themselves (*rufang* 乳房) where it exits as milk, the womb (*zigong* 子宮, *xuehai* 血海) where it flows down and gathers, and the vagina (*pinhu* 牝戶) where it exits the body as menstruation (*jing* 經). All these fluids and loci, as well as the practices involving those fluids and loci (breast massage, disappearance of the menstrual flow), are discussed in great detail in the texts. Based on these differences, the three-step process described above is also modified: while for men we have the transformation of *jing* to *qi*, for women, we have the transformation of blood (*xue* 血) into *qi*, through a similar circulation process. In women, this process starts in a different location than the male practice, the place between the breasts (*ruxi*) and not the lower cinnabar field (*dantian* 丹田), continues downwards to the uterus, to the coccyx and up the spine. The following two steps are essentially the same for men and women. The final ascendance to the skies is, however, more challenging for women, who retain traces of the pollution they worked so hard to eliminate. The refinement of blood into a less heavy, less polluted and more ethereal substance, is central to female alchemy self-cultivation and the discourse of the difficulty in dealing with female blood and its complex multifarious presence mirrors medical discourses on female physiology.

At the cosmological level, there is a parallel transformation. While the *Qian* ☰ and *Kun* ☷ *Yijing* trigrams symbolise male and female at the primordial level, *Kan* ☵ and *Li* ☲ trigrams are two of its offspring, and they have special significance in female alchemy. *Kan* ☵ symbolises water and female, *Li* ☲ symbolises fire and male. *Kan* is the image of the female, with two *yin* broken lines on the outside and a *yang* unbroken line inside, and *Li* ☲ is the image of the male, with two unbroken *yang* lines on the outside, and one broken *yin* line on the inside. The two *yin* broken external lines of *Kan*, the female, are directly related, in the texts, with water and the menstrual cycle. Once the menstrual cycle is refined, those two *yin* lines will also revert to unbroken ones, forming the pure *yang* trigram, *Qian* ☰. The trigrams are thus not only cosmological symbols, but they are embodied in the practitioner and transformed through the physiological process.[6] This is underlined further by descriptions of the process of formation of the female embryo in utero in female alchemy texts: the blood of the mother enveloping the semen of the father: this mirrors the Kan structure, *yin* outside and *yang* inside.

The cosmological change from *Kan* to *Qian* is an embodied process. The cosmological symbol *Kan* signifies and is the body of the menstruating woman, which is created in that form at conception. The outer expression of the female body is the physical representation of the broken lines of the Trigram Kan; their transformation into unbroken lines, the repairing of *Kan* into *Qian*, is parallel in time with the physical disappearance of the menses and the shrinking of the breasts in female practitioners, and the female body becomes more androgynous. The physicality of the female process of transformation is evident: there is a direct relationship between the broken lines and the external features of the female body. As in the *neidan* process described above, the final goal of the practice, at the cosmological level, is still to recreate *Qian*, the purely *yang* trigram and hexagram, therefore both genders have to revert to the primordial *yang*, male, symbol.

The process of self-refinement and transcendence is thus much more embodied for women, and this makes it easier to recognise and understand through the lens of medical literature, which already has a mapped physiology for women. This is a useful way to explain the differences in the female body, which are difficult to explain otherwise.

Thus, Chinese medical beliefs about the difference between male and female physiology, and the importance of blood as the essential energetic substance for a woman, are definitely central to the understanding of the female body and the changes it undergoes as a result of the process of self-cultivation. The aim of the two disciplines is, however, very different. In medicine, blood (*xue* 血) is, together with *qi* (氣), one of the two main energetic bases for the female body. It is also the main culprit for many of the illnesses typical of female physiology, all linked to blood stagnation, depletion and blockage. Thus, in the traditional Chinese medical view of female physiology, blood needs to be appeased, conquered and its negative influence on the female body counteracted. From this point of view, however, blood when well regulated is also a positive force of generation and the basis of the gestation process that produces children. For *nüdan*, blood is also the main energetic base of the female body. It is an element that, more than any other in the female body, can and should be refined. This, though, does not lead to a better, unhindered and healthy flow, but to a radical transformation. This change, into ethereal energy (*qi*, *shen* and then *xuwu*, as in the traditional *neidan* sequence), leads to the formation and nourishment of the immortality embryo. Thus, blood is certainly not a generative force leading to the production of children, but quite the opposite, its transformation and eventual disappearance into a spiritual energy leads to the negation of traditional fertility and maternity, and to the formation of an immortal embryo instead. In contracts to discussions of medical traditions, then, the goal of these very physical/bodily changing practices, their efficacy, was not a question of health, but of transcendence of the ordinary world. As will be clarified below, however, health and wellbeing were an important pre-requisite for starting the practice, especially for women, who were defined in medical treatises as difficult to treat because of their physiology.

The sources I will use below are Daoist texts dating from the Song to the Republican period, with a focus on the Qing dynasty, when female alchemy flourished. I will be particularly concerned with passages discussing the female body, her essences, her illnesses, her health; thus, for the specific purposes of this chapter, I will not focus on the origins of the texts or their social context, which I have discussed elsewhere (Valussi 2008a, 2008b).

Literature

Until very recently the tradition of female alchemy was generally ignored by early scholars of Daoism, even though there is a long history of the study of inner alchemy in China and in the West. This is due to several different reasons. First of all, it is a late tradition, and often dismissed as 'popular', thus not sophisticated enough to be taken into serious consideration. No female alchemy texts were included in the fundamental Daoist compendium, the *Daozang* 道藏, because they were all composed later, as part of a period of intense scripture production starting in the seventeenth century and tied to momentous changes in the religious landscape of China. Large eschatological and rebellious movements appear on the horizon and, in an effort to find individual salvation from impending disaster, lay groups start to establish their own altars where they receive direct scriptural transmissions from the Gods through a technique called spirit writing (*fuji* 扶乩) (Clart and Goossaert, forthcoming). These scriptures have been marginalised as syncretic, without a traceable origin, and connected to a 'superstitious' practice, and they have not, therefore, received a lot of scholarly attention until very recently (Goossaert 2022; Schumann and Valussi forthcoming). Further, within Daoist studies, focusing on gender and specifically on women and female bodies has long been considered a niche and unimportant area. Practices involving women became interesting when they also involved men, thus there are a variety of sources on sexuality and sexual hygiene, from the early to the modern period, often connected to the field of *yangsheng*.[7] Sexual practices with a soteriological goal also have a specific niche.[8] Solo female cultivation was, however, less interesting. Probably the first book in Chinese or Western languages to deal with this tradition was Despeux's (1990) ground-breaking *Immortelles de la Chine Ancienne*. Its English language adaptation was less historically grounded but still important (Despeux and Kohn 2003). My own work has revealed and described the depth and variety of the sources; has provided a grounded historical perspective; and has discussed their provenance from a spirit-written milieu and a much-needed gender analysis (Valussi 2008a, 2008b, 2009).

The importance of this tradition has not, however, been fully and widely acknowledged in China or in the West. While it is fruitful to connect this tradition to traditional studies of *neidan* and of Chinese cosmology, as I do initially below, the overwhelming presence of the female body, and of its physiological processes at the centre of this tradition, requires us also to connect it deeply to, and be inspired by, critical ideas emerging from the field of women's medicine in China, in combination with works on gender, medicine, religion and the body in the West.

Cosmology

As mentioned above, *Yijing* cosmology and the symbolism of *yin-yang*, the five agents, etc. is very strong in *neidan* as well as in *nüdan*.

Pregadio (2006: 149) writes eloquently about the complex symbolism that *neidan* incorporates, the ingenious use of correlative cosmology, of 'various sets of cosmological symbols' (the five agents, the three cinnabar fields, *yin-yang*, the trigrams and hexagrams, the pre-celestial and post-celestial cosmogonic arrangements…) to describe the path to transcendence and immortality, and all of these elements are present in *nüdan*. While Pregadio has focused extensively on the discursive level of inner alchemy, and not so much on its embodied practices, Steavu (2016) has recently discussed the embryological metaphors deeply embedded in early inner alchemy. He indicates that, since the early formation of *neidan* in the Song, the lines between medical and Daoist views of the body were not clear, and that soteriological discourses always included medical understanding. Even though the metaphor of the embryo is obviously related to a process that can only happen in the female body, however, there are no mentions of specific gender differences in the early medieval texts he surveys, and specific bodily practices are not extensively described. For a later period, Despeux (2016: 168) describes how Daoist writers continue to discuss the symbolic embryo formation in the bodies of non-gendered practitioners as a spiritual and non-physical process; one writer attains the 'spiritualisation of the reproductive process' by synchronising the stages of embryo development with the stages of Buddhist meditation leading towards nirvana. Thus the inherent 'femaleness' of the gestation process is elided and we can say that the physicality of the *neidan* process is not central to the achievement of transcendence.

Women's medicine

For female alchemy, however, the body is present and central and discussed in detail. Comparing female alchemy texts and standard alchemy texts from the same period, it is clear that in female alchemy texts, the terminology is powerfully linked to the physical body and its gender-specific attributes. As Lee Jen-der (2008) points out in the introduction to her book *Xingbie shenti yu yiliao shi* 性別、身體與醫療史 (Gender, Body and Medicine), Chinese medicine has traditionally seen the male body as the model and standard for illness and health, and the female body as a special case, therefore it is actually easier to identify the specific characteristics of the female body, its health and illness, than those of the male body. The same can be said for female alchemy. As I mentioned above, the emergence of female alchemy in the late Ming and Qing gendered inner alchemy, and revealed quite clearly that the previous practices were mostly taking the male body as the model, the standard of practice. Further, in female alchemy we see a much more specific attention to the physical body, the most obvious locus of difference, than in standard alchemy, where the physical body of the (male) practitioner is not central to the process.

The narrative of the female body as ruled by blood, chronically depleted and weak, and the need to counteract it in order to restore health, is pervasive in Chinese primary sources on women's medicine (*fuke* 婦科), and has been widely addressed in secondary literature, as discussed below. In discussing female physiology in female alchemy texts, these pre-existing medical metaphors and narratives are widely used, from embryogenesis, to life cycles, to the role of blood, both in its energetic sustaining role and in its problematic role in blood-related illnesses. Well-known passages on female health and illness are quoted verbatim or adapted in female alchemy texts. For this reason, it is useful here to discuss works on the conceptions of the body in women's medicine, in order to make more sense of the physicality of the female body in *nüdan* texts. Wilms (2005) describes how important a gendered understanding of the bodies becomes in the period from the Han to the Song, where blood and menstruation become central to the discussion of health and illness. Women's illnesses were categorically different from male illnesses, and this new perception gave way to the creation of a medical field specialised in those illnesses, *fuke* or gynaecology, in the Song. Physiological as well as psychological factors, often related to the female's reproductive functions, were part of what made women more difficult to cure. Despite the generative and energetic power of blood in the female body, it also was the substance most connected with female illnesses, due to depletion, stagnation, blockage and general irregularity. In the Song, menstruation became a paramount concern to physicians and menstrual regulation the goal to achieve, in order to ensure healthy reproductive capacities in women (Wilms 2005). Women were described as ten times more difficult to cure than men because of blood, whose effects on the female body also made it more vulnerable to external factors like wind and cold.

Emotions also had an effect on the female body and negative emotions, like sadness and rage, were especially related to blood irregularities. Furth's (1986) analysis of the development of *fuke* in the Song and Ming further describes how blood continued to be of central concern in medical discussions of women; blood was not only menstrual blood, but pervaded the female body in many guises (breast milk, nourishment for the fetus, energetic basis), and caused a variety of health problems. Li Shizhen 李時珍 (1518–1593), famous doctor and pharmacologist of the seventeenth century, wrote about the role of blood in women, 'before conception, it descends as menses, after conception, it nourishes the embryo, after birth, red transforming into white, it becomes milk'.[9] At the same time, blood is also responsible for the deficiency and complexity of female physiology, causing serious illnesses. Both Yang Shi-Yin, a physician in the Southern Song, and Li Shizhen, acknowledged the importance and pervasiveness of blood in a woman's body: 'Males and females both have blood and *qi*, and yet people say that in women blood is fundamental. Why? Because their blood is in ascendancy over *qi*. It is stored in the liver system, flows through the womb and is ruled by the heart system; it ascends to become breast milk, descends to become menses, unites with semen to make the embryo'.[10] 'Before conception it appears as menses below, during pregnancy it provides nourishment for the fetus, after birth, red changing to white, it ascends as milk' (Furth 1986: 46). Chen Ziming 陳字明 (1190–1270), a famous Song gynaecologist, says, 'In men one regulates *qi*, in women one regulates blood' and 'Men think of the bedroom when their essence (*jing*) is exuberant, women crave pregnancy when their blood is exuberant'.[11]

All of these descriptions are commonly used in female alchemy texts to justify a different, gendered, practice. Yi-li Wu (2010), in her work on Qing dynasty gynaecology, focuses on female illnesses and their relation to menstruation and blood; she also discusses the uterus and the breasts as essential parts of female physiology and describes in detail the functions of these organs and how they are dealt with in Chinese medicine. They are central also in female alchemy practice. While acknowledging, however, that there is, certainly from the Song onwards, a strong understanding of women as drastically different from men, Wu insists on the fact that, in the Late Imperial Period, the female body is not seen any longer as categorically different from the male, apart from the gynaecological ailments, and she maintains that Chinese medical doctrine saw androgyny and gender difference as two sides of the same coin (Wu 2010: 231). In her work (Wu 2016) on the seventeenth century Korean doctor, Ho Chun, Wu further questions the insistence on the generative organs in the construction of gender and proves that in the work of this doctor, the womb is a generative organ for both men and women, and that Chinese preoccupation with the menses as the fundamental cause for female illnesses was different from other East Asian medicines, and it was an 'intellectual orientation that needed to be constructed and sustained' (Wu 2016: 52). Androgyny is a fundamental concept when discussing female alchemy too: while the physiological differences are great at the beginning of the practice, as the work progresses, grosser features disappear to give way to a more androgynous body.

The narrative in female alchemy never, however, completely leaves the specificity, and deficiency, of the female body behind, which, while overwhelming at the beginning of the practice, resurfaces at the end of it. In female alchemy, the female body and its gendered components, especially blood, is still central, it is populated by blood, it is manipulated through massage of the breasts and abdomen, the results of the practice are tested by checking the colour of the menses. This understanding of the female body in female alchemy is very different from the non-gendered body in standard alchemy, where *jing*, as opposed to blood, is present but not overwhelming, and where cosmology does not relate in such a strong and powerful way to physiology. And, even though female alchemy manuals say that, after the first step, the rest of the practice is the same for men and women, the first step is exceedingly difficult for women and fraught with dangers; these dangers are due to illnesses that result from female physiology and especially blood-related complications. These dangers and complications, clearly influenced by Chinese medical descriptions of the female body and its ailments, continued to be the same all the way to the contemporary period.

This is confirmed by anthropological work describing the power and pollution of menstrual blood within the family boundaries, in religious rituals, and in medical practice. Ahern (1975) discusses the power that women derive from the polluting nature of their menstrual blood, and how it is perceived and utilised within the family boundaries. She contends that, in order to rationalise women's social inferior status, women's sexuality and physiology is rendered negatively, 'Once the polluting nature of the sex act, ... menstrual blood, ... and childbirth ... is established, the source of a woman's power is obscured, if not rendered invisible, by a layer of negative sentiment' (Ahern 1975) Seaman (1981) applies this concept to his analysis of the polluting power of blood in the ritual of the 'bloody pond'; in this ritual, a son goes through extreme trials and tribulations in order to rescue his mother from hell, where she is confined because of the pollution caused by the blood she shed giving birth to him. Seaman (1981: 381) describes 'a ritual that shows gratitude and pity for women's fate on the one hand while dramatising women's pollution on the other'. Social and religious taboos, traditionally and today, prevent menstruating women from entering temples and worshipping gods, for fear of offending them. Women themselves have internalised these beliefs and continue to transmit them, while Furth and Ch'en (1992) found that these beliefs are not necessarily perceived negatively by women themselves. The overarching belief about the defiling and polluting nature of female blood is one of the main reasons for the need to transform it in the female alchemy process.

Sources

Mentions of specific self-cultivation for women in Daoist sources do not appear until the Song dynasty, in parallel with the development of *neidan*. While the *neidan* discourse is well organised and sophisticated by the early Song, however, it incorporates elements from *Yijing* cosmological theory, and the theory of *yin-yang* and the five agents, there are only very few and very vague references to the self-cultivation of women. It is important to identify these sources in the *Daozang*, the largest collection of early Daoist sources, which was compiled in 1444. The references we have indicate that the different physiology of men and women is acknowledged, even though in a minority of texts. The tradition of female alchemy had not yet developed, but I will highlight below examples in which the male and female body are indeed described differently, according to their dissimilar physiology, how the female constitution might lead to ill health, and what the self-cultivation process for eliminating illness looks like for different bodies. These primary sources are mostly from Daoist compendia, not from medical ones, even though in the Ming dynasty there are two examples of prominent doctors experimenting with alchemical techniques and describing specific ones for healing gynaecological diseases. While most of the sources that I will review below are clearly categorised as Daoist, they take full advantage of contemporary medical understanding of the body, and often quote from medical texts or refer to well-known medical beliefs, to support their construction of the female alchemical body and its workings. The opposite does not seem to be true; especially in the late imperial period, there is not such a widespread use of alchemical ideas in medical texts.

Early Daoism

The earliest example of physiologically based gender differentiation in Daoist practices is found in the *Daozang*. The *Chongyang zhenren jinguan yusuojue* 重陽真人金關玉鎖訣 (Instructions Concerning the Golden Bar and the Jade Lock),[12] is attributed to Wang Chongyang 王重陽 (1113–1170):

> It was asked: Why is it that men and women suddenly fall sick and die?
>
> it is because their heart/minds like pleasures… men damage their *jing*, women damage their blood. During the day they continuously have indescribable vexations, and at night they cannot stop the three corpses and the *yin* spirits.[13]
>
> If men nurture the *jing* and women nurture the blood, the ten thousand evils are corrected, the ten thousand illnesses do not arise; only then can the *dantian* be pure and calm.[14]

In the above examples, what is discussed are illnesses and how male and female bodies can respond to them differently. With a gendering of the bodily fluids, men lose their *jing*, women lose their blood. For men *jing* is the energetic base that needs to be safeguarded, and in women blood is the energetic base that needs to be safeguarded. The solution, for both men and women, is maintaining purity and calm, which will replenish the male *jing* and the female blood.

The *Taixuan baodian* 太玄寶典, dated to the Song, again highlights separate but correlated practices:

> Men are endowed with the Dao from Heaven, receive the *yang qi,* which gives birth to the kidneys (where the semen is produced). Women are endowed with the Dao from Earth, receive the *yin qi* which gives birth to blood and to the heart. For this reason, men refine the *qi* to become 'perfected', and protect their *jing*. Women refine the blood to become 'perfected', and protect their *shen*. The transformations of *yin* and *yang* have their differences.[15]

While the previous examples connected the preservation of *jing* and blood in men and women to avoiding illnesses and death, this passage clearly pushes the goal of self-cultivation further to transformation into a Perfected. Here we see a more comprehensive understanding of the male and female 'systems': the cosmological connection between men, Heaven and *yang* is also represented physiologically by men's production of sperm (*jing*). Women, cosmologically connected to Earth and to *yin*, are pervaded by blood. Both men and women attempt, through different self-cultivations that involve physiology and cosmology in parallel, to become Perfected.

The attention to the breasts noted above, and the differentiation of the elements to be refined in men and women are important. Whereas women need to practice to refine their blood and refine their bodies, men will have to work on their *qi*, a more ethereal entity.

Ming dynasty – the self-cultivation milieu

As we move towards the late imperial period, the descriptions in Daoist sources become more and more detailed and complex. Inner alchemy texts become more specific about the physiological effects of the practice. As explained by Chen Hsiu-fen (2009), there is a growing interest in health regimens for late Ming literati, who incorporated self-cultivation into their daily activities. Her discussion of the popularity of *yangsheng* treatises, their simple language and useful illustrations, may help us situate the literature discussed in this section. *Yangsheng* manuals were extremely popular and wide-spread in the late Ming, their audience was, however, in fact intended to be male, as the pictures depict male practitioners and the practice generally does not have any specific instructions for female physiology. As mentioned above, *yangsheng* ideas had been part and parcel of *neidan*, bringing attention to physical processes of healing and wellbeing.

From the Ming onwards, the female body emerges very strongly from the pages of female alchemy texts, in many different ways, and in ways not seen in standard non-gendered alchemy:

1. clear description of external bodily parts and attention to the menstrual cycle, its cyclicity, its pains and aches;
2. specific practices (self-manipulation of breasts and abdomen, inner visualisations);
3. body changes related to that practice (menses changing colour, breasts shrinking);
4. emotions related to that practice (sexual arousal, confusion, dizziness);
5. practical ways to check the progress of the practice (inserting silk into the vagina).

All of this indicates that the body is central; it is a certain kind of body, the *xing* 形, the form, the body of materiality, the body symbolised by the menstrual blood; it is from this 'external' body that the practices start. Once its grosser elements, which are also what might cause illnesses, are transformed, the rest of the practice is similar to the male practice.

Here, I want to discuss the work of two late Ming doctors and alchemists, Fu Shan 傅山 (1606–1684) and Cao Heng 曹珩 (ca. 1632), who combined interest in healing and meditation and straddled the semantic fields of medicine and alchemy. Unlike the majority of authors at this time, they discuss self-cultivation specifically for women, and meditation techniques to cure gynaecological illnesses. In these texts, there is an interesting admixture of medical concerns and practices with religious practices and goals; the authors, medical doctors, do not distinguish the two realms.

The first text is the *Duan Honglong* 斷紅龍 (Cutting the Red Dragon) by Fu Shan, who was a successful doctor and author of several medical books, including one on male medicine, *Fu Qingzhu nanke* 傅青主男科, one on gynaecology *Fu Qingzhu nüke* 傅青主女科, and one on children's ailments *Fu Qingzhu youke* 傅青主幼科. At the same time, he was also a Daoist adept, possibly a Quanzhen convert, and follower of hermit Lü Danting 盧丹亭, or Danting zhenren

丹亭真人, from whom he received several instructions on inner alchemy and on healing different illnesses through meditation practices (Xiao 1956–1983). One of these texts includes the *Duan Honglong*, a health practice for women which involves the gradual transformation of the menses. In this text, the focus is on the blood, the breasts and the womb. The explicit aim is to refine the menses into a less polluting and offending substance, and thus to improve the health of the female practitioner. There are very specific instructions, from the meditating position, to the movements to implement, to the rhythm and timing of the practice; the specificity is very physical, as is the way the results of the practice are confirmed, by inserting silk into the vagina, checking for the volume and colour of the menses. All of this allows us to perceive the embodied experience of the female practitioner. Interestingly, the practice is offered as a healing method, and not as a way to immortality.

A similar, and even more specific guide to healing female illnesses through meditation is the *Nügong quebing* 女功卻病 (Women's Practices for Repelling Illnesses), written by Cao Heng in 1632.[16] The *Nügong quebing* is a section in the work *Baosheng miyao* 保生祕要 (Essential Secrets for Conserving Life), collected in the second section of the *Daoyuan yiqi* 道元一氣 (Unitary *Qi* of the Origin of the Dao), a work at the intersection between medicine and inner alchemy. The *Baosheng miyao* is not gender specific, and it describes various kinds of meditations, applying them as cures to common ailments. In the same way, but specifically targeting female illnesses, the *Nügong quebing* offers different kinds of meditation practices in order to cure problems like blood congestion, pre- and post-natal problems, menstrual irregularity, etc. The female body, its loci, processes and fluids, and its transformations are all described in great detail.

These are the earliest full-fledged texts of female alchemy, which present the beginning of a coherent formulation of the *nüdan* process. They appear to be the first clearly composed solely for the benefit of women; they exhibit the technical language and the contents of *nüdan*, and were published by physicians, as part of medical collections. They state in clear terms the existence of a way to self-refinement for women, and are the beginning of an expanding field of interest in female meditation techniques. One example is from the *Nügong quebing*, a guide to healing female illnesses through meditation. The first of these meditation techniques focuses on the breasts and on Slaying of the Red Dragon (cutting the menses):

> As for women's true refinement, it is always necessary to gather the *qi* within the breasts; as for the circulation (of the *qi*), it is also necessary to concentrate the strength there; (in this way) it will be possible to slay the Red Dragon. [...] If you refine the *qi* and calm the heart, and focus your attention on the sea of *qi* slowly it ascends in a revolving motion; first move it to the right breast in the chest and revolve it ten times; return and apply to the *qihai*, from the beginning until it starts the revolution (*zhou*); up and down between the chest and belly (*Nügong quebing*, 1a).

Then the text moves on to meditation practices intended to cure specific female illnesses. The categorisation is very reminiscent of Song dynasty doctor Chen Ziming's *Good Prescriptions* (*Furen daquan liangfang* 婦人大全良方). However, as in Fu Shan's case, the healing is not done through herbal prescriptions but through a repertoire of practices coming directly from inner alchemy. The titles indicate the medical concerns:

'Pacifying the fetus' (*An tai* 安胎); 'Successful Birth' (*shun chang* 順產); 'Difficult birth' (*nanchang* 難產); 'Oedema during pregnancy' (*yunnü xuezhong* 孕女血腫); 'The many illnesses of pregnant women' (*yunfu duobing* 孕婦多病); 'Ghost fetus and ectopic pregnancy' (*guitai xueqiu* 鬼胎血毬); 'Accumulation of blood clots' (*ji xuekuai* 積血塊); 'Fright caused by wind after the birth' (*chanhou jinfeng* 產後驚風); 'Post-partum frightened chills' (*chanhou weihan* 產後畏寒); 'Endomethriorrhagia' (*xuebeng* 血崩); 'Leucorrhea' (*baidai* 白帶); 'Reverted the menses' (*nijing* 逆經); 'Irregular menses' (*jing budiao* 經不調) and 'Regulating the menses' (*diaojing* 調經). The section closes in this way: 'For all other illnesses, the healing methods are the same as for men. But you need to work hard on the breasts'.

The practice involves concentration on the umbilicus as well as on the breasts, visualisation of the energies circulating through the body, the use of internal and external observation. The text itself says that all other illnesses, not related to menstrual irregularity, are to be healed in the same way as for men, but with particular attention to the breasts. However, it is not surprising to see that, for the female body, illnesses related to pregnancy, postpartum, blood deficiency and obstruction are so central. The female body is still defined by its specific fluids and loci. Cao Heng and Fu Shan gender diseases related to blood, and their discourse is clearly reflected in female alchemy texts, where the discourse of female depletion due to blood ailments is obvious.

Qing compendia

As argued by Yi-li Wu (2016: 43–5), the late imperial period saw an epistemological shift in the understanding of women's bodies in medical sources. While in earlier periods women were seen as categorically different from men in their physiologies, and they had illnesses specific to their female bodies, in the late imperial period this description started to change, moving away from a narrative of difference towards a narrative of sameness, except for gestational illnesses. This interpretation gave more importance to social and not physiological factors, in the explanation of disease in women. This shift is not perceptible in the female alchemy texts that start emerging at this time. In fact, for female alchemy, it seems to be the opposite, and the understanding of the female body and its processes exemplified in these Qing manuals is an expansion and a systematisation of the previous references discussed above. By the Qing, there seems to be a hardening of the belief in the clear-cut and embedded distinction between male and female physiology, in the connection between it and deficiency and illness, in the reality that illnesses are due to the overwhelming presence and influence of blood, and in the need to resolve illnesses connected to female physiology before starting the practice. The cosmological foundation of this physiological reality lends further authority to the claim. This is clearest in the preface to the *Nüdan hebian* 女丹合編 (Collection of Female Alchemy) edited by He Longxiang 賀龍驤, which offers a detailed comparison between male and female self-cultivation in terms of Innate Nature (*bingxing* 秉性), Form and the Structure (*xingti* 形體) and Methods of the Practice (*gongfa* 功法). Here is the first section only:

> The man is *yang*, and *yang* is pure (*qing*); the woman is *yin*, and *yin* is impure (*zhuo*). Male Nature is unyielding, female Nature is flexible. A man's feelings are excitable, a woman's feelings are tranquil. Male thoughts are confused (*za*), female thoughts are clear (*chun*). The man is fundamentally in movement, and movement facilitates the

> loss of *qi*; the woman is fundamentally quiet, and quietness facilitates the accumulation of *qi*. The man is associated with the trigram *li* and, like the Sun, he can complete a whole rotation in one year; the woman is associated with the trigram *kan* and, like the Moon, she can complete a whole rotation in one month. For a man, *qi* is difficult to submit (*fu*); for a woman, *qi* is easy to submit.
>
> These are the differences concerning Innate Nature.[17]

This collection, published in Sichuan, in 1906, is the culmination of the discourse on female alchemy that had developed during the previous two centuries.[18]

In terms of female physiology, then, Qing female alchemy texts often provide specific descriptions of personal bodily perceptions of the menses. The *Nüjindan* (Female Golden Elixir) says:

> Knowing the time (*Zhishi* 知時).
>
> You need to start practising just before the 'message' has arrived. The *Sanming pian* says: the message of the menses, it is not the monthly message of when the menses actually arrive. The word 'message' is like when a person is outside and has not arrived home yet, but a message (announcing his arrival) arrives first. The day when the message arrives, you know it by yourself: the hips and legs hurt, the head and the eyes are restless, you do not feel like eating or drinking; this is the message arriving, and then it will transform into blood.[19]

It is this embodied knowledge that allows the practice, and the recovering of *yang*, to take place at the right time.

Throughout the female alchemy corpus, we find many similar references to the connected levels of cosmology and physiology: *yin*, *Kun*, blood. Further, as hinted above, both at the cosmological and at the physiological level, femaleness is polluting, dangerous, challenging, close to illness and death. This is confirmed, for example, in the following excerpt from the *Niwan Li zushi nüzong shuangxiu baofa* 泥丸李祖師女宗雙修寶筏 (Precious Raft on Paired Cultivation of Women by Master Li Niwan):

> It is said that blood is the energetic basis of the woman. Her nature is inclined toward the yin, and the nature of *yin* is to enjoy cold (*xiliang*). If a woman does not avail herself of massage, helping through it the *qi* mechanism (*qiji*) to circulate subtly, she will easily

> sink into Pure *yin*. *Yin* is cold, cold is ice-like. If you do not activate it through the revolving motion, this may result in illnesses such as congestion and blood obstruction, and the practice would be difficult to implement.[20]

This correlation is made even more explicit in this excerpt from the *Jinhua zhizhi,* a rare text that provides female and male alchemy side by side. This particular chapter is called 治病 *Zhi bing* (Cure illnesses):

> As for those women who have an honest heart and seek the Dao, there is no doubt that their monthly water is the cause of their illnesses and makes it difficult for them to practice; [...]. First you need to eliminate the illness's symptoms, and only then can you implement the refinement. As for female's illnesses, in some of them the blockage of the menses results in illness, in others it is childbirth which causes disasters, in others again the collapsing of the uterus and leuchorrhea cause the illness. There are many different kinds [of illnesses], and I have three main methods to cure them: the first method cures the illnesses that develop before the child is born or after childbirth; [...]. Another (method) treats those illnesses begotten as a result of blood loss from the vagina not connected to the period. [...] Another (method) cures the blockage of menses followed by the release of blood and sedimentous bloody clots.[21]

Comparing the male and female sections of this text, several elements appear: first, there is no corresponding section on curing illnesses in the male section, even though it has a larger number of chapters. There is also not the same amount of reference to body parts, to massaging or touching those body parts, or to fluid transformation. The clear implication is that the female body has a congenital deficiency, is prone to illness, is in need of healing, and that the healing involves concentrating and exerting pressure on physical body parts and transforming fluids. The embodied experience of these illnesses is manifested in the specificity of the description. Finally, the three categories of illnesses identified (a) Pre- and post-partum (b) Blood loss (c) Blood clots and stagnation, are not only the same categories that we see in medical treatises from Sun Simiao to Chen Ziming, but also resemble closely the kinds of illnesses targeted by Cao Heng in the healing meditation above.

Republican period – modernisation and scientisation

In the Republican period, Western scientific ideas influenced not only medicine but also inner alchemy. A good example is Chen Yingning 陳櫻寧 (1880–1969), a Daoist intellectual who re-interpreted the classical alchemical canon through the lens of Western science and medicine.[22] He published the 1936 collection *Nüzi daoxue xiao congshu wuzhong* 女子道學小叢書五種 (Small Encyclopedia in Five Books on the Female Learning of the Dao). Promoting a scientific, rational, approach to the investigation of alchemy was central to Chen's writings, by providing a spiritual practice devoid of overtly religious elements. Chen reinterpreted and annotated the pre-existing *nüdan* canon according to his own ideas about Daoism and *xianxue* 仙學 (the study of immortality), as well as contemporary notions of modernisation, scientific experimentation, and gender equality. He criticised, ridiculed and even deleted references to the divine nature of the scriptures, asserting their human origins. He added detailed notes about the physiological processes involved in, and the bodily changes that would result from, the practice of female alchemy, explaining the process from a Western scientific, medical point of view. Moreover, he criticised previous authors for their negative portrayal of women' physiology as burdensome, and affirmed the equality between male and female access to immortality, introducing a gender equality perspective. Chen's 'rediscovery', reformulation and wide dissemination of Daoist practices for women was thus influenced by contemporary perceptions of gender relations, the anti-superstition campaign, and, importantly, he used modern Western medical concepts to explain the transformation inside the female body. In the preface to his collection of female alchemy texts, Chen feels the need to explain, to the female practitioners he was writing for, some 'basic understanding of medicine', lest they encounter problems. These basic understandings, and the trouble that might ensue if women do not follow them, all relate to gynaecological disorders:

> If women want to enter the Dao, it is necessary to first clarify some basic understandings of medicine, and only then is it possible to practice... . If your own body does not have the capability of producing a common embryo, it also does not have the hope of creating an immortal embryo. The principles of creating a person and

> of becoming immortal are not separate. They only separate in terms of 'going along' (*shun* 順) or 'reverting the course' (*ni* 逆)… . As for 'beheading the Red Dragon', it is created by reverting the course. But if your own body does not have the capability to create, and you mistakenly take the fact that you do not have the menses as a proof that you can become immortal, then in the case of women who are over 50 and their menses are stopping naturally, can they really all have the qualifications to become immortals?… Similarly, contemporary young women who ask doctors for an operation to remove the uterus and the ovaries, their menses also naturally stop, but how can we call that 'beheading the Red Dragon?[23]

Chen transforms the tradition, eliminating most of the religious elements and exchanging them for Western medical interpretations, he translates in medical language the religious process of self-cultivation. At the basis of this transformation, however, is the necessity for female health, and health for women is still directly related to the absence of illnesses pertaining to their gestational body, and this is clear in Chen's mention of embryo creation, menstruation and menopause, and illnesses requiring the removal of the ovaries and uterus. No other processes or illnesses are ever mentioned in these texts. Therefore, even in the Republican period, with a definite stronger attention to gender equality, the female body is still reduced to a gestational body, and health in women still means menstrual regularity, absence of blood stagnation and the ability to conceive.

In more modern times, female alchemy has been subsumed under the *qigong* category, stripped of all religious and spiritual characteristics and presented as a health practice for women.

Analysis

This chapter is particularly concerned with the physicality of the female body, its fluids, its loci, its health and illness, and how this physicality relates, expresses itself, and corresponds to cosmological processes, to self-cultivation and to transcendence. Thus this study does not only concern itself with a discursive arena, but an arena of actual practices which women use to modify their physical and cosmological bodies.

My questions: how is the female body represented in these texts? What of the contemporary medical understanding and treatment of the female body is represented in them? How important are physical and psychological health in the religious belief and practice towards immortality? And how does gender play in this interaction? In order to answer these questions, in combination with critical works on Daoism, *neidan* and Chinese gynaecology then, comparisons with works on gender, medicine, religion and the body in the West have proved very fruitful.

Embryology and cosmology

Selby (2009), in her analysis of gestation metaphors in Ayurveda, discusses the intersection between religion and medicine, and how the cosmic language of conception and that of clinical observation go hand in hand in the texts she covers. Cosmogonic ideas make sense of what happens in the moment of conception. In female alchemy texts, cosmology and physiology are parallel, intertwined and they co-explicate the processes of transformation and birth. Whereas in earlier Daoist sources embryogenesis was described as a meditative process creating an immortal embryo, the way in which embryology is represented in female alchemy sources is very close to that of medical sources, where the blood of the mother surrounds the sperm of the father and forms a female embryo, *yin* on the outside and *yang* on the inside. Selby's (2009: 44) observation that 'the cosmic language of conception and that of clinical observation are augmented by a third category of information composed of descriptions of what is happening on the outer bodily surface of the woman herself' evokes the interpenetration of cosmology, internal fluid transformation and the recognition of external changes, expressed in the description of changes in the size of the breasts or in the colour of the menstrual fluid.

The female body

Focusing on the corporeality of the female alchemy process, it may be possible to get to what Duden (1991: 6) indicates as the 'life inside the body', the 'hidden sphere beneath the skin' of women practitioners. Walker Bynum (1987), in her study of medieval female religious practices, points out the emergence of numerous ways of manipulating one's body in order to be nearer to God, such as flagellation and all kinds of self-inflicted sufferings; amongst these, cases of psychosomatic manipulation are almost exclusively female. Phenomena sometimes called paramystical or hysterical, such as trances, levitations and catatonic seizures, are confined to women. The phenomenon of holy anorexia – the inability to eat anything apart from the eucharistic host – is a peculiar trait of female believers as well. This form of anorexia led, in the accounts, to other miraculous bodily closures as the blockage of menstruation and of excretion. Miraculous lactation and mystical pregnancy were other manifestations of an extreme physiological way to approach holiness and sanctity. Incorruptibility of the cadaver (parts of it or the whole) was a necessary requirement for female sanctity up to the modern period (especially virginity). Another kind of bodily experience, illness and recurrent pain, was given religious significance in women's lives more than in men's (Bynum 1987: 166). While suffering was not central to the female alchemy practice in China, it sees the same kind of attention to the female body, to bodily secretions such as lactation and menstruation, to illness, and to eventual bodily transformation.

Cadden (1993) discusses sex differences in the Middle Ages, and how medical and scientific notions related to societal and cultural changes. Her study points to some fundamental questions that also emerge, if in different ways, in works of female alchemy, and are discussed in contemporary Chinese medical texts on women. These are, for example, the contribution of a woman to conception and to the sex of the child, the basic coldness and dampness of the female constitution, as opposed to the male's activity and warmth, the relationship between pleasure and reproduction (a topic much discussed by Chinese physicians, but not mentioned in *nüdan* texts), the insistence on the negative influence and polluting nature of menstrual blood.

Female alchemy texts also remind us of what Duden (1991) has highlighted about Western concepts of the female body emerging in the nineteenth century: 'the naturalistic reality of the body was created as the object of investigation and treatment' (Duden 1991: 22). The advent of female alchemy, and the emergence of the female body as categorically different from the male body, allows for a more specific investigation of its workings, of its health and illnesses, of its transformations and of the correct way to cultivate it. The self-cultivation, the understanding, the challenges and the different way to enlightenment, however, all seem to be determined by the writers of the texts, intellectual men. My investigation is, therefore, also inspired by what Duden has described as the birth of gynaecology, an 'enforcement of male power over the female body', while at the same time creating a 'new kind of corporeality', 'isolating the female organs from the traditional undefined body' (Duden 1991: 17–18). In this way, not only female but male bodies were re-defined. Laqueur (1986) and Martin (1987) have, in different ways, reinforced this concept by asserting that, by the eighteenth century, men's and women's bodies were seen as fundamentally different, based on their distinct physiologies. Medical knowledge of the gendered body was essentialised in a biology of two incommensurable sexes. Laqueur's focus on the genital organs has been questioned in favour of a wider perspective on sexual differences, one that includes not only the genitals, but also 'every part of the flesh' (King 2013: 48); this indeed is true for female alchemy, for which it is not the genital area that defines gender difference, but the whole body, its physiology and its cosmology. For Martin (1987), gender difference is culturally and intimately tied to menstruation, and female health and illness to menstrual regularity.[24] Further, she says, men are associated with activity, energy, passion, and women with passivity, stability, sluggishness and coldness (Martin 1987: 33). In the same way, female alchemy texts present men and women as fundamentally different from a physiological and emotional perspective; men are active, strong and in movement, women are passive, weak and quiet, and this determines their health, the way they practice, their access to immortality. Insistent presence of the female body and its metaphors of deficiency, coldness, insufficiency, and the need to re-build a *yang*, pure, strong and invincible body, is reminiscent not only of work on pre-modern Western societies, but also of contemporary understanding of embryogenesis. Discussing modern scientific descriptions of sperm and egg, their structures and behaviours, Martin retraces how the stereotypes of 'heroic males and passive females... are now being written at the level of the cell' (Martin 1991: 500). While these works help us to contextualise the definition of the body as female, the medicalisation and subjugation of the female body, with all that this definition entails, what *nüdan* contributes is the idea that the female body can and does transcend this world and gender differences through a physical, but at the same time also spiritual, practice. This particular religious practice, strongly anchored in the female body, in its peculiar processes and in its perceived deficiencies, invites us to rethink both the process of salvation and the process of bodily transformation in a gendered way.

Conclusion

In the above examples, the 'difference' of the female is highlighted in different ways: cosmological, physiological, structural.

This is necessary because the texts themselves speak of a body saddled with illnesses that are difficult to treat, and almost always relate the process of transcendence to women's gestational bodies. In discussing these female bodies in transformation, I draw comparisons with the contemporary discourses on the female body in the Chinese medical tradition, and show how Daoist and medical traditions represent the female body in very similar ways, and how they interact and borrow from each other. In fact, in some cases, it is hard to define our sources as either medical or religious, and therefore even the concept of interpenetration of these two fields loses its power. The more relevant question here is how both medical and religious texts contribute to the creation of a gendered body, which is transformed through both medical and soteriological practices to reach immortality. While immortality is definitely a religious goal, it is made very explicit that, without the medical understanding of the female body and the medical interventions on the female body, that goal would be impossible to attain. Medical understanding and intervention on the female body are, therefore, necessary to the religious goals.

Finally, as all of these texts are composed by men, the insistence on the categorical differences, cosmological and physiological, the fact that these differences mostly manifest through challenging gynaecological disorders, the need to practise being aware of those differences, implies an univocal understanding of women, and portrays a confidence in the ownership of knowledge about female bodies, treatment of their illnesses, and ways to their transcendence.

Notes

1 On different ideas of immortality in Daoism, see Pregadio (2018).
2 For an exhaustive introduction to early *neidan* sources and the earliest emergence of the term *neidan*, see Baldrian-Hussein (1989–1990: 163–90, 2008: 762–6). A good introduction to the subject is Pregadio (2014).
3 Li Daochun 李道純 (late thirteenth century), translated in Pregadio (2019: 169).
4 The *weilu, jiaji* and *yuzhen* passes are *loci* on the spinal column (respectively at the coccyx, in the middle of the spine, and at the base of the neck) through which the energy passes on the way to the *niwan*, a point on the crown of the head. From there, the energy descends through the front of the body, and continues to cycle.
5 *Nüdan hebian* 女丹合編 1b, introduction to collection by He Longxiang 賀龍驤 (1906).
6 For an anthology of translations of important *neidan* works, see Pregadio (2019).
7 Interest in sexual practices has a long history in both academic and practitioners' circles. One of the earliest works in the West on sexual practices in China is van Gulik (1966, reprinted 2003). Harper (1987) has investigated early sexual practices. Often in these descriptions, as well as in later novels, women are accessories to men's pleasure and refinement. Late Imperial medical manuals are also replete with references to sexual hygiene (Furth 1988).
8 On early Daoist sexual practices, see Raz (2008). For later Daoist sexual manuals, see Wile (1992). For contemporary practitioners, Mantak Chia ((2005 [1986]) has brought together several earlier traditions and added his own teachings in China. For a review of contemporary publications on female self-cultivation techniques in the US, see Valussi (2010).
9 *Bencao gangmu*, 52.2950.
10 Translated in Furth (1999: 73).
11 Translated in Wilms (2005: 202).
12 *Daozang* 1156 (fasc. 796). For an introduction to this text, see '*Chongyang zhenren jinguan yusuojue*', in Schipper and Verellen (2004: 1185).
13 *Chongyang zhenren jinguan yusuojue* 10a–b.
14 *Chongyang zhenren jinguan yusuojue* 3a.
15 *Taixuan baodian*, *juan shang* 2a-b. This section of the text is called *Yinyang zaohua* 陰陽造化 (*Yin* and *yang* cyclical transformations). This text is discussed in Schipper and Verellen (2004: 785).

16 The first edition of this work is dated 1636. For more on Cao Heng's life, see Liu, unpublished manuscript.
17 A full translation of this important passage is given in Valussi (2008b: 259–61).
18 Earlier texts were published by Daoist patriarchs Min Yide 閔一得 (1758–1836), and Liu Yiming 劉一明 (1734–1821), and by Daoist practitioner Fu Jinquan 傅金銓 (fl. 1820), who also compiled the first full-fledged female alchemy compilation, the *Nüjindan fayao* 女金丹法要 (Essential Methods for the Female Golden Elixir) in 1813, as part of his larger alchemy collection *Jiyizi zhengdao mishu shiqizhong* 濟一子道書十七種 (Seventeen Daoist Books by Jiyizi), in *Zangwai daoshu* 藏外道書 11: 1–720. On these different collections, see Valussi (2008).
19 *Nüjindan* 女金丹, by Yongzhong Zhenyizi 用中貞一子, preface dated 1892, in *Nüdan hebian* 21b–22b.
20 *Niwan Li Zushi nüzong shuangxiu baofa*, in *Zangwai daoshu* 10.540–6, 540.
21 *Jinhua zhizhi* 24a–24b.
22 For a masterful introduction to Chen Yingning, see Liu (2009).
23 *Nüzi daoxue xiao congshu wu zhong* 女子道學小叢書五種 (Small Encyclopedia in Five Books on the Female Learning of the Dao) 4a–4b.
24 A discussion of the relationship between menstrual regularity, fertility and ideal womanhood in China is found in Bray (1997: 317–34).

Bibliography

Ahern, E. (1975) 'The Power and Pollution of Chinese women', in M. Wolf and R. Witke (eds) *Women in Chinese Society*. Stanford: Stanford University Press, pp. 193–214.

Baldrian-Hussein, F. (2008) 'Neidan', in Pregadio, F. (ed.) *Encyclopedia of Taoism*, vol. 2. London: Routledge, pp. 762–6.

Andreeva A. and Steavu, D. (eds) (2016) *Transforming the Void: Embryological Discourse and Reproductive Imagery in East Asian Religions*. Leiden: Brill.

Baldrian-Hussein, F. (1989–1990) 'Inner Alchemy: Notes on the Use of the Term Neidan', *Cahiers D'extreme Asie*, 5: 163–90.

Bencao gangmu 本草綱目 (Systematic *Materia Medica*) (1596), Li Shizhen 李時珍 (1518–93) (1975). Beijing: Beijing renmin weisheng chubanshe.

Bray, F. (1997) *Technology and Gender: Fabrics of Power in Late Imperial China*. Berkeley, CA: University of California Press.

Cadden, J. (1993) *Meanings of Sex Difference in the Middle Ages: Medicine, Science and Culture*. Cambridge: Cambridge University Press.

Chen Hsiu-fen 陳秀芬 (2009) *Yangsheng Yu Xiushen: Wan Ming de Yangsheng Wenhua Yu Wenren Shenghuo* 養生與修身: 晚明的養生文化與文人生活 (Nourishing Life and Cultivating the Body: Writing the Literati's Body and Techniques for Preserving Health in the Late Ming). Taipei: Dawshiang.

Chia, M. (2005 [1986]) *Healing Love through the Dao: Cultivating Female Sexual Energy*. Rochester, VT: Destiny Books.

Chongyang zhenren jinguan yusuojue 重陽真人金關玉鎖訣 (Instructions on the Golden Chain and the Jade Lock), *Daozang* 1156 (fasc. 796).

Clart, P. and Goossaert, V. (forthcoming) 'Spirit-Writing', in S. Kory (ed.) *Handbook on Chinese Divination Techniques*. Leiden: Brill.

Despeux, C. (2016) 'Symbolic Pregnancy and the Sexual Identity of Taoist Adepts', in A. Andreeva and D. Steavu (eds) *Transforming the Void: Embryological Discourse and Reproductive Imagery in East Asian Religions*. Leiden: Brill, pp. 147–85.

Despeux, C. (2008) 'Yangsheng', in F. Pregadio (ed.) *Encyclopedia of Taoism*, vol. 2. London: Routledge, pp. 1148–50.

Despeux, C. and Kohn, L. (2003) *Women in Daoism*. Magdalena, NM: Three Pines Press.

Despeux, C. (1990) *Immortelles de la Chine ancienne. Taoïsme et alchimie féminine*. Puiseaux: Pardès.

Duden, B. (1991) *The Woman Beneath the Skin, a Doctor's Patients in Eighteenth Century Germany*. Boston: Harvard University Press.

Furen da quan liang fang 婦人大全良方 (All-inclusive Good Prescriptions for Women) 1227, Chen Ziming 陳自明 (1190–1270), revised in 1284, Yu Yingao 余瀛鳌 (ed.) (1985). Beijing, Renming weisheng chubanshe.

Furth, C. (1986) 'Blood Body and Gender: Medical Images of the Female Condition in China', *Chinese Science*, 7: 43–66.

Furth, C. (1988) 'Androgynous Males and Deficient Females: Biology and Gender Boundaries in Sixteenth- and Seventeenth-Century China', *Late Imperial China*, 9.2: 1–31.

Furth, C. and Ch'en Shu-yueh (1992) 'Chinese Medicine and the Anthropology of Menstruation in Contemporary Taiwan', *Medical Anthropology Quarterly*, 6.1: 27–48.

Furth, C. (1999) *A Flourishing Yin, Gender in China's Medical History: 960–1665*. Berkeley, CA: University of California Press.

Goossaert, V. (2022) *Making the Gods Speak: The Ritual Production of Revelation in Chinese Religious History*. Harvard: Harvard University Press.

Harper, D. (1987) 'The Sexual Arts of Ancient China as Described in a Manuscript of the Second Century B.C.', *Harvard Journal of Asiatic Studies*, 47.2: 539–593.

Hu Daojing 胡道靜, Chen Yaoting 陳燿庭, Duan Wengui 段文桂, Ling Wanqing 林萬清 *et al.* (eds) (1992–1994) *Zangwai daoshu* 藏外道書. Chengdu: Bashu shushe.

Jinhua Zhizhi 金華直指 (Direct Instructions on the Golden Essence) (1804). Unpublished manuscript in the author's collection.

Jiyizi zhengdao mishu shiqizhong 濟一子道書十七种 (Seventeen Daoist books by Jiyizi), in Fu Jinquan 傅金銓 (fl. 1820) (ed.) (1994) *Zangwai daoshu* 藏外道書 (Daoist Texts Outside the Canon). Sichuan: Bashu shushe, vol. 11, pp. 1–720

King, H. (2013) *The One-Sex Body on Trial, The Classical and Early Modern Evidence*. Farnham; Burlington VT: Ashgate Publishing.

Kory, S. (ed.) (forthcoming) *Handbook on Chinese Divination Techniques*. Leiden: Brill.

Laqueur, T. W. (1986) 'Orgasm, Generation and the Politics of Reproductive Biology', *Representations*, 14: 1–41.

Lee, J.D. (2008) *Xingbie shenti yu yiliao shi* 性別, 身體與醫療史 (Gender, Body, and Medicine). Taipei: Lianjing chubanshe.

Liu, X. (n.d.) *Late Ming Women's Practices for Repelling Illnesses*, unpublished manuscript.

Liu, X. (2009) *Daoist Modern; Innovation, Lay Practice and the Community of Inner Alchemy in Republican Shanghai*. Cambridge, MA: Harvard University Asia Center.

Martin, E. (1987) *The Woman in the Body: A Cultural analysis of Reproduction*. Boston: Beacon Press.

Martin, E. (1991) 'The Egg and the Sperm: How Science has Constructed a Romance Based on Stereotypical Male-Female Roles', *Signs*, 16.3: 485–501.

Niwan Li Zushi nüzong shuangxiu baofa 泥丸李祖師女宗雙修寶筏 (Precious Raft on Paired Cultivation of Women by Master Li Niwan), in Min Yide 閔一得 (1758–1836) (ed.) *Zangwai daoshu* 藏外道書 (Daoist Texts Outside the Canon). Sichuan: Bashu shushe, vol. 10, pp. 540–6.

Nüdan hebian 女丹合編 (Combined Collection of Female Alchemy), He Longxiang 賀龍驤 (ed.) (1906). Chengdu: Er xian'an.

Nügong quebing 女功卻病 (Women's Practices for Repelling Illnesses), Cao Heng 曹珩 (or Cao Shiheng 曹士珩), 1632, in *Baosheng miyao* 保生祕要 (Essential Secrets for Conserving Life), collected in the second section of the *Daoyuan yiqi* 道元一氣 (Unitary *Qi* of the Origin of the Dao) 1634; in Tao Bingfu 陶秉福 (ed.) (1990) *Dao yuan yi qi*. Beijing: Beijing shifan daxue chubanshe, pp. 371–520.

Nüjindan 女金丹 (Female Golden Elixir) 1892, Yongzhong Zhenyizi 用中貞一子, in He Longxiang 賀龍驤 (ed.) (1906) *Nüdan hebian*, Chengdu: Er xian'an, pp. 21b–22b. Reprinted in Tao Bingfu 陶秉福 (ed.) (1989) *Nüdan jicui* 女丹集萃 (A Treasury of Female Alchemy). Beijing: Beijing Shifan daxue chubanshe, pp. 53–122.

Nüjindan fayao 女金丹法要 (Essential Methods for the Female Golden Elixir) 1813, Fu Jinquan 傅金銓 (ed.) (1971). Taipei: Ziyou chubanshe.

Nüzi daoxue xiao congshu wu zhong 女子道學小叢書五種 (Small Encyclopedia in Five Books on the Female Learning of the Dao), vol. 2, Chen Yingning 陳攖寧 (ed.) (1936). Shanghai: Yihuatang.

Penny, B. (ed.) (2006) *Daoism in History, Essays in Honor of Liu Ts'un-Yan*. London: Routledge.

Pregadio, F. (2006) 'Early Daoist Meditation and the Origins of Inner Alchemy', in B. Penny (ed.) *Daoism in History, Essays in Honor of Liu Ts'un-Yan*. London: Routledge, pp. 121–58,149.
Pregadio, F. (2008) 'Waidan', in F. Pregadio (ed.) *Encyclopedia of Taoism*, vol. 2. London: Routledge, pp. 1002–4.
Pregadio, F. (ed.) (2008) *Encyclopedia of Taoism*. London: Routledge.
Pregadio, F. (2014) *The Way of the Golden Elixir: An Introduction to Taoist Alchemy*. Mountainview, CA: Golden Elixir Press.
Pregadio, F. (2018) 'Which is the Daoist Immortal Body?', *Micrologus*, XXVI: 385–407.
Pregadio, F. (2019) *Taoist Internal Alchemy: An Anthology of Neidan Texts*. Mountainview, CA: Golden Elixir Press.
Raz, G. (2008) 'The Way of the Yellow and the Red: Re-examining the Sexual Initiation Rite of Celestial Masters Daoism', *Nannü*, 10: 86–120.
Robinet, I. (2008) 'Yijing', in Pregadio, F. (ed.) *Encyclopedia of Taoism*, vol. 2. London: Routledge, pp. 1161–4.
Schipper, K. and Verellen, F. (eds) (2004) *The Taoist Canon: A Historical Companion to the Daozang*. Chicago: University of Chicago Press.
Schumann M. and Valussi, E. (forthcoming) *Communicating with the Gods: Spirit-Writing in Chinese History*. Leiden: Brill.
Seaman, G. (1981) 'The Sexual Politics of Karmic Retribution', in Ahern, E. and Gates H. (eds) *The Anthropology of Taiwanese Society*. Stanford: Stanford University Press, pp. 381–96.
Selby, M.A. (2009) 'Between Medicine and Religion: Discursive Shifts in Early Ayurvedic Narratives of Conception and Gestation', in *Divins remèdes: Médecine et Religion en Asie du Sud*. Paris: Éditions de l'École des Hautes Études en Sciences Sociales, pp. 41–63.
Steavu, D. (2016) 'Cosmos, Body and Gestation in Taoist Meditation', in A. Andreeva and D. Steavu (eds) *Transforming the Void, Embryological Discourse and Reproductive Imagery in East Asian Religions*, Leiden: Brill, pp. 111–146.
Taixuan baodian 太玄寶典 (Precious Canon of the Greatest Mystery), *Daozang* 1034 (fasc. 703).
Valussi, E. (2008a) 'Female Alchemy and Para-text: How to Read *Nüdan* in a Historical Context', in *Asia Major*, 21.2: 153–93.
Valussi, E. (2008b) 'Men and women in He Longxiang's *Nüdan hebian* (Collection of Female Alchemy)', *Nannü*, 10.2: 242–78.
Valussi, E. (2009) 'Blood, Tigers, Dragons: The Physiology of Transcendence for Women', *Asian Medicine*, 4: 46–85
Valussi, E. (2010) 'Women's Qigong in America: Tradition, Adaptation and New Trends', *Journal of Daoist Studies*, 3: 187–201.
van Gulik, R.H. (1966, reprinted 2003) *Sexual Life in Ancient China: A Preliminary Survey of Chinese Sex and Society from ca. 1500 B.C. till 1644 A.D.* Leiden: Brill.

Walker Bynum, C. (1987) *Holy Feast and Holy Fast: The Religious Significance of Food to Medieval Women*. Berkeley, CA: University of California Press.

Wile, D. (1992) *Art of the Bedchamber: The Chinese Sexual Yoga Classics including Women's Solo Meditation Texts*. Albany: New York State University Press.

Wilms, S. (2005) 'Ten Times More difficult to Treat: Female Bodies in Medical Texts from Early Imperial China', *Nannü*, 7.2: 182–215.

Wolf, M. and Witke, R. (eds) (1975) *Women in Chinese Society*. Stanford: Stanford University Press.

Wu, Y. (2010) *Reproducing Women, Medicine, Metaphor and Childbirth in Late Imperial China*. Berkeley, CA: University of California Press.

Wu, Y. (2016) 'The Menstruating Womb, A Cross-Cultural Analysis of Gender in Ho Chun's Precious Mirror of Eastern Medicine, 1613', *Asian Medicine*, 11: 21–60.

Xiao Tianshi 蕭天石 (ed.) (1956–1983) *Daozang jinghua* 道藏精華 (Essential Splendors of the Taoist Canon). Taipei: Ziyou chubanshe.

Zhengtong Daozang 正統道藏 (The Daoist Canon of the Zhengtong Reign) 1444–1445, Bai Yunji 白雲霽 and Qiu Changchun 丘長春 (eds) (1985). Taipei: Xinwenfeng chuban gongsi.

Part II

South Asia

4

Religion and medicine in Sanskrit literature: the *Rāmāyaṇa* and the politics of an epic plant

Anthony Cerulli

Background

There is medicine in premodern Sanskrit literature, if by 'medicine' we mean that a type of mental and/or physical restorative process, a kind of healing in the broadest sense, including surviving sickness and recovery of safety or wellbeing of spirit and/or body, is involved. Likewise, there is religion in premodern Sanskrit literature, if by 'religion' we mean that some form of authoritative discourse (often considered transcendent) is at play, from which distinct practices, communities and institutional hierarchies derive.[1] Medicine and religion also coexist in this literature, sometimes as overlapping and ostensibly complementary, and other times as opposing epistemes. Medicine and religion, of course, are English language categories that scholars use to understand and interpret premodern Sanskrit literature. They are also colloquially pervasive words in the English-speaking world and, because of their ubiquity, without some qualification and contextualisation these words are often used variously and imprecisely, and thus can be misleading and misunderstood.

If the words medicine and religion and the contexts they entail can arouse any number of objects, relationships and meanings in people's minds, I would like at the outset of this chapter to underscore a simple and perhaps obvious point to illuminate how I use the terms: medicine and religion are analytic categories. The category of religion helps us explain why, how and where people congregate and invest their energies in certain cosmologies and ethical systems and not in others. The category of medicine points to reasons why certain body types and behaviours are considered defective, optimal or otherwise and qualifies methods for changing and/or maintaining people's individual and social conditions. Medicine and religion are not things (barring the use of *medicine* as a synonym for *drugs*). They are attributive expressions that help us point to, classify and describe historical and cultural processes and events; human activities, behaviours and relationships; and locations and organisations where events occur and human communities come together. In an academic context, we often use these terms to articulate our 'readings' or interpretations of literature, history and societies. If the research involves ethnography, since fieldwork affords access to people involved with medicine and religion, we might also adduce data about medical and religious beliefs, intentions and expectations.

If the intended uses of medicine and religion are clear – to researchers, at least, since practitioners will have different relationships with the terms – and the meanings they convey are polythetic and adaptable, then these categories can benefit comparative and interdisciplinary analysis in the human sciences, comprising textured examinations of human intentions, worldviews and institutions. In such a context, the language researchers use to explain medicine and religion can be useable in historical, anthropological and literary studies, and it may be applied in multiple locations. Medicine and religion need not be viewed as epistemically or inescapably antithetical, as Mark Noll and David Livingstone remind us, even though they are frequently portrayed in popular culture and by practitioners and scholars that way.[2] Religious and medical practitioners contribute to, draw from, and thereby cultivate human cultures, and in some cases the work they do informs and even complements one another. Medicine and religion are not always linked, however. Healing is not necessarily a religious practice. Yet if we look at medicine and religion as cultural components, associated or not, we might see that the domains of one are similar to the domains of the other, and we can examine both through similar lenses to illuminate human history and behaviour.

In Indology and South Asian Studies, medicine and religion can be useful to examine and explain premodern Sanskrit literature. Thus, let's now consider Hanumān's medicine journey in the

Rāmāyaṇa and probe how a well-known classical Sanskrit text simultaneously implicates pharmaco-botany and Ayurveda (medicine) and key Hindu principles (religion), *dharma* (social-legal-moral 'duty') and *bhakti* ('devotion').

Literature

In the centuries before and after the turn of the Common Era, new ideas about healing appeared in South Asia in an exhaustive Sanskrit medical work called the *Carakasaṃhitā* (*Caraka's Collection*). It became the foundation of classical *āyurveda*, 'life science' (or more inelegantly, 'knowledge for long life'), and it has informed the teaching and practice of the medical tradition known as Ayurveda ever since.[3] Scholars usually consider the *Carakasaṃhitā* to be the oldest of a threesome of classical sources, the 'great trio' (*bṛhattrayī*), which also includes the *Suśrutasaṃhitā* (*Suśruta's Collection*) and the *Aṣṭāṅgahṛdaya* (Vāgbhaṭa's *Heart of the Eight Parts [of Medicine]*). *Caraka's Collection* is the most comprehensive of the trio; it is the first work concentrating on medical matters in Sanskrit that covers a wide array of topics about illness, healing and wellbeing; and it often discusses these topics in ways that engage other fields of knowledge, such as astrology, astronomy, philosophy and ethics. To get an idea of what medicine in South Asia was like before it, Dominik Wujastyk observed, 'we are reduced to searching through books on other – mainly religious – subjects, looking for oblique references which may tell us something about the position of medicine at the time' (Wujastyk 2003: 3).[4] By mentioning 'oblique references', Wujastyk seems to be gesturing to older Vedic texts like the *Ṛg Veda* and *Atharva Veda*, whose ideas about healing and curative modalities Kenneth Zysk amply explored and analysed in the 1980s and '90s (Zysk 1985, 1996). More direct in its healing intent, the Buddhist *Tripiṭaka* is likewise germane to the discussion of what medicine in South Asia before *Caraka's Collection* looked like.[5]

The idea of healing in *Caraka's Collection* rests on three vital factors: the aid of divinities; a doctor's capacity to assess patients; and patients' mental health.[6] Healing that involves deities is perhaps the most obvious convergence of medicine and religion in this premodern Sanskrit work, for it includes therapies such as mantras, physical austerities, ritual performance, sacrifice and pilgrimage. Like the other Sanskrit medical classics, *Caraka's Collection* is essentially a manual for doctors. It is therefore reasonable to interpret medicine that relies on divine assistance as part of the doctor's craft. Bearing in mind *Caraka's* term for this type of medicine, *adravyabhūta*, healing 'consisting of nothing' (i.e., no medicaments), this type of medicine likely hearkened back to the forms of healing in the *Ṛg* and *Atharva Vedas* that recognised the potent effect of transcendent powers on human welfare.[7] The eleventh-century commentator, Cakrapāṇidatta, explained that healing reliant on divine aid can eliminate human disease. But its efficacy, he said, came from the power of the gods, not doctors or patients.[8] To use the central categories of the present volume, it appears that both Cakrapāṇidatta and *Caraka's Collection* acknowledge a type of healing that is more religious than empirically verifiable, in the scientific sense that bases the treatment of illness on observation and experience. *Caraka's Collection* distinctly frames healing concerns, however, so that classical life science (*āyurveda*) moves beyond palliative modalities of the *Vedas* that take recourse in divine aid, and thus in this foundational Ayurvedic text and later works like Cakrapāṇidatta's commentary, the *Āyurvedadīpikā*, the abilities of doctors and the conditions of patients vis-à-vis prospective treatments receive more attention than *adravyabhūta*.[9]

The other two principles of healing in *Caraka's Collection* include the Ayurvedic doctor – known variously as a *bhiṣaj*, *vaidya* and *cikitsaka*[10] – and the patient, *rogin*, literally 'diseased one'. A doctor's examination looks at the patient's overall condition in addition to her or his manifest symptoms. It can include an evaluation of the patient's likes and dislikes, family life, temperament and social class. The literature says that doctors should also assess the associations patients have with the lands and environments they inhabit, which can reveal the nutrient quality of the soil in the regions where they live, whether or not known diseases have been reported in those areas, food habits of people in those regions, and so on (Kakar 1982: 228). By gathering these data, a doctor tries to get a full picture of the patient's life that can then be used as the socio-individual and body-mind contexts in which to understand the disease that prompted the patient to seek treatment in the first place.

The compilers of *Caraka's Collection* and later commentators evinced categories of medicine parallel to the spiritual-religious/empirical-medical divisions in modern scholarship. They distinguished between different healing modalities, such as divine and non-divine, non-botanical and botanical. But these are often contiguous within the larger agenda of healing in the text. At many turns, in fact, *Caraka's Collection* suggests they overlap and perhaps even blur these curative purviews. Describing the nature and structure of the human body, for example, *Caraka's Collection* considers it to be an independent system with an ordered structure and standard working components that is at the same time distinct from, and yet part of, a much greater cosmological body.

> The person is of the same measure as the universe. As much as there is elemental diversity in the universe, in equal measure there is elemental diversity in the person. As much as there is elemental diversity in the person, in equal measure there is elemental diversity in the universe.[11]

The human body is a miniature cosmos, one among many microscopic counterparts within a macroscopic universe, and the material components of the one are constitutive elements of the other.

> Earth comprises the solid form of the person. Water makes up the moisture. Fire is the heat. Wind is the breath. Atmosphere constitutes the hollow parts. The interior self is *brahman*.[12]

In every single body the three humors (*doṣa*s) of wind (*vāta*), bile (*pitta*) and phlegm (*kapha*) circulate, determining a person's health. When they are excessive or deficient in certain areas of the body, they foment maladies and dysfunction. Ailing bodies of patients have become misaligned in some way that extends beyond their individual lives. The humoral landscapes of patients might have been distressed, and discord in the social lives of patients may have upset their constitutions. In an earlier study of the body and embodiment in the Sanskrit medical classics, I explained that South Asia's classical life science attempts to re-calibrate affiliations existing between patient, society and environment (Cerulli 2016). When that is done effectively, the execution of *āyurveda* can synchronise and, in so doing, restore a patient's physical, psychological and social planes of being in the world.

Ideas about healing and wellbeing in life science at the turn of the Common Era in South Asia, around the time of the Sanskrit *Rāmāyaṇa*, thus acknowledged the earlier Vedic period but also fixed new models for understanding and treating the body. Before studying how Hanumān's medicine journey and some of its retellings illuminate the association of medicine and religion in premodern Sanskrit literature, let's briefly look at the *Rāmāyaṇa* and its general place in the study of South Asia. Few treatments of the *Rāmāyaṇa* rival the seven-volume annotated English translation led by Robert Goldman and Sally Sutherland Goldman, *The Rāmāyaṇa of Vālmīki: An Epic of Ancient India*.[13] I refer to this collection many times in this chapter, especially Book 6, the 'Battle Book' (Yuddhakāṇḍa), where Hanumān's medicine journey takes place.

The Sanskrit *Rāmāyaṇa* that we have today was produced around the same time as the other, much longer Sanskrit epic, the *Mahābhārata*. Both texts are colloquially called 'epics', as I refer to them here, although Indian tradition refers to them in narrower terms: the *Rāmāyaṇa* is India's first poem (*kāvya*), and the *Mahābhārata* is history (*itihāsa*).[14] The *Rāmāyaṇa* has major recensions in north and south India. 'All existing recensions and subrecensions', Robert Goldman argued, 'are ultimately to be traced to a more or less unitary archetype' (Goldman 1984: 6), which he cautiously dates somewhere between the seventh and fifth centuries BCE (1984: 22–3). Many scholars suggest that the *Rāmāyaṇa* available today was composed over the course of four centuries, beginning before and ending in the Common Era, with a range of about 200 BCE–200 CE (Doniger 2009: 325ff). Wherever in history one places its composition, scholars generally agree that many hands were involved in its production over multiple generations, despite the common attribution of authorship to the poet Vālmīki.

The *Rāmāyaṇa's* seven books (*kāṇḍas*) recount the life and times of Rāma, the legendary prince of Ayodhyā, eldest and most celebrated son of King Daśaratha and his co-wife Kausalyā, though we, the audience, also know that Rāma is an avatar of the Hindu god Viṣṇu. The story covers Rāma's disinheritance of his father's throne; his exile for 14 years in the wilderness; his wife

Sītā's abduction by Rāvaṇa, the ten-headed demon-king of Laṅkā (Sri Lanka); and then, with the aid of his half-brother Lakṣmaṇa, the monkey warrior Hanumān, and other forest animals, Rāma's rescue of Sītā. From there the story returns to Ayodhyā, where Rāma and Sītā become king and queen. Their reunion in Ayodhyā is only temporary, however, for Rāma banishes Sītā, pregnant with twins, to the forest, when he panics in the face of gossip that she was unfaithful to him while Rāvaṇa held her captive.

Some historians have proposed that the *Rāmāyaṇa* simultaneously conveys mythic and geo-historical data. Romila Thapar, for example, has argued that the text celebrates Lord Rāma's suffering and triumphant victory over evil and narrates usable social and economic development of urban areas and the political arrogation of lands in north India in the Gangetic plain and around Ayodhyā (Thapar 1978). If Thapar attempted to deconstruct the literary and historical layers of the epic, in 'Three Hundred *Rāmāyaṇas:* Five Examples and Three Thoughts on Translation' A. K. Ramanujan inspired a generation of scholars to read beyond Sanskrit texts when exploring India's literary cultures and discuss the richness, range and diversity of vernacular storytelling in South Asia (Ramanujan 1991). Paula Richman's edited volume about the epic's retellings and fluidity, *Many Rāmāyaṇas: The Diversity of a Narrative Tradition in South Asia*, is a classic example of the path that Ramanujan paved for literary studies of the region.[15] Her subsequent publications further challenged long-held beliefs about the hegemony of Sanskrit literature in everyday or lived Hinduism by exploring examples of non-Sanskritic iterations of the epic and retellings in non-Indo-European languages, from locations outside of South Asia, and among non-Hindu communities (Richman 2001, 2008).

Ramanujan's essay was ground-breaking. By drawing attention to the lives of vernacular and non-Hindu *Rāmāyaṇa* traditions, he destabilised the scholarly penchant through much of the twentieth century to query South Asian (specifically Indian) literature and Hinduism from a position that assumed the supremacy and fixity of Sanskritic traditions and Hinduism in the development of culture and religion in India and the South Asian region. Scholars of Ayurveda have been slower than scholars of religion in South Asia to apply this lesson in their research. The Sanskrit medical classics have endured as the sine qua non markers of the Ayurvedic tradition through two millennia. But a similar vernacular reading of the medical tradition has been slow to arrive. Studies of parallel healing traditions in South Asia, such as Unani, Siddha and Nature Cure, have appeared with increasing frequency in the twentieth and twenty-first centuries, and in these comparative explorations scholars are often observant of language use and influence.[16] A thorough re-consideration of the authority of Sanskrit medical sources in the development of Ayurveda through the reading of vernacular and popular literatures has yet to be done, however.

The multiple lives of the *Rāmāyaṇa* continue to drive innovative research about the links between oral, performative and written narrative traditions. To this end, Pika Ghosh echoed studies by Robert Goldman, Mandakranta Bose, Monika Thiel-Horstmann and Vidya Dehejia, by pointing out that the name of Vālmīki attached to the Sanskrit version should be taken as a generic ascription rather than the name of a specific author of an individual text. Many of the *Rāmāyaṇa* retellings that came after the Sanskrit version, she explains, 'can hardly be considered translations, but rather are creative adaptations and variations that must be acknowledged as independent works in their own right'.[17] This observation is germane to the study of medical literature and history in South Asia in that even if the names attached to the classics – Caraka, Suśruta and Vāgbhaṭa – referred to actual people, their hands were surely not the only ones that produced the collections (*saṃhitās*) associated with them today. Unlike variation and retelling of the *Rāmāyaṇa* in South Asia and elsewhere, the 'lives' of the Sanskrit medical classics developed largely through commentary traditions, which are interpretations per se of the root texts, not retellings in the narrative sense that the epic has been retold.

The *Rāmāyaṇa* conveys numerous model social and religious virtues, such as self-sacrifice, filial piety, perseverance and heroism. For Hindus, Rāma's story (*rāmakathā*) overflows with examples of Hindu *dharma*, and many characters in the epic are celebrated dharmic exemplars. Rāma, for example, exemplifies the *dharma* of an obedient son, and by wilfully surrendering his kingdom to honour his father's earlier pledge to one of his co-wives, he further embodies sacrifice. Sītā models the dharmic qualities of an ideal wife, and Hanumān lives and breathes the dharmic features of the loyal servant and ally. At the same time, the *Rāmāyaṇa* is an important early record of Hindu *bhakti*, especially Vaiṣṇava *bhakti*, devotional worship of Viṣṇu, expressed nowhere more clearly than in the exploits of Hanumān, the model *bhakta* or 'devotee'.

Sources

Hanumān is a standout warrior in the army of Kiṣkindhā *vānaras* – 'forest animals', typically depicted as monkeys – that help Rāma rescue Sītā. Among his many heroic acts in the epic, one of the most fêted, retold and represented is his journey to the Himalayas to obtain healing plants (*oṣadhis*) to revitalise soldiers injured by Rāvaṇa and his son, Indrajit. By enthusiastically making the voyage, Hanumān demonstrates his devotion to Rāma and his family. The apparent distance he travels – 'across the seas and beyond the mountains where the sun rises' (Sattar 2016: 174) – is astounding: from Laṅkā to the north Indian state of Uttarakhand (approximately 1600 miles). And he was also under great pressure. To prevent Lakṣmaṇa from dying, Hanumān had to complete the roundtrip mission before the first light of the next day hit Laṅkā's skyline.

I consider several versions of Hanumān's medicine journey in this chapter. But I begin with the Sanskrit *Rāmāyaṇa*, where Hanumān's association with revitalising flora is so special that in the Battle Book the trip is mentioned three times (Goldman, Sutherland Goldman, and van Nooten 2009: 65). The first reference appears in chapter 40, although the mission never actually happens. After Indrajit immobilised Rāma and Lakṣmaṇa with serpent-arrows, the *vānara* doctor Suṣeṇa remembered that Bṛhaspati, teacher of the gods, once used a mixture of herbs and incantations to restore the health of the gods after the demons had thrashed them. So, he assembled a task force that included Hanumān, and he told them to travel to the Ocean of Milk to collect healing plants from Mt. Candra and Mt. Droṇa, referencing two plants by name: 'the divine restorer of life and the healer of arrow wounds, which the gods created'.[18] But before the errand could commence, Viṣṇu's avian vehicle, Garuḍa, swooped onto the scene and frightened the serpentine arrows that beset Rāma and Lakṣmaṇa, causing them to flee. A mere touch of Garuḍa's wings then healed the princes' wounds and their health immediately improved.

The two plants Suṣeṇa requested, *saṃjīvakaraṇī* (aka *saṃjīvanī*) and *viśalyā*, are cited elsewhere in Sanskrit literature. The same plants are used to remove arrows from Yuddhiṣṭhira in the *Mahābhārata*, for example.[19] Classical and medieval medical sources also mention *viśalyā*, which purportedly grows in the Himalayas.[20]

The second reference occurs in chapter 61, where Hanumān and one of his allies, Vibhīṣaṇa – who is actually Rāvaṇa's brother, but has turned against his *rākṣasa* kin and joined Rāma's corps – are surveying a gloomy and bloodstained battlefield. Indrajit had crushed Rāma, Lakṣmaṇa, and most of the monkey army. Amid the casualties, Vibhīṣaṇa found Jāmbavān, wise old king of the bears who inhabited the forests during Rāma's exile. He was blinded and badly injured, but he managed to say that Hanumān could restore the fallen soldiers by going to the Himalayas and locating the glowing mountain of healing plants situated between Mt. Ṛṣabha and Mt. Kailāsa. There he should collect four plants: *mṛtasaṃjīvanī*, restorer of life to the dead; *viśalyākaraṇī*, healer of arrow wounds; *sauvarṇakaraṇī*, restorer of a golden glow; *saṃdhānakaraṇī*, joiner of limbs.[21] Hanumān promptly flew northward across India to the Himalayas. He located the correct mountain but couldn't find the specific plants he was sent to get. The plants were there. But they sensed the purpose of Hanumān's visit and, not wanting to be uprooted, made themselves invisible. Frustrated, Hanumān let out a roar and ripped off the mountain's peak. As he flew south back to Laṅkā, holding the mountain's peak in his hand, its plants glimmered like the sun. The image of the monkey warrior sailing through the air or marching towards the battlefield carrying the flora-rich mountaintop, like a nimble waiter carrying a tray of drinks, permeates Hanumān imagery in South Asia and around the world and exhibits his dutiful ingenuity, strength and devotion.

Back at the battlefield, where Rāma and the others lay wounded, Vālmīki's text affirms the potency of the healing plants and explains that Hanumān's mission from Laṅkā to the Himalayas was actually a double roundtrip:

> As soon as both human princes smelled the fragrance of those powerful healing plants, their arrow wounds instantly healed. All the others, too, the heroic tawny monkeys, stood up.

> Then that immensely powerful tawny monkey [Hanumān], son of the wind-god Vāyu, bearer of scents, quickly took the mountain of healing plants back to the Himalayas, and then again he rejoined Rāma.[22]

The third reference to Hanumān's expedition occurs in chapters 88–90 of the Battle Book. As we approach the end of the epic's sixth book (which ends at chapter 116) and Rāma's ultimate triumph over Rāvaṇa, the warfare becomes more and more remarkable. A spectacular battle unfolded, as Lakṣmaṇa and Vibhīṣaṇa clashed with Rāvaṇa. Lakṣmaṇa protected Vibhīṣaṇa against his brother's onslaught, prompting Rāvaṇa to threaten the Ayodhyā prince: 'Because you, so boastful of your strength, saved Vibhīṣaṇa like this, this spear that freed the *rākṣasa* will kill you. After breaking your heart, this blood-stained spear, hurled by the iron mace that is my arm, will exhaust your life breaths'.[23] Rāvaṇa hurled the weapon, and it sank in Lakṣmaṇa's chest. Seeing his brother collapse, drenched in blood, Rāma begged the gods not to let Lakṣmaṇa die and he cursed Rāvaṇa. He was forlorn and hopeless. But this quickly turned into rage, and he removed the spear from Lakṣmaṇa's chest and boldly snapped it in two.

As Rāma knelt clutching his brother, Rāvaṇa continued to attack. Yet Rāma appeared not to notice. He was fantasising about transcending his many sufferings – the loss of his kingdom, his exile, Sītā's kidnapping, clashes with *rākṣasa*s, and more. He managed to press on, resolving to end his battle with Rāvaṇa then and there. 'I swear to you monkeys', he forecast, 'that not long after this moment, you shall see a world that is either without Rāvaṇa or without Rāma'.[24] He instructed Hanumān and Sugrīva to look after Lakṣmaṇa's body, and he continued: 'Today let the three worlds along with the *gandharva*s, gods, seers, and celestial bards observe in my battle the Rāma-ness of Rāma'.[25]

But Rāma's confidence soon waned as he and Rāvaṇa fought. He confessed to Suṣeṇa that he wanted to quit the battle because his brother appeared to be dying, and neither the prospect of regaining his kingdom nor a reunion with Sītā could bring him joy or make life worth living. When Rāma expressed his wish to die, Suṣeṇa tried to ease his desperation by assuring him that Lakṣmaṇa wasn't actually dead: 'his face is not altered, nor has it darkened. Look at his face. It is splendid and bright. The palms of his hands are like lotus petals, and his eyes are very clear. This is not the look, O Lord, of people whose life breaths have left them. Therefore, do not despair, heroic conqueror of enemies. He is still living'.[26] Although this reassured Rāma, Suṣeṇa knew that Lakṣmaṇa's injury was terminal if left untreated. So, he gave Hanumān an urgent assignment:

> Go quickly, gentle one, to the stone mountain of healing plants Jāmbavān told you about previously. From its southernmost peak bring back the great healing plant known as *viśalyakaraṇī*, healer of arrow wounds, and *sauvarṇakaraṇī*, restorer of a golden glow. O excellent one, to revitalize the hero Lakṣmaṇa, you must also bring back *saṃjīvakaraṇī*, restorer of life, and the powerful plant *saṃdhānī*, joiner of limbs.[27]

Hanumān sprung into action and flew to the mountain of healing plants. The reference to the mountain 'Jāmbavān told you about previously' (in chapter 60) underlines the fact that the mountain is not named here. Suṣeṇa simply calls it an *oṣadhiparvatam*, 'healing plant mountain', and Jāmbavān earlier said it was located between Mt. Ṛṣabha and Mt. Kailāsa in the Himalayas. M. N. Dutt identifies the *oṣadhiparvatam* as Mt. Mahodaya in a parenthetical note in his Sanskrit edition of the *Rāmāyaṇa*; Sako and Mohan call it Droṇagiri; and Vaidyanath and Nishteswar refer to it as Kailasa.[28] Retellings of premodern Sanskrit literature are often the products of many generations of accumulative composition that sometimes simplify or smooth over uncertainties and contradictions. These retellings, editions and interpretations – even within one source, as in Vālmīki's text – shed light on the reception and adaptation of Rāma's story. It is useful to explore later and alternative interpretations and identifications – of healing plant mountain, of the plants' medicinal powers, and so on – not to establish an *Ur*-source of the episode, but to consider how the variations reaffirm and/or influence our own readings of the text today. In this particular episode, we can also examine the confluence of healing, *dharma*, and *bhakti* in premodern India and see how institutions of religion and medicine that we identify and define now draw from the epic and adapt its characters and *materia medica* to new religious and medical ideas and agenda.

When Hanumān returns to Suṣeṇa, everyone sees him carrying something massive in his hand. 'I couldn't find the healing plants', he explains, 'so I brought the entire mountain peak'.[29] Suṣeṇa found and picked the four restorative plants. He crushed one of them and held it under Lakṣmaṇa's nose, and the aroma revived him instantly. The monkeys cheered and as a teary-eyed Rāma hugged his brother, he declared that Lakṣmaṇa was raised from the dead.[30] Suṣeṇa's medical role in this story extends beyond resuscitating Lakṣmaṇa. By healing Rāma's brother, he alleviated the discord and distress that blanketed Rāma and those waged in battle against Rāvaṇa. Re-establishing health in one body, in other words, reunified the entire community, recalibrated their soldierly focus, and ultimately empowered them to defeat Rāvaṇa and retrieve Sītā.

Hanumān's medicine journey is a mini-epic in its own right, with numerous vernacular tracts in South Asia and elsewhere celebrating Hanumān as the devotee par excellence, as Philip Lutgendorf's research on the *Hanumāyana*, *Hanumān-nāṭaka*, *Hanumān jīvan caritra*, and other stories attest (Lutgendorf 2007: 147–8; 208–11). Modern versions of the *Rāmāyaṇa* come in comic, graphic novel, cinematic, televised, choreographic and theatrical forms. It is most commonly associated with Hinduism, yet Buddhists, Jains and Muslims have their own versions too. In Buddhist retellings in Pali, Thai and Lao literature, the Buddha is the epic's narrator and Rāma is a *bodhisattva* who embodies equanimity and compassion and promotes Buddhist values. In the Jain version, preserved in Prakrit, Sanskrit and Apabhramsa manuscripts, Rāma is an evolved Jain whose austere commitment to non-injury (*ahiṃsā*) means he cannot kill Rāvaṇa; Lakṣmaṇa thus performs the deadly act, allowing Rāma to maintain his pacifist vow. The Muslim version, the *Mappila Rāmāyaṇaṃ*, is in Malayalam and is named after the Mappila Muslim community in Kerala that produced it. Rāvaṇa is the Sultan of Laṅkā in this version, and the story offers lessons in Sharia Law.

I first read a translation of the Tamil version of the *Rāmāyaṇa* in college. My first live encounter with Rāma's story was among a Hindu community, not in India, but at a mask dance performance of the epic in Bali, Indonesia. When the actors performed Hanumān's medicine journey, and the monkey warrior brought the healing plants from the Himalayas to help the Ayodhyā princes, the crowd roared with delight. Hanumān's resolute devotion to Rāma, his *bhakti* and mindful awareness of a devotee's *dharma*, augured good things to come, and the audience clearly understood the layered impact of the episode. The sudden reversal of the princes' misfortune would lead to Rāvaṇa's demise, Sītā's rescue and Rāma's enthronement.

Hanumān's medicine journey conveys the general message that medicine, healing and the restoration of individual and social wellbeing begets the opportunity to realise religious pursuits. It also drives the epic's grand narrative to report the triumph of good over evil.[31] These expressions align with a trope in Sanskrit medical literature that infirm bodies cannot attend to religious obligations in the same ways healthy bodies can, and sometimes they cannot at all. People need to know and understand who they are, the nature of their relationships in families and societies, and what their bodies are capable of doing in view of their circumstances. This entails a personal commitment to maintaining the health of one's own body and, at times, a public duty to contribute to the wellbeing of the sociopolitical body to which one belongs. Elsewhere I described this as the body *dharma* principle, which 'involves actively and at all times living a healthy life through one's social, religious, and environmental endeavors' (Cerulli 2012: 158).[32] To upkeep individual and social bodies is a context-dependent endeavour, with obligations that reflect the social and religious interests and needs of particular people and institutions at specific periods. The *Rāmāyaṇa* performance I saw in Bali years ago was a distant relative of Vālmīki's Sanskrit text, and I don't know how apparent South Asian history or Sanskrit literature were in the minds of the Balinese people in attendance. Surely the episode when Hanumān fetched the healing plants was a Balinese story that evening, and it illustrated Balinese models of Hindu devotion and duty, as well as ideas about the confluence of medicine and religion in Balinese culture.

The proliferation of the *Rāmāyaṇa* throughout the world and across history prompted Ramanujan to state boldly that in South and Southeast Asia 'no one ever reads the *Rāmāyaṇa* or the *Mahābhārata* for the first time' (Ramanujan 1991: 46). The epics are 'always already' there, he asserted, in children's books, theatrical and dance performances, and grand Bollywood re-imaginings.

Generations have grown up with Rāma stories in the Amar Chitra Katha comics (est. 1967) – where Hanumān's medicine journey appears in the issue, 'Hanuman to the Rescue' – like children in the US have learned about Aquaman and Elektra in DC and Marvel comic books. Recent generations have more video and animated options to take in Rāma's story than earlier ones did. Each form presents a unique take on the old tale, teaching new cohorts about the importance of qualities like ingenuity, devotion, perseverance, duty, and so much more. The index of uses of the epic is sprawling, diverse and ever-expanding; so in this chapter I have, for the sake of convenience, limited my 'archive' to what I could find on the bookshelf in my son's bedroom. I realise this collection is patently unique in *Rāmāyaṇa* studies but, nevertheless, I believe it can illustrate the elasticity of the medicine journey episode and point us in fruitful directions to explore how divinity and devotion merge with healing through the different lenses of South Asian texts and communities.

Some accounts on my son's bookshelf are quite short, as in Sanjay Patel's illustrated novel, *Ramayana: Divine Loophole*, which has a one-page chapter entitled, 'Mountain of Medicine'. Patel emphasises Hanumān's resourcefulness when he can't locate the herbs he was sent to get: 'Hanuman did the only thing he could think of. In a cloud of snow and dirt, the massive vanara uprooted the entire mountain and balanced it in the palm of his hand. He shot across the sky, racing against time to return to Lakshman'. As he neared the battlefield,

> a strong onshore wind blew toward Lanka and across the hillside of medicine, carrying the smell of the life-restoring herbs straight to Lakshman's nose. He revived, and when Hanuman landed, they wasted no time in gathering the herbs to restore him back to perfect health. Rama thanked the shrewd vanara and instructed him to harvest plenty of medicine before returning the mountain to its home (Patel 2010: 104).

Arshia Sattar's translation offers a traditional, albeit abridged, interpretation of Hanumān's hunt for healing plants. After Jāmbavān says 'bring back the sanjeevani, Hanuman, you are our only hope', Sattar underscores Hanumān's might and shapeshifting abilities. He grows in size, leaps into the air, and expeditiously flies to the Himalayas. When he cannot find the *saṃjīvanī*, knowing that he is running out of time, he decides to take the mountain's summit back to Laṅkā, breaking it off 'as easily as if he were snapping a twig' (Sattar 2016: 174). Travelling 'faster than the wind, swifter than thought', he reached Rāma's dying brother in time for Suṣeṇa to crush up the plant, mix it with oils, and apply it to Lakṣmaṇa's forehead and around his eyes. And just like that 'Lakshamana's pale face flushed, his eyelids fluttered, and he began to breathe' (Sattar 2016: 175).

My son's bookshelf also holds a copy of the Indo-Japanese anime collaboration of Yugo Sako and Ram Mohan, *Ramayana: The Legend of Prince Rama*. This animated version presents the healing narrative unhurriedly and focuses on Hanumān's pleasure in carrying out Suṣeṇa's assignment. Hanumān is resplendent as he sails through the sky, grinning, thinking about Rāma at every turn. The mission appears effortless, and Hanumān's abilities even seem to exceed the feats of Rāma. Hanumān is 'a kind of normative ego-ideal for South Asian society that is perhaps more compelling than even that of his omnipotent master', Goldman and Sutherland Goldman (1996: 86) observed of Rāma's paradigmatic devotee. Tulsidās conveyed this sentiment clearly in a final verse of the *Rāmcaritmanas*, his magnum opus, exalting Hanumān's exemplary devotion: 'My heart, Lord, holds this conviction: Greater than Rama is Rama's servant' (this is also the epigraph of Lutgendorf's masterful 2007 study of Hanumān: vi). By highlighting model aspects of Hindu *bhakti*, including Hanumān's obvious delight in serving Rāma and his determination not to disappoint his lord, Sako and Mohan link religion and medicine: Hanumān's devotion to Rāma enables the restoration of injured bodies and a broken soldierly regiment. Once the collective is restored, their mission can resume and ultimately succeed.

Ramanand Sagar's 1987–88 televised series, *Ramayan*, is perhaps the most famous visual rendering of Rāma's story (loosely based on the Sanskrit version of Vālmīki and the Avadhi version of Tulsidās). The DVD collection of the *Ramayan's* 78 episodes I got for my son years ago is now widely available on YouTube (and it was re-aired on Doordarshan's flagship station, DD National, during the 2020 COVID-19 lockdown). In this televised version, Suṣeṇa says that *saṃjīvanī* cannot simply be harvested and used.

He explains that one must pray to the Hindu god of healing, Dhanvantari, and to the *saṃjīvanī* plant itself, thanking them for their assistance. *Saṃjīvanī* is also called Ayurvedic, and as part of Ayurveda's *materia medica*, Sagar's *Ramayan* gestures to this medical tradition as a homegrown, precolonial, and Hindu Indian science.[33] The alignment of *saṃjīvanī* with Dhanvantari places the plant in the orbit of Vaiṣṇava *bhakti*, since Dhanvantari is an avatar of Viṣṇu. Suṣeṇa also calls Lakṣmaṇa 'an adherent of *dharma*', and he prays for *saṃjīvanī*'s healing blessing to cure him. The shimmering and luminous plant responds approvingly to Suṣeṇa's appeal, and it offers itself to the doctor for preparation with a mortar and pestle. He drops three teaspoons of *saṃjīvanī* juice (*ras*) into Lakṣmaṇa's mouth, reviving the prince, and Rāma conspicuously credits Hanumān with his brother's recovery.

Hanumān's medicine journey appears in countless other places and forms than the foregoing ones. The triumphant image of Hanumān in this episode is evoked in various types of literature, plays and songs, Philip Lutgendorf (2016: 148) has shown, and it is also 'the subject of one of his most popular and ubiquitous icons, both in sculpture and in painting'. For many Hindus, Hanumān represents the principle of *bhakti-śakti*, worshipful devotion and energy – for Vaiṣṇavas as well as Śaivas, who began to regard Hanumān as the eleventh avatar of Rudra-Śiva around the start of the second millennium CE (Lutgendorf 2007: 44). Hanumān's devotion energises his commitment to do whatever he can to ensure the welfare of the Ayodhyā princes. His story illustrates the multidimensional nature of *dharma*, which suffuses all of life and is critical to support the welfare of a community, even the universe, in addition to one's own wellbeing. The *dharmaśāstra* works of Manu, Yājñavalkya and Viṣṇu go to great lengths to show the many sides of *dharma*, including its social, legal and religious facets. The idea that there are thought to be in every person's life multiple obligations to the health of personal, social, political and global bodies – to body *dharma* in all its forms – and these obligations are fundamental to other types of dharmic activity, is an under-discussed aspect of Hindu *dharma*. Yet body *dharma* is helpful when we try to make sense of premodern Sanskrit texts today, whether we label those texts Ayurvedic, mythological, poetical or something else. It is a hermeneutic device that enables us to:

> begin to see that the interest and aim to heal – to heal ailing bodies and broken hearts, deluded minds and inept leaders, fractured armies and crumbling fortresses, and countless other areas and examples – have been and still are central components of South Asian cultures that at times inform, structure, and soothe other cultural domains. That is, the drive to heal, mend, and stabilize that we are accustomed to seeing most clearly in medicine is much more than a strictly medical matter in South Asia (and we can extend this observation elsewhere as well). The drive to heal, that is, in many ways subtends many aspects of South Asian cultures. (Cerulli 2020: 191–2)

Because the tale of Hanumān's hunt for healing plants has been so popular throughout the centuries, his successful procurement of *saṃjīvanī* and other medicinal herbs from the Himalayas, ensuring Lakṣmaṇa's survival, has also established the monkey warrior as more than just a model devotee in contemporary South Asia. He is sometimes regarded as a healer in his own right, a patron deity of Ayurveda, and he has even become the mascot and logo for a modern Indian courier company, ABT Parcel Service (Lutgendorf 2016: 156). Retellings of the medicine journey in multiple media keep discussions and imagery of Hanumān as a healer and devotee in the zeitgeist of the twenty-first century. On occasion, people with religious and political interests in the *Rāmāyaṇa* also treat the Sanskrit epic as an historically factual resource for practical use in the present day.

Analysis

If Rāma's story continues to express models of Hindu *dharma* and *bhakti* today, the epic's story of *saṃjīvanī* has also inspired scientific research in the twenty-first century. In recent decades government officials in the north Indian state of Uttarakhand – where Vālmīki's text tells us that Hanumān acquired the plants that saved Lakṣmaṇa – have applied for government funds to study and harvest plants in the state's mountains they suspect are the same *saṃjīvanī* plants mentioned in the *Rāmāyaṇa*. Such proposals raise several questions about the associations between myth and history and religion and medicine in modern India. Is it possible, we might ask, that the story of Hanumān's medicine journey was informed by Ayurvedic pharmaco-botany, *dravyaguṇa*? What is the place of *saṃjīvanī* in classical and contemporary *dravyaguṇa*? And how have Ayurvedic doctors and researchers responded to the possibility of harvesting and using 'epic medicine' in India today?

In 2016, *The New York Times* published an article, 'Medicinal Herb or Myth? Indian Official Proposes Hunt for Sanjivani of Lore', in a series called *What in the World?* (Venkataraman 2016). The author, Ayesha Venkataraman, told the story of Surendra Singh Negi, minister for alternative medicine in Uttarakhand, who was concerned that forest fires in the Himalayan foothills in his state were destroying valuable plants, most notably *saṃjīvanī*. Negi hadn't actually seen the plant, he confessed. But 'you can tell that the hills of Uttarakhand are abundant in medicinal plants', he told Venkataraman, 'from the fragrant smoke that fires give off' (Venkataraman 2016). In the *Rāmāyaṇa*, *saṃjīvanī* revives fallen soldiers simply by its smell, thus Negi's attentiveness to the fires' fragrance is possibly useful. While doing fieldwork in south India, I have been told by Ayurvedic doctors that the aromas of herbal decoctions and salves they prescribe can be essential to caring for the sick. A foul smell indicates putrefaction and foretells futility in treatment. I have also observed Ayurvedic doctors in Kerala describe to their patients that the medicines they prescribe should smell certain ways. Which is all to say that the odors of botanical remedies are not insignificant to the treatment of illness in Ayurveda.

Nevertheless, Venkataraman's article raises healthy skepticism about the extent to which Negi's remarks were influenced by Hanumān's epic medicine journey vis-à-vis science. For, based largely on his olfactory observations, he had proposed that the Uttarakhand government spend 250 million rupees (roughly US$ 3.75 million) to send researchers into the mountains to find the source of the aromatic smoke he detected and try to link it to the epic *saṃjīvanī*. A similar plan was proposed in Uttarakhand in 2009, but was not funded. In 2016, Negi's hope of success was buoyed by the Uttarakhand's Ayurvedic adviser, Mayaram Uniyal, who confirmed that 'a real-life version of the legendary sanjivani has been seen growing on the slopes of Dunagiri, a mountain in northern Uttarakhand' (Venkataraman 2016). He said the plant had yellow flowers and secreted a yellowish milk, and he corroborated Negi's remark about its smell. He furthermore suggested that it has a unique lustre that 'lights up in the night', recalling the glow of the mountain peak Hanumān carried to the *Rāmāyaṇa* battlefield, which Vālmīki described as shining like the sun. One also wonders if this putative feature of the plant provoked the *New York Times* to accompany its online version of Venkataraman's article with a picture of an iridescent green plant, digitally enhanced so that it appeared to glitter and pulsate.

Uniyal offered additional botanical information to support Negi's proposal, saying that the plant 'has been used extensively by the local shepherds when someone is unconscious, in pain or even under stress', clearly linking the epic plant's effects on the human body and the plant he and Negi claimed was growing in the Himalayas (Venkataraman 2016). Although both men were optimistic that the project's medical result could be great, Uniyal noted that 'no one expects it to have one ability that the Ramayana ascribes to *sanjivani*: resurrecting the dead' (Venkataraman 2016). As we saw, the *Rāmāyaṇa* has diverging reports about this power of *saṃjīvanī*. In the third reference to Hanumān's medicine journey, for example, Suṣeṇa assured Rāma that Lakṣmaṇa was not really dead, and thus the plant didn't restore Lakṣmaṇa's life. Yet, in the second reference, the plant is called *mṛta-saṃjīvanī*, meaning restorer of life to the 'dead', *mṛta*, and appears to belie the third reference and align with Uniyal's comment.

The prospect of identifying a modern-day *saṃjīvanī* and potentially drawing a pharmaco-botanical link to Vālmīki's *Rāmāyaṇa* has interested many scientists, too. Ganeshaiah, Vasudeva and Shaanker (2009) mined the Indian Bioresource database for the name *saṃjīvanī* and associated synonyms and phononyms in eighty Indian languages, looking for references to features of the plant mentioned in the *Rāmāyaṇa*. The motivation for their study was to give the famed plant a scientific examination before simply dismissing it as a mythic fabrication of Vālmīki. It might be the case, they hypothesised, that *saṃjīvanī* is a particular plant or it might refer to a collection of plants with corresponding properties. They were open to the possibility that the name *saṃjīvanī* has served as a metonym for centuries for several kinds of 'good medicine', perhaps a *rasāyana*-type elixir. Initially they found seventeen Linnaean-named species, which they reduced to six potential options. Of the six, three stood out for their healing qualities and frequent associations with the Sanskrit plant name *saṃjīvanī*: *Cressa cretica*, *Selaginella bryopteris* and *Desmotrichum fimbriatum* (Ganeshaiah *et al.* 2009: 485). Since Hanumān finds *saṃjīvanī* in the Himalayas, they decided to rule out *Cressa cretica*, since its primary habitats include backwaters, salt lakes, dry plains and moist deciduous forests. It is not a mountainous plant, and it is mostly found in areas common to the dry Deccan plateau and lowland areas in Andhra Pradesh, Karnataka, Maharashtra and Tamilnadu. The bioprospecting possibilities of these areas did not look enough like the geography of the *Rāmāyaṇa* to consider it further (Ganeshaiah *et al.* 2009: 486).

Ganeshaiah, Vasudeva and Shaanker then invoked the homeopathic dictum 'like cures like' (*similia similibus curantur*), the Law of Similars, which says that any plant (or drug) capable of producing certain symptoms in healthy individuals will relieve similar symptoms that occur as an expression of disease, to choose between the remaining two plants. Epic *saṃjīvanī*, they wrote, 'had the ability of resurrecting itself from a state of near-death situation and hence the ancient doctors, on the principle of "similar cures similar" used it to cure Rama, Lakshmana and others' (Ganeshaiah *et al.* 2009: 486–7).[34] Based on habitat and the Law of Similiars, they identified *Selaginella bryopteris* as the closest botanical relative of the plant known as *saṃjīvanī* in the *Rāmāyaṇa*, even though *Desmotrichum fimbriatum* also met several criteria. In the end, language use ended up being a key determining factor for the researchers. *Desmotrichum fimbriatum* is not consistently called *saṃjīvanī* in Sanskrit and other Indian languages, whereas *Selaginella bryopteris* is.

Some researchers classify *Selaginella bryopteris* as a poikilohydric lithophyte, meaning it can 'resurrect' from an almost dead-dry state to a normal condition upon hydration, at which point it can bloom and become quite vibrant in colour (Antony and Thomas 2011: 933). Others take it to be a pteridophyte and/or other allied species (Pandey *et al.* 2017: 11; Ganeshaiah, Vasudeva and Shaanker 2009). Sah *et al.* (2005) tested the plant on rats subjected to ultraviolet radiation and oxidative stress and reported cases of resuscitative recovery. But to date, there are no documented cases of the plant being used on humans. *Selaginella bryopteris* is found in hilly regions, including, according to Varma (2015: 41), 'on the hills of tropical areas, particularly the *Arawali* mountain terrains'.

The Aravalli Mountains, however, run southwesterly from Delhi into Rajasthan and Gujarat, suggesting that *Selaginella bryopteris* is not indigenous to the Himalayas. The plant is also somewhat rare nowadays, though it has been reported in the hills of both tropical and moist deciduous forests (Ganeshaiah, Vasudeva and Shaanker 2009: 487). Perhaps because of the associations the plant has garnered with epic *saṃjīvanī*, *Selaginella bryopteris* is sometimes found for sale at Hindu pilgrimage sites in north India, such as Rishikesh, Haridwar and Varanasi.

Where does this leave us with respect to medicine and religion in Vālmīki's *Rāmāyaṇa*, Minister Negi's expensive hunt for *saṃjīvanī*, and ongoing botanical research on epic medicine? Apart from conjecture that *Selaginella bryopteris* is the most likely contemporary form of *saṃjīvanī*, no one has decisively identified modern flora with the healing capacity of the epic plant that could lend scientific credibility to Vālmīki's story. Even if a proposal like Minister Negi's appears worthwhile in theory – a life-saving drug would be useful in any society – some people, even those deeply invested in the success of contemporary Ayurveda, have criticised these types of efforts for drawing attention away from more pressing social needs. When, for example, I shared the *New York Times* article and three articles from Indian news sources (Mudur 2005; Balasubramanian 2009; Pande 2016) with two Ayurvedic doctors I know in south India, both wondered why large sums of money should be used to search for mythological plants instead of funding what they consider to be reliable Ayurvedic projects and products that have been used for centuries. One rhetorically asked why a state minister of Uttarakhand, which suffers from a shortage of good doctors (of any medical tradition), would consider investing money in a *saṃjīvanī* project instead of giving health care to Uttarakhand's people now and, more long term, building a better medical education system for future generations. The other doctor, who is also a professor of *dravyaguṇa*, suspected that because research funding in India is so difficult to get, people tend to take wild liberties with their imagination when writing grant proposals.

Modern-day attempts to corroborate the historicity and/or scientificity of premodern Sanskrit texts are not new in South Asia. Comparatively, one might think of Christians who espouse Intelligent Design and assert the historical validity of the Genesis creation stories as opposed to evolution and the Big Bang Theory. There is also an element of decolonising nuance at play in the modern search for *saṃjīvanī*. The association of this powerful plant with classical life science (*āyurveda*) and the modern institution of Ayurveda puts it in a botanical lineage going back to *Caraka's Collection* that predates not just British and French biomedicine in South Asia, but also the Mughals and Delhi Sultans, who advanced Unani medicine throughout much of the second millennium CE. It is well-known that conservative Hindu groups in recent decades have mobilised millions of proponents of Hindu nationalism and Hindutva ('Hindu-ness') under the banner of the *Rāmāyaṇa*'s true history, often with devastating results. The Bharatiya Janata Party (BJP) and Sangh Parivar, for example, levelled historically baseless claims in the 1980s and early 1990s that a temple memorialising Rāma's birthplace had been in the city of Ayodhyā until it was desecrated by the construction of the Babri Masjid in the sixteenth century. This rhetoric incited mobs of Hindus to raze the mosque in 1992 and prompted riots and Hindu–Muslim violence across India that lasted for years (Pollock 1993).[35] The Ram Setu controversy is another example of Hindutva objections to meddling with religious symbols tied to the *Rāmāyaṇa*. In this case, the Sangh Parivar protested plans of the Tamilnadu state to dynamite the shallow waterway between India and Sri Lanka to build a shipping channel on the grounds that Rāma and the *vānara* army built a bridge there, now long-submerged, to give them safe passage into Rāvaṇa's kingdom on their mission to rescue Sītā. The victimisation claimed by Hindus was targeted not at Muslims this time, but at the Tamil government and, rather than citing outrage over the destruction of a religious symbol, Sangh Parivar leadership cited strategic and economic reasons for defending the historical bridge to Sri Lanka (Jaffrelot 2008).

The politics of the *Rāmāyaṇa* notwithstanding, to what extent can we discuss the therapeutic nature of *saṃjīvanī*? Does the plant have a genuine place in Ayurvedic pharmacology? Both doctors I contacted about the *New York Times* and Indian newspaper articles told me that while *saṃjīvanī* is mentioned in the *materia medica* literature of Ayurveda, it is uncommon in Ayurvedic therapies today. I asked the *dravyaguṇa* professor if he could comment on the confluence of healing and religious discourse in the *Rāmāyaṇa*. 'The *Rāmāyaṇa* is not Ayurvedic science', he said. 'But every year at least one student asks me if the *saṃjīvanī* Hanumān brought from the Himalayas to save Lakṣmaṇa is real. Most Indians know the *Rāmāyaṇa* and most don't know about Ayurvedic drugs. So, new students often see a connection between the stories they've heard all their lives and the medical career they are beginning. The plant is a bridge, and they wonder if it's possible that Hindu literature has scientific value'. He also told me that during his college days he recalled hearing that *saṃjīvanī* grew in the evergreen forests of his Karnataka hill-station campus. Now, as a professor, he does not teach *saṃjīvanī*, although he does introduce his students to *Selaginella bryopteris*, which is sometimes called *saṃjīvanī* in Indian languages and which is part of the BAMS and MD *dravyaguṇa* syllabus set by the Central Council for Indian Medicine. He told me that '*saṃjīvanī* is probably a type of spike moss or possibly a fern which I've seen studies link to *Selaginella*', adding: 'the plant's medicinal properties seem to be inflated nowadays. I have even heard of a few cases where people got duped by dishonest medicine men claiming they could cure all diseases with *saṃjīvanī*, which they brewed in concoctions containing a plant that was probably *Selaginella*'. Notably, this professor also owns an Ayurvedic pharmaceutical manufacturing plant, and over the many years he has run it, he has never used a recipe from the classical literature that has *saṃjīvanī* as an ingredient. Similarly, the other doctor flatly told me that 'nobody takes it seriously and it is not a common ingredient in any of our major remedies. I think *The New York Times* has gone overboard with the story and its glowing *Selaginella* graphics'.

Conclusions

The two Ayurvedic doctors I asked about Minister Negi's 2016 proposal to find *saṃjīvanī* in the Himalayas questioned whether Negi and his colleagues actually believed their claims about the reality of a life-saving plant, and they doubted the appropriateness of their proposal on a scientific platform. Their doubt brings to mind Clifford Geertz's observation that religion, and in this case one of India's most widely known religious stories, can be such a totalising ideology that it can subsume science. It has the capacity to capture the human imagination, he said, by establishing 'powerful, pervasive, and long-lasting moods and motivations in [people] by formulating conceptions of a general order of existence and clothing these conceptions with such an aura of factuality that [the] moods and motivations seem uniquely realistic' (Geertz 1973: 90). Like other theorists in the last quarter of the twentieth century, Geertz was keen to extend Ricoeur's hermeneutics of suspicion and to encourage others to read against the grain and between the lines to reveal unfavourable truths, important exclusions, and contradictions that are not readily apparent on the surface.[36] And, as true as his observation about the totalising nature of religious ideology might still be today, almost fifty years later, we should take care not to reject proposals like Minister Negi's out of hand simply because the so-called science has yet to say, irrefutably, that Vālmīki's *saṃjīvanī* is a specific plant that grows in a specific area.

That is, suspicion is important and can be useful. But it need not be our only approach. Instead, we would do well, as Felski (2015: 175) advises, to allow ourselves the opportunity 'to wiggle out of the straightjacket of suspicion' that so often motivates investigations of religions generally and scientific explorations of religious healing, and take seriously recent studies like one led by Sandeep Pandey's research team. In addition to a pharmacological analysis, Pandey *et al.* (2017: 13) offer a brief study of *saṃjīvanī* and ethnomedicine, where the scholars assert that a plant most researchers presume is linked to epic *saṃjīvanī* is used among indigenous (tribal) communities in Gond, Bhil, Korku and other parts of Madhya Pradesh to treat urinary and gynaecological disorders. This observation urges us not to see 'an aura of factuality' superimposed on a religious text or 'to diminish or subtract from the reality of texts we study but to amplify their reality' in step with Felski's postcritical method (Felski 2015: 185). In this way, we can manoeuvre between various material relations, such as the plants and people interested in the historical data of Vālmīki's epic, and semiotic markers like the concepts of medicine and religion with which we began this chapter. This requires a willingness to jettison assumed epistemic priorities and privileges and re-focus our concepts – medicine and religion – on the various configurations of different times, places and peoples. Religion has affective power. In modern India this power often drives national and local politics, and yet the text that is at stake for Minister Negi is not even a story for just one religion – it is also a Muslim, Jain and Buddhist story. It is not even entirely religious. It is *kāvya* (poetry), which spans religious, mythic, historical and literary spheres. The postcolonial dimensions that arise in the alignment of the *Rāmāyaṇa* with Ayurveda also form a partly religious and partly nationalistic kind of allegiance, based on ostensible marginalisations by political-intellectual powers perhaps not fully understood and the loss of control among local communities over their natural resources. It is a veritable tangle of referential knottiness.

Efforts to validate classical stories like Hanumān's medicine journey, whether they are grounded in deep belief or not, teach us less about people's aspirations to legitimate epic events, plants and technologies and, instead, provide us with depth and historical texture for making sense of the ways people struggle to preserve the legitimacy, relevance and constancy of their classical traditions amid contemporary social changes and challenges. By examining how some Hindu communities, researchers and politicians read Hanumān's medicine journey today, practical uses of old texts emerge. The *Rāmāyaṇa* story of Hanumān and *saṃjīvaṇī*, on the one hand, expresses central Hindu principles like *bhakti* and *dharma*. On the other hand, the story lies at the heart of scientific studies and costly proposals that subtly and at times unambiguously connect the future progress of Ayurveda, as an important indigenous medicine in the competitive and diverse South Asian medical marketplace, to technologically enticing visions of Ayurveda's past.

Notes

1 The four interlinked domains comprising religion mentioned here – discourse, practice, community and institution – are drawn from Bruce Lincoln's intervention in the longstanding conversation about what constitutes religion and the religious (2004: 5–7).

2 Riffing on Steven Shapin's famous turn of phrase about the Scientific Revolution, in their introduction to *The Warfare Between Science & Religion*, Mark Noll and David Livingstone explain that even though 'there has never been systemic warfare between science and theology… the notion nonetheless lives on' (2018: 1).

3 In this chapter I use the words '*āyurveda*', 'Ayurveda' and 'Ayurvedic' to draw distinctions about the healing tradition that developed following the *Carakasaṃhitā*. The term *āyurveda* is a Sanskrit compound meaning 'life science'. The term Ayurveda is a proper noun that denotes the title of the modern Indian medical profession that is based on *āyurveda* and in many ways has extended it. I use the term Ayurvedic as the adjectival form of *āyurveda*. When qualifying a noun, it implies that the noun in some way, even if remotely, relates to classical Indian life science (i.e., Ayurvedic college, Ayurvedic pharmacy, Ayurvedic doctor, and so on). This is not a Sanskrit word, but an English neologism, not to be confused with the more expansive Sanskrit word *āyurvedika*, 'acquainted or familiar with *āyurveda*', which sometimes serves as a synonym for a doctor of *āyurveda*.

4 There are several good publications that succinctly present, contextualise and explain the literature of Ayurveda, among which the most exhaustive is Jan Meulenbeld's five-volume, *A History of Indian Medical Literature* (1999–2002). Three of my publications (2010; 2012: 13–48; forthcoming) offer thorough accounts of the Sanskrit classics and aspects of healing and wellbeing in Ayurveda. Dominik Wujastyk's *Roots of Ayurveda* (2003) remains a solid introduction to, and partial translation of, the most well-known Sanskrit medical literature.

5 This is a topic that Zysk explored directly in *Asceticism and Healing in Ancient India* (1991).

6 *Carakasaṃhitā*, Sūtrasthāna 11.54.

7 *Carakasaṃhitā*, Vimānasthāna 8.87.

8 *Āyurvedadīpikā* on *Carakasaṃhitā*, Sūtrasthāna 11.54.

9 A late-classical Sanskrit collection about the health of women and children, the *Kāśyapasaṃhitā* (*Kaśyapa's Collection*, seventh to eighth century CE), reduced the three categories of healing in *Caraka's Collection* down to two: botanical therapies (*auṣadha*) and non-botanical therapies (*anauṣadha*), the latter of which is broadly termed *bheṣaja*, 'healing' (Indriyasthāna 1.3–4), and seems to be a re-naming of *adravyabhūta*. Both *bheṣaja* and *adravyabhūta* echo remedies in India's Vedic era, where cures for mental and physical ailments tend to be explained via mythologies and treated with spells, talismans, rituals and mantras.

10 We find all three terms in *Caraka's Collection*. Based on an expansive collection of medical and non-medical Sanskrit literature, Patrick Olivelle's translation of the premodern 'medical professional' in Sanskrit literature is drawn from these three terms, which he parses as 'physician' (*bhiṣaj*), 'doctor' (*vaidya*) and 'medic' (*cikitsaka* – 2017: 3

fn.4). For the sake of clarity and simplification, throughout this chapter I use only the term doctor.

11 *Carakasaṃhitā*, Śārīrasthāna 5.3: *puruṣo 'yaṃ lokasaṃnitaḥ ityuvāca bhagavān punarvasurātreyaḥ / yāvanto hi loke bhāvaviśeṣāstāvantaḥ puruṣe yāvantaḥ puruṣe tāvanto loke* (NB: translation of this and subsequent primary sources is the work of the author unless otherwise noted).

12 *Carakasaṃhitā*, Śārīrasthāna 5.5: *tasya puruṣasya pṛthivī mūrtiḥ āpaḥ kledaḥ tejo 'bhisantāpaḥ vāyuḥ prāṇaḥ viyat suṣirāṇi, brahma antarātmā*.

13 Goldman and Sutherland Goldman translated volume 1 (Bālakāṇḍa 1984); Sheldon Pollock translated volume 2 (Ayodhyakāṇḍa 1986) and volume 3 (Araṇyakāṇḍa 1991); Rosalind Lefeber translated volume 4 (Kiṣkindhākāṇḍa 1994); Goldman and Sutherland Goldman translated volume 5 (Sundarakāṇḍa 1996); Goldman, Sutherland Goldman, and Barend van Nooten translated volume 6 (Yuddhakāṇḍa, 2009); and Goldman and Sutherland Goldman translated volume 7 (Uttarakāṇḍa 2017).

14 Wendy Doniger observed that the *Mahābhārata* actually refers to itself as a form of didactic story or communication (*ākhyāna*) about *dharma* more often than history (2009: 302).

15 Contributors to Paula Richman's *Many Rāmāyaṇas* were asked to read Ramanujan's essay and, she explains in the book's Preface, 'each chapter can be seen, in some way, as a response to some of the questions that Ramanujan raises' in his seminal essay (1991: xi).

16 See, for example, Lisa Brooks, Anthony Cerulli, and Victoria Sheldon's introduction and Cerulli's epilogue to a special issue of *Asian Medicine* about memory and medicine in South Asia (2020).

17 Ghosh (2016: fn. 1, 10). See also Goldman (1984, introduction to the *Bālakāṇḍa*); Bose (2004); Thiel-Horstmann (1991); and Dehejia (1994).

18 *Rāmāyaṇa* YK 40.30: *saṃjīvakaraṇīṃ divyāṃ viśalyāṃ devanirmitām*. The Ocean of Milk (*kṣīrodam sāgaram*), 'where the nectar of immortality was churned' (*Rāmāyaṇa* YK 40.31), is a frequently recurring place in Indian mythology that involves themes of resuscitation and renewal. It is thus an appropriate source of these 'supreme plants' (*paramauṣadhī*).

19 *Mahābhārata* 8.58.21; Pagani (1999: 1662).

20 *Aṣṭāṅgahṛdaya* 1.84, 6.38, 15.28, 22.69; *Bhāvaprakāśa* 3.7; *Rājanighaṇṭu* 3.14, 5.158, 6.127.

21 *Rāmāyaṇa* YK 61.28–33. Goldman, Sutherland Goldman, and van Nooten note that the literal meanings of these herbs would be

'reviving the dead', 'making arrow-less', 'making golden' and 'joining' (2009: 1091–2), and their translations, which I have adopted here, are derived from *Rāmāyaṇa* commentators' explanations of the plants.

22 *Rāmāyaṇa* YK 61.67–8: *tāvapyubhau mānuṣarājaputrau taṃ gandhasmāghrāya mahoṣadhīnām / babhūvatustatra tadā viśalyāvuttasthuranye ca haripravīrāḥ // sarve viśalyā virujāḥ kṣeṇena haripravīrāśca hatāśca ye syuḥ / gandhena tāsāṃ pravaroṣadhīnāṃ suptā niśānteṣviva saṃprabuddhāḥ // 67 // tato harigandhavahātmajastu tamoṣadhīśailamudagravegaḥ / nindruya vegāddhimavantameva punaśca ramena samājagāma // 68 //* D. P. Mishra argued that the location of Laṅkā in the *Rāmāyaṇa* is not modern-day Sri Lanka, but was instead an island off the east coast of the Indian peninsula near the Godavari Delta (1985: 63–4).

23 *Rāmāyaṇa* YK, 88.28–9: *mokṣitaste balaślāghinyasmādevaṃ vibhīṣaṇaḥ / vimucya rākṣasaṃ śaktistvayīyaṃ vinipātyate // 28 // eṣā te hṛdayaṃ bhittvā śaktirlohitalakṣaṇā / madbahuparighotsṛṣṭā prāṇānādāya yāsyati // 29 //*

24 *Rāmāyaṇa* YK 88.45: *asmin muhūrte na cirātsatyaṃ pratiśṛṇomi vaḥ / arāvaṇamarāmaṃ vā jagaddakṣyatha vānarāḥ //*

25 *Rāmāyaṇa* YK, 88.52: *adya paśyantu rāmasya rāmatvaṃ mama saṃyuge / trayo lokāḥ sagandharvāḥ siddhagandharvacāraṇāḥ //* Goldman, Sutherland Goldman, and van Nooten translate *rāmasya rāmatvaṃ* as 'what makes Rāma Rāma' (2009: 415).

26 *Rāmāyaṇa* YK, 89.10–11: *nahyasya vikṛtaṃ vaktraṃ na ca syāmatvamāgatam / suprabhaṃ ca prasannaṃ ca mukhamasya nirīkṣyatām // 10 // padmapatratalau hastau suprasanne ca locane / nedṛśaṃ dṛsyate rūpaṃ gatāsūnāṃ viśāṃ pate / viṣādaṃ mā kṛthā vīra saprāṇo 'yamariṃdama // 11 //*

27 *Rāmāyaṇa* YK, 89.14–16: *saumya śīghramito gatvā śailam oṣadhiparvatam (parvataṃ hi mahodayam) / pūrvaṃ tu kathito yo 'sau vīra jāmbavatā tava // 14 // dakṣiṇe śikhare jātāṃ mahauṣadhimihānayaḥ / viśalyakaraṇīṃ nāmnā sāvarṇyakarṇīṃ tathā // 15 // saṃjīvakaraṇīṃ vīra saṃdhānīṃ ca mahauṣadhīm / saṃjīvanārthaṃ vīrasya lakṣmaṇasya tvamānaya // 16 //*

28 Dutt (1998: 309); Sako and Mohan (1992); Vaidyanath and Nishteswar (2007: 40).

29 *Rāmāyaṇa* YK 90.21: *auṣadhīrnāvacchāmi tā ahaṃ haripuṅgava / tadidaṃ śikharaṃ kṛtsnaṃ girestasyāhṛtaṃ mayā //*

30 *Rāmāyaṇa* YK 89.27: *maraṇāt punar āgatam.*

31 The triumph of Rāma over Rāvaṇa and rescue of Sītā in the *Rāmāyaṇa* is a common motif of good vanquishing evil commemorated every autumn (October–November) in Diwali celebrations.

32 See also Cerulli (2012: 147–160; 2016: 81–2).
33 Meera Nanda (2003, 2005) has written at length about the modern history of Hindu nationalists' attempts to portray Ayurveda as India's precolonial Hindu science.
34 It is worth noting that Ayurveda does not generally work on this homeopathic principle, but rather tends to operate on the theory that opposites cure (e.g., vitiating *kapha*-diseases with *pitta*-heavy drugs, countering cold and heavy illness with hot and light drugs, etc.), which is the fundamental meaning of allopathy, or treating symptoms of illness with drugs that have the opposite effects (from the Greek *állos*). This is somewhat curious, given that Ayurveda has been, and often still is, positioned in scholarship and popular conversation in opposition to biomedicine, which in India is colloquially called allopathy.
35 On November 9, 2019, the Indian Supreme Court ruled that the area where the Babri Masjid had been standing, since the first Mughal emperor, Babur, had the mosque built, would be given to Hindus who wanted to build a Rāma temple there. The ruling reserved an alternate location to be given to Muslims for their own place of worship (Pandey 2019).
36 Ricoeur (2008: 32); see also Ricoeur's elaboration of these three masters of suspicion (2008: 32–6).

Bibliography

Antony, R. and Rini T. (2011) 'A Mini Review on Medicinal Properties of the Resurrecting Plant *Selaginella Byropteris* (Sanjeevani)', *International Journal of Pharmacy and Life Sciences*, 2.7: 933–9.

Aṣṭāṅgahṛdaya: A compendium of the Ayurvedic System Composed by Vāgbhaṭa, with the commentaries (Sarvāngasundarā) of Aruṇadatta and (Āyurvedarasāyana) Hemādri. Annā Moreśwar Kunte, K.R. Śāstrī Navre, and B.H. Parādkar Vaidya (eds), 6th edition (1939). Bombay: Nirnaya-sāgar Press.

Balasubramanian, D. (2009) 'In Search of the Sanjeevani Plant in the Ramayana', *The Hindu*, September 10.

Bhāvaprakāśa of Bhāvamiśra, with Hindi *Vidyotinī-Nāmikayā Bhāṣāṭīkayā Saṃvalitaḥ*. 2 vols. Brahmaśaṅkara Miśra and Rūpalāljī Vaiśya (eds), 10th edition (2002). Varanasi: Chaukhambha Sanskrit Bhawan.

Bose, M. (2004) *The Rāmāyaṇa Revisited.* New York: Oxford University Press.

Brooks, L., Cerulli, A. and Sheldon, V. (2020) 'Introduction: Medicines and Memories in South Asia', *Asian Medicine*, 15.1: 3–9.

Carakasaṃhitā of Agniveśa, with the Āyurveda-Dīpikā Commentary of Cakrapāṇidatta. Jādavjī Trikamjī Āchārya (ed.) 5th edition (1992). New Delhi: Munshiram Manoharlal.

Cerulli, A. (2010) 'Āyurveda', in K.A. Jacobsen, H. Basu, A. Malinar and V. Narayanan (eds) *Brill's Encyclopedia of Hinduism*, Vol. II, *Texts, Rituals, Arts, and Concepts*. Leiden: Brill (revised online ed., 2013), pp. 267–80.

Cerulli, A. (2012) *Somatic Lessons: Narrating Patienthood and Illness in Indian Medical Literature*. Albany: State University of New York Press.

Cerulli, A. (2016) 'Body, Self, and Embodiment in the Sanskrit Classics of Āyurveda', in B. Holdrege and K. Pechilis (eds) *Refiguring the Body: Embodiment in South Asian Religions*. Albany: State University of New York Press, pp. 59–88.

Cerulli, A. (2020) 'Epilogue: Healing Concerns in South Asian Texts, Histories, and Societies', *Asian Medicine*, 15.1: 183–96.

Cerulli, A. (forthcoming) 'Early Indian Medical Literature', in J. Hegarty and L. Greaves (eds) *Oxford Handbook of Hindu Literature*. Oxford: Oxford University Press.

Dehejia, V. (1994) *The Legend of Rama: Artistic Visions*. Bombay: Marg Publications.

Doniger, W. (2009) *The Hindus: An Alternative History*. New York: Oxford University Press.

Dutt, M.N. (1998) *Rāmāyaṇa of Vālmīki: Sanskrit Text and English Translation*, Vol. III *Yuddha-kāṇḍa*, Ravi Prakash Arya (ed.) Delhi: Parimal Publications.

Felski, R. (2015) *The Limits of Critique*. Chicago: University of Chicago Press.

Ganeshaiah, K.N., Vasudeva, R. and Shaanker, R.U. (2009) 'In search of *Sanjeevani*'. *Current Science*, 97.4: 484–9.

Geertz, C. (1973) *The Interpretation of Cultures: Selected Essays*. New York: Basic Books.

Ghosh, P. (2016) 'A Ramayana of One's Own', in F. McGill (ed.) *The Rama Epic: Hero, Heroine, Ally, Foe*. San Francisco: Asian Art Museum, pp. 1–19.

Goldman, R.P. (1978) 'Fathers, Sons, and Gurus: Oedipal Conflict in the Sanskrit Epics', *Journal of Indian Philosophy*, 6: 325–92.

Goldman, R.P. (2016) 'Hero of a Thousand Texts', in F. McGill (ed.) *The Rama Epic: Hero, Heroine, Ally, Foe*. San Francisco: Asian Art Museum, pp. 23–33.

Goldman, R.P. and Sutherland Goldman, S. (1984–2017) *The Rāmāyaṇa of Vālmīki: An Epic of Ancient India*. Princeton: Princeton University Press.

Goldman, R.P., Sutherland Goldman, S. and van Nooten, B.A. (trans.) (2009) *The Rāmāyaṇa of Vālmīki: An Epic of Ancient India*, Vol. VI *Yuddha-kaṇḍa*. Princeton: Princeton University Press.

Jaffrelot, C. (2008) 'Hindu Nationalism and the (Not So Easy) Art of Being Offended: The *Ram Setu* Controversy', *South Asia Multidisciplinary Academic Journal*, 2: 1–17.

Kakar, S. (1982) *Shamans, Mystics, and Doctors: A Psychological Inquiry into India and Its Healing Traditions*. Chicago: University of Chicago Press.

Kāśyapasaṃhitā of Vṛddhajīvaka (microfiche), Vaidya Jādavjī Trikamjī Āchārya and Somanāth Śarmā (eds) (1938). Kathmandu: Nepal Sanskrit series, no. 1.

Lutgendorf, P. (2007) *Hanuman's Tale: The Messages of a Divine Monkey*. New York: Oxford University Press.

Lutgendorf, P. (2016) 'Ally, Devotee, Friend', in F. McGill (ed.) *The Rama Epic*. San Francisco: Asian Art Museum, pp. 147–95.

Lincoln, B. (2004) *Holy Terrors: Thinking about Religion after September 11*. Chicago: University of Chicago Press.

Meulenbeld, G.J. (1999–2002) *A History of Indian Medical Literature*. 5 vols. Groningen: E. Forsten.

Mishra, D.P. (1985) *The Search for Laṅkā*. New Delhi: Print India.

Mudur, G.S. (2005) 'Sanjeevani Maybe, Maybe Not: Experts – Herb Under Hyderabad Scanner'. *The Telegraph*, September 29.

Nanda, M. (2003) *Prophets Facing Backward: Postmodern Critiques of Science and Hindu Nationalism in India*. New Brunswick: Rutgers University Press.

Nanda, M. (2005) *The Wrongs of the Religious Right: Reflections on Science, Secularism, and Hindutva*. Delhi: Three Essays Collective.

Noll, M.A. and Livingstone, D.N. (2018) 'Introduction', in J. Hardin, R.L. Numbers and R.A. Binzey (eds) *The Warfare Between Science & Religion: The Idea That Wouldn't Die*. Baltimore: Johns Hopkins University Press, pp. 1–6.

Olivelle, P. (2017) 'The Medical Profession in Ancient India: Its Social, Religious, and Legal Status', *eJournal of Indian Medicine*, 9: 1–21.

Pagani, B. (1999) *Le Rāmāyaṇa de Vālmīki*. Canto 6: La Guerre, M. Biardeau (ed.). Paris: Gallimard.

Pande, M. (2016) 'The Sanjivani Quest: An Uttarakhand Village Hasn't Forgiven Hanuman for Defacing Their Holy Mountain'. *Scroll.in*, July 31.

Pandey, S., Shukla, A., Pandey, S. and Pandey, A. (2017) 'An Overview of Resurrecting Herb 'Sanjeevani' (*Selaginella Byropteris*) and Its Pharmacological and Ethnomedical Uses', *The Pharma Innovation Journal*, 6.2: 11–14.

Pandey, V. (2019) 'Ayodhya verdict: Indian top court gives holy site to Hindus', *BBC Online* https://www.bbc.com/news/world-asia-india-50355775, accessed 5 May 2022.

Patel, S. (2010) *Ramayana: Divine Loophole*. San Francisco: Chronicle Books.

Pollock, S. (1993) '*Rāmāyaṇa* and Political Imagination in India', *Journal of Asian Studies*, 52.2: 261–97.

Ramanujan, A.K. (1991) '300 *Rāmāyaṇas*: Five Examples and Three Thoughts on Translation', in P. Richman (ed.) *Many Rāmāyaṇas: The Diversity of Narrative Tradition in South Asia*, Berkeley, CA: University of California Press, pp. 22–49.

Richman, P. (ed.) (1991) *Many Rāmāyaṇas: The Diversity of a Narrative Tradition in South Asia*. Berkeley, CA: University of California Press.

Richman, P. (ed.) (2001) *Questioning Ramayanas: A South Asian Tradition*. Berkeley, CA: University of California Press.
Richman, P. (2008) *Ramayana Stories in Modern South India: An Anthology*. Bloomington, IN: Indiana University Press.
Ricoeur, P. (2008) *Freud and Philosophy: An Essay on Interpretation*, D. Savage (trans). Delhi: Motilal Banarsidass.
Sagar, R. (dir.) (1987–88) *Ramayan*. Mumbai: Sagar Art Enterprises and Doordarshan.
Sah, N.K., Singh, S.N.P., Sahdev, S., Banerji, S., Jha, V., Khan, Z. and Hasnain, E. (2005) 'Indian herb '*Sanjeevani*' (*Selaginella bryopteris*) can promote growth and protect against heat shock and apoptotic activities of ultra violet and oxidative stress', *Journal of Biosciences*, 30 (September): 499–505.
Sako, Y. and Mohan, R. (dirs) (1992) *Ramayana: The Legend of Prince Rama* (ラーマヤーナラーマ王子伝説 *Rāmayāna: Rāma-Ōji Densetsu*). Nippon Ramayana Film Co.
Sattar, A. (2016) *Ramayana for Children*, illustrated by Sonali Zohra. New Delhi: Juggernaut Books.
Thapar, R. (1978) *Exile and the Kingdom: Some Thoughts on the Rāmāyaṇa*. Bangalore: The Mythic Society.
Thiel-Horstmann, M. (1991) *Rāmāyaṇa and Rāmāyaṇas*. Weisbaden: Otto Harasowitz.
Vaidyanath, R. and Nishteswar., K. (2007) *A Hand Book of History of Ayurveda*. Varanasi: Chowkhamba Sanskrit Series Office.
Varma, D. (2015) 'Medicinal Plants Used During the Period of Ramayana', *International Journal for Exchange of Knowledge* 2.1: 41–4.
Venkataraman, A. (2016) 'Medicinal Herb or Myth? Indian Official Proposes Hunt for Sanjivani of Lore', *New York Times*, September 26.
Wujastyk, D. (trans.) (2003) *The Root of Ayurveda: Selections from Sanskrit Medical Writings*. Reprint edition. London: Penguin Books.
Zysk, K. (1985) *Religious Healing in the Veda: With Translations and Annotations of Medical Hymns in the Ṛgveda and the Atharvaveda and Renderings from the Corresponding Ritual Texts*, Transactions of the American Philosophical Society 75, no. 7. Philadelphia: American Philosophical Society.
Zysk, K. (1991) *Asceticism and Healing in Ancient India: Medicine in the Buddhist Monastery*. New York: Oxford University Press.
Zysk, K. (1996) *Medicine in the Veda: Religious Healing in the Veda*, Reprint ed. Delhi: Motilal Banarsidass.

5

From ‘medical men’ to ‘local health traditions’: the secularisation of medicine in portrayals of health care in India

Helen Lambert

Background

My analysis explores how the ‘medical’ domain in India has been understood and documented, with special reference to Rajasthan, a north Indian region brought under indirect rule by the British Government of India in the early nineteenth century. Rajasthan is a semi-arid area south-west of Delhi that borders present-day Pakistan to the west and Gujarat to the south. Known as Rajpootana by the British, the province was a patchwork of ‘native states’ and, throughout the colonial period, British presence was very limited. Following military action against a local ‘predatory tribe’, the Mers, in 1822 Ajmer-Merwara became the first and only district of Rajpootana to be brought under direct Government authority and a regiment that became known as the Merwara Battalion was established there (Woolbert 1905). The British also signed a series of treaties with the rulers of Rajpootana native states in 1821, after which the Jeypore Political Agency (Jaipur being the largest and wealthiest of these states) was established and the first Agent to the Governor-General of India arrived at Jaipur. A medical presence was first established in Ajmer-Merwara, perhaps initially to cater to the health needs of European officials and the Merwara Regiment, but also to respond to epidemic threats; in 1837 Lt. Col. Irwin, the first Indian Medical Service (IMS) officer posted to the region, submitted a detailed report on his investigation of ‘the plague at Jalia’ on the orders of Lt. Col. Alves, Agent to the Governor General (Government of India 1837). Irvine’s report describes his attendance on the victims, features of the disease and measures for its containment, including the posting of guards on roads in and out of the town at the behest of the cooperative local ruler. Official correspondence about the outbreak includes consideration of a military 'cordon sanitaire' to prevent northward spread into areas under direct British rule (GOI 1830–1839). This option was rejected and the outbreak eventually died down. Subsequently the identity of the 'Pali plague' as true plague was vigorously (though judging by Irvine's lucid description, erroneously) disputed by commentators on plague in India.

Generally, however, the introduction of European medicine focused on providing treatment and later on disease prevention, in the form of vaccination, for the native population. Other than Ajmer-Merwara, all Rajpootana districts remained under the authority of (mostly Hindu) local rulers and administrative relations with the Government were handled through the Foreign Department. This included arrangements for establishing medical facilities and the posting of salaried officers of the Indian Medical Service (IMS) to serve the local population (and, on a private basis, members of the royal courts). The establishment of European forms of medical care in this region therefore not only takes on a highly political cast, being dependent upon the cooperation of local rulers, but provides an interesting window into understandings of 'medicine' during a period of change.

Contrary to some accounts of 'imperial medicine' in India, British support for the development of medical facilities in this region cannot plausibly be attributed to a desire to protect the wellbeing of the British, since there were few European residents. The period following the establishment of the Political Agency saw a gradual expansion of medical facilities, as local rulers became persuaded of the value of establishing dispensaries and subsequently, hospitals for their subjects. Their investment was required to cover the costs of medical facilities, public health initiatives and non-IMS medical personnel, as part of local state expenditure. Regular returns from the medical facilities were produced from 1856 onwards and the first report on 'the present condition and the last year's progress of the Rajas' dispensaries in Rajputana' by Dr. Ebden, Agency Surgeon, details the operation of eight dispensaries, with efforts being made to establish three more. The returns show steadily increasing numbers of 'pauper sick' (denoting free medical care) being treated, from 33,500 in 1855 and 58,942 in 1866 to 68,030 in 1858, despite the closure of two dispensaries in 1857 due to the 'disturbed state of the Country' at that time (Rajputana Political Agency 1857).

Over the second half of the nineteenth century, IMS 'civil surgeon' posts were established at the capitals of all the major native states to oversee medical work in these districts, though opportunities for IMS officers to increase their income through private practice were reportedly rare, due to the lack of a European population and the relative conservatism of the 'native' population (GOI 1864). Official correspondence also attests to the difficulties of procuring high-quality 'Native Doctors' and assistants to staff the dispensaries. Some reports refer to a demand for (British) medical aid or explicitly lay claim to its political value in 'impressing the local population' (Hendley 1895). Between 1850 and 1890, at least 19 hospitals were opened in cities across Rajpootana (Government of Rajasthan 1996) and, by 1900, European medicine dispensaries were operational in all state capitals. This health care system continued to develop across the province until 1949, when the princely states were dissolved and Rajasthan became a state within the Indian federal union. Primary care continued to expand and, by 1996, there were 125 urban and 450 rural dispensaries across the state in addition to district and city hospitals. The structure of health services in postcolonial India is relatively uniform, although the budget for health is devolved to State level. There is a degree of variability in the extent to which States support non-biomedical health services; in Rajasthan, Ayurvedic dispensaries at panchayat level form part of the formal health sector.

Literature

In late nineteenth and early twentieth century India both the colonial administration and missionaries carried out ethnological surveys, with a particular focus on caste, but early ethnographers of India focused on so-called 'primitive' peoples; thus Rivers conducted research among the Toda, an Adivasi (tribal) people of the Nilgiri Hills, while Radcliffe-Brown studied the Andamanese. Notably, the posthumously published seminal contribution of Rivers (1924) to the comparative study of medicine and religion did not explicitly draw on his ethnographic work in India, which focused on genealogy. Little of this early anthropological work focused on medical or health-related phenomena. Once social anthropological interest shifted to the Hindu, Muslim and Buddhist populations of the subcontinent in the 1940s, the Indian village became the chosen unit for synchronic studies of social relations (cf. Burghart 1985) and it was only after this that health-related aspects of social life started to be documented, albeit mostly as a secondary focus.

Following Independence, anthropologists working in India started to take an interest in modernisation and development in line with more general post-Second World War trends. One aspiration was to contribute to development initiatives, given the pervasive assumption among policy makers and international health experts that the continuing use of non-biomedical forms of treatment in developing countries could be explained by cultural 'barriers' to the use of biomedicine (and the study of culture was anthropology's domain). Another was simply a desire to document the implications and consequences of the introduction of modern (bio)medicine into local understandings and management of illness. The importance of religion as an explanatory idiom for all forms of misfortune, including illness, was already well known in the discipline (cf. Evans-Pritchard 1937); anthropologists were interested in documenting shifts in aetiological understandings and treatment-seeking practices consequent on the introduction of new forms of care. Many studies (e.g. Opler 1963) offered explanations of observed preferences for 'traditional' forms of treatment in terms of what Sujatha and Abraham describe as 'cultural resistance' (2012:14), although other authors documented the interplay of faith and treatment, described hierarchies of resort between indigenous and biomedical forms of therapy, or explored the political economy of health at work in medically plural situations (e.g. Carstairs 1955; Djurfeldt and Lindberg 1975; Beals 1976). Questions of interpretation aside, anthropological research into the medical domain between the 1950s–1970s mainly focused on lay people's aetiological concepts and practical actions relating to treatment of illness, sometimes designating their subject as 'folk medicine' (Khare 1963; Jaggi 1973). These accounts either explicitly (Mandelbaum 1970; Carstairs 1955) or otherwise positioned their material in relation to local religious practice but did not situate themselves as studies of Indian 'medicine'. That domain had come to be understood as the province of Indologists studying the 'classical' texts underpinning the codified traditions of Ayurveda and, to a lesser extent, Unani and Siddha.

The anthropological accounts of local treatment formations overlapped extensively with studies of affliction and ritual healing, especially with respect to spirit possession, that were rooted in local cosmologies. They were portrayed as aspects of the 'little traditions' (Marriott 1955) that were seen as locally variable and associated with village society, in contrast to the unitary 'great tradition' associated with Sanskritic Hindu beliefs and practices. Studies of both traditions were mainly concerned with 'religion' but encompassed, particularly in respect of 'little tradition' folk practice, research on phenomena such as spirit and divine possession and treatment at shrines broadly understood as concerned with illness and its management (such as Opler 1958; Carstairs 1961; Freed and Freed 1964; Fuchs 1964). Thus Carstairs, an anthropologist and psychiatrist, described *bhakti* worship before turning to *bhopa* who officiate and treat illness at regional shrines through possession, village gods, veneration of ancestors and 'supernatural beliefs', under which he considered omens, evil spirits and ghosts and witches to whom illnesses were commonly attributed. While contributing to the understanding of local therapeutic practices and the cultural management of ill health, these accounts were not described as being about 'medicine'.

In the 1970s, two shifts occurred in social science approaches to the study of the medical sphere, one empirical, the other analytic. First, Indian sociological and public health commentators began to argue that biomedicine was readily accepted and that the continuing use of other therapies was less a matter of 'cultural barriers' than a response to the relative inaccessibility and poor quality of biomedical care in rural areas (Banerji 1973). In reality, preferment of 'English medicine' – as biomedicine is termed in Hindi – for the treatment of certain complaints had been evident from at least the late nineteenth century (Lambert 1995, 1997). Other sociologists and anthropologists began to study biomedicine and aspects of the formation of modern health services (Madan 1969, 1972; Minocha 1980; Jeffery 1988). However, most anthropological scholarship retained a focus on local responses to illness and cultural dimensions of therapy and paid relatively little attention to the political economy of health care provision or to differentials in access to the range of medical forms.

At this time, anthropologists interested in indigenous approaches to the management of health problems began to deploy sets of distinctions that were becoming well established in the newly developing field of medical anthropology, such as those between 'disease' and 'illness' and between 'curing' and 'healing', as well as the concept of 'medical pluralism'. Lengthy debates over these terminologies occupied a large volume of print space in the general medical anthropological literature of the 1980s and 1990s. Their salience to the Indian context is demonstrated by the inclusion of a largely theoretical paper on the illness/disease distinction by US medical anthropologist Robert Hahn in a special issue of *Contributions to Asian Studies* otherwise devoted to 'South Asian systems of healing'. Apart from a paper by Daniel on the pulse in Siddha medicine, the other seven papers all concerned ritual and spiritual forms of treatment. The underlying rationale for this is evident in the guest editors' introductory remarks to Claus's study of Tulu spirit possession, which considers, 'a theme which resonates through the other essays, namely, that spirit possession is a religious phenomenon and a complex mode of personal experience which cannot be adequately described as a medical phenomenon in the biomedical sense' (Daniel and Pugh 1984: IX). Most subsequent anthropological work across the globe has continued to pursue these approaches, on the basis that biomedicine's individualist focus gives insufficient weight to intersubjective meaning and the individual sufferer's positioning in a social world. However, such attempts to resist biomedical reductionism effectively ceded 'medicine' as a category entirely to *bio*medicine. This has been reinforced by the preferment of the term 'healing' solely to describe non-biomedical treatment, even while studies of the relationships between indigenous and biomedical forms of treatment in different settings increasingly came under the overarching rubric of 'medical pluralism' (Leslie 1980). The refusal to recognise the possibility of 'healing' as contained in all medical encounters including biomedical ones has, in the Indian setting, produced a terminological inconsistency between anthropological approaches to (non-biomedical) 'healing' and scholarship on the codified traditions of Indian 'medicine'.

From the late 1970s onwards, in part due to Louis Dumont's use of Indological materials and his emphasis on the civilisational character of Indian culture in his seminal work on caste (1970), anthropologists began turning away from village-based studies that included the empirical study of 'folk' (including religious) aspects of therapy to focus on social and cultural institutions that could be seen as part of mainstream Indian civilisation. The seminal contribution of Charles Leslie (1976) reinforced the emphasis on attending to textual authority as manifest in the 'classical', textually based or 'codified' medical traditions. Most anthropological research on medical traditions in India since the 1980s has focused on the codified 'systems' of Ayurveda, Unani and Siddha (see e.g. Langford 2002; contributions to Leslie 1976; Leslie and Young 1992; Sujatha and Abraham 2012; Zimmerman 1982), despite the fact that these forms of medicine, at least until recently, only served an elite minority of the population. Anthropological scholarship on the codified traditions has increasingly converged with that of historians of Indian medicine to document selective processes of legitimation ongoing since at least the 1860s, whereby these indigenous medical traditions have been reformulated into professionalised and accredited knowledge systems (Leslie 1976; Langford 2002; Attewell 2005, 2007; Banerjee 2009; Hardiman 2009).

Sources

Apart from the published ethnographic literature reviewed in the previous section, my sources are mainly government documents from British and Indian national and regional archives and contemporary policy documents. My reading of these secondary sources is broadly informed by a background of long-term ethnographic research work since 1984 conducted primarily in the erstwhile Jeypoor State, both in Jaipur city and in a rural area which is now part of Tonk District. My initial research in the 1980s sought to document *all* forms of popular therapeutic practice used by ordinary local people in that part of Rajasthan (Lambert 1989), with the initial aim that I would thereby be characterising the local 'healthcare system' (Kleinman 1980). The diverse array of diverse therapeutic forms that I found to be in use did not, though, appear to be integrated in any coherent 'systemic' form, although I discerned coherent cultural logics underlying many of these approaches to the management of health problems (Lambert 1992, 2013). The therapeutic formations and treatment trajectories I documented as responses to illness in Jaipur and in and around a multi-caste, predominantly Hindu village with a few Muslim and tribal families, included (in no particular order) the widespread use of *mantra*, *jhara* (ritual sweeping) and/or herbal medicines from lay specialists and religious officiants for a wide range of health problems; treatment at local shrines from deities who regularly became embodied in their shrine priests including for snakebite (the specialist domain of the deity Tejaji) and miscarriage (caused by the spirit of a dead foetus, or witchcraft); injections, saline drips and pharmaceuticals from private, mostly unqualified, practitioners of allopathy; local manipulative procedures to treat abdominal discomfort (see Lambert 2012a) and sprains; the occasional use of cautery for infant pneumonia; the occasional use of Ayurvedic medicines from the poorly attended government Ayurvedic dispensary; and some use of antenatal care and family planning offered by the local auxiliary nurse-midwife (summarised in Lambert 1996).

In earlier analyses of this ethnographic material and of documentary accounts from the colonial period I sought to unsettle the conceptions of 'folk medicine' that dominate the literature described in the previous section, that portray local therapeutics as essentially religious and largely unaffected by secular trends. I showed that the establishment of European dispensaries and hospitals preceded the decline of folk specialists in surgery (*sathiyas* or couchers, *jarrahas* or barber surgeons, lithotomists) (Lambert 1995, 1997b).

Further background source material that broadly informs the analysis of this chapter was gathered during more recent field research (2009–2010) in Jaipur on vernacular practitioners known as 'bone doctors' (Lambert 2012a, 2012b) and in national and regional archives in Delhi and Jaipur pursuing early British accounts of medicine in Rajasthan. I also conducted some subsequent archival work in the Africa and Asia archives (previously the India Office) of the British Library in London. Archival sources included all documents pertaining to Rajpootana, medicine and associated entries in the National Archive of India Foreign Department Registers from 1830–1912 and the Rajpootana Dispensary Returns from 1864 onwards (appearing from 1875 as combined annual Rajpootana Dispensary, Vaccination, Jail, and Sanitary Reports once these facilities and procedures had been established at the provincial capitals), and eight 'medico-topographical' accounts by Indian Medical Service officers serving in various Rajpootana provinces that were published between 1895–1912 at the behest of Civil Surgeon Col. T.H. Hendley, as well as Hendley's own *General Medical History of Rajputana* (1900). An obvious limitation of these archival sources is that they include few indigenous documents. Official documents pertaining to the former Jaipur State in Rajputana are not accessible, as the state archives have been closed for some years due to an inheritance dispute within the erstwhile royal family. However, these and the Rajasthan State archives at Bikaner contain material only up to the end of the colonial period and thus have limited relevance to the present discussion. Moreover, my focus is primarily on the ways in which public depictions of 'medicine' in governmental and scholarly accounts have changed in the modern period, rather than in local portrayals. The following sections thus draw on analysis of the available archival sources from British observers of the regional scene, mostly by Indian Medical Service officers, of local medical formations and on publicly available Government of India policy documents.

Analysis

British accounts of 'medicine' in Rajputana

Of greatest import for this analysis is that in all colonial records and accounts reviewed for the last half of the nineteenth century, all forms of treatment for ill health are characterised as 'medical'. No distinctions are drawn between the 'medical' and the 'religious' in relation to the source or content of the therapeutic procedure. Thus, the section on 'Medical Aid' in Archibald Adams's book-length account of the western Rajputana States (1899) lists 'four main classes of medical men' including, 'I Sadhs or Ascetics [...], II Baids or Hindu practitioners [...], III Hakims or Mahomdean physicians [...], IV Pansaris or Attars [who] are prescribing chemists [...]' (1899: 54). Surgery is described as mainly in the hands of barbers, but also to some extent 'Zarrahs or Mohamedan surgeons, and amputations were often performed by Rajput swordsmen…' (Adams 1899: 255); Sojat Sathias practised couching and 'village specialists' treated guinea worm, while the actual cautery was used to treat rheumatic ailments.

Likewise, the description of 'Medical Aid' in Hendley's *Medico-topographical account of Jaipur* (1895) lists seven types including 'Baids, or Hindu physicians', 'Jain priests or *jaties*, and other priests', 'Hakims or Mohammedan physicians', '*Jarrahs* or barber-surgeons', 'Sathyas or couchers', 'Bairagis or Hindu, and fakirs or Musalman, devotees; wise women; clever persons who drive out diseases by aid of the jharu or broom and charms', and 'Pansaris or druggists' (see Lambert 1995, 1997 for a fuller account).

Other reports by officers of the Indian Medical Service vary widely in the numbers and types of practitioners described and in the degree of detail provided, but none distinguish therapies or practitioners with a religious dimension or designation from 'medical' ones, even when (as in at least two cases) the authors indicate detailed knowledge of specific Ayurvedic or Unani therapeutics. Regardless of writers' opinions as to the efficacy of the treatments described, there was no hesitation to describe the work of (for example) Jain priests or the use of 'charms' as 'medical'. What, then, needs to be accounted for is the fact that a half-century later, the compass of what is officially described as 'medicine' had narrowed to refer exclusively to those procedures and practitioners that are non-religious in character.

Post-independence official accounts of medicine and health services in Rajasthan

The District Gazeteers published by each State offer a glimpse into postcolonial characterisations of the content of the medical domain. The 1964 Gazeteer for Bundi (a district of Rajasthan) includes a chapter on 'Medical and public health services' that begins with a section on 'Early History'. This appears to be transcribed directly from (though unattributed to) the 1899 medico-topographical account by Adams excerpted in the previous section; *vaidyas*, *hakims*, *pansaris* and *fakirs* or *Bairagi sadhus* are described as the 'four classes of medical men' upon whom the populace depended, as well as barbers and *jarrahs* who practised 'crude surgery'

(Dhoundiyal 1964: 248). A section headed 'Traditional Remedies' then observes that, 'Besides the *ayurvedic* and *unani* systems of medicine, which were scientific, the following old methods of treatment were followed...', and lists *Agnikaran Chikitsa* (referred to in earlier accounts as *gul* or actual cautery), *Seengadi* (blood-letting), *Khangi* ('an oil massage used in cases of dislocated bones and strained muscles', p. 249) and '*mantras* (incantations), *tantras* (spells), *jharas* (exorcism) and *phoonka* (charms)', the use of amulets for preventing disease, and visits to specific shrines, listed by name and Tehsil. This officially sanctioned rendering of the medical domain differs from the colonial accounts of the turn of the century that it reproduces in only one respect. It separates off Ayurveda and Unani as 'scientific' 'systems of medicine' from other 'old methods', which include both faith-based and non-religious modes of treatment. This segregation of certain Indian codified traditions as 'scientific systems of medicine' alongside biomedicine is a likely consequence of the espousal of Ayurveda and (to a lesser extent) Unani as part of the nationalist project (Khan 2006), together with the requirement to represent India as a modern nation-state.

A more recent Gazeteer for Rajasthan State (Government of Rajasthan 1996) provides a detailed account of 'Medical and public health services' that notes India's fortune 'in having an indigenous system of medicine even in the beginning of the Christian era' (1996: 302) but goes on to observe that, 'in the remote areas of the State, even now', disease is often attributed to 'a variety of supernatural forces, the wrath of gods, the work of demons, malefactory influences exerted by the stars on human lives or malicious acts of magic and witchcraft'. It describes faith in the efficacy of exactly the same list of remedies given in the 1964 Gazeteer and elaborates on that account by noting that 'Religion is closely associated with healing and the priest is not infrequently also the medicine man', before going on to note the attribution of small pox, chicken pox and measles to feminine deities and how these are dealt with, as well as listing some of the rituals undertaken to ward off evil planetary influences. A subsequent section entitled, 'Medical History of Rajputana' reproduces the seven-fold categorisation of medical aid from Hendley's *General Medical History* (1900) verbatim but additionally attributes to this source three further categories that do not appear in the original account: '8, *Syana, Bhopa, Abhona* (persons said to be possessed by a god or goddess), 9, Massagists and Bone Setters [...] and 10, Snake charmers (or *Saperas*) [...]' (1996:304). It then gives an overview of the introduction and development of European medicine drawing on sources cited in the previous section of this chapter and a selection of Annual Dispensary Returns. The section concludes that even those in remote villages:

> have come to understand the usefulness of allopathy. The Ayurvedic system of medicine has also been receiving government's attention. It is generally accepted that the system is useful one and should be given due recognition and encouragement. Accordingly, Ayurvedic dispensaries have been opened. ... The *Unani* system of medicine has got a serious setback following the migration of most of the Hakims, and only a few *Hakims* and *Attars* prescribe Unani medicines now. (1996: 308–9)

The remainder of the chapter exhaustively records all biomedical hospitals and dispensaries in Rajasthan by province. Thus, while providing a rather comprehensive overview of the diverse treatments and practitioners to which the Rajasthan population have had recourse, in this late twentieth-century account, all those that are not part of the European, Ayurvedic or Unani 'systems of medicine' are firmly situated as part of medical *history*.

Health policy and the portrayal of medicine in contemporary India

Contemporary accounts of health care in India mostly adopt a similar approach to that described in the last section as emergent in post-Independence official documents. 'Indian medicine' is taken to consist of the institutionalised codified medical traditions, primarily those that are indigenous (Ayurveda, Unani and Siddha) although most of the indigenous 'systems' of medicine are themselves not unitary and include both college-trained, qualified practitioners and 'traditional' providers who have acquired expertise through informal transmission of knowledge and practice (cf. Sebastia 2012; Jansen 2011). In addition to these, health care in India includes the introduced traditions of biomedicine or 'allopathy' and homeopathy. Throughout the second half of the twentieth century Indian government policy concerning non-biomedical forms of health care remained consistent in recognising three 'Indian Systems of Medicine' (ISM), originally defined as Ayurveda, Unani and Siddha, to the exclusion of all non-textually based and other traditions. In 1995, the Ministry of Health and Family Welfare (MOHFW) created a Department of Indian Systems of Medicine & Homeopathy (ISM&H) to oversee non-biomedical elements of the formal health system.

A significant shift occurred at the start of the present century, however, when in 2003 the MOHFW renamed the Department of ISM&H the Department of Ayurveda, Yoga and Naturopathy, Unani, Siddha and Homeopathy, or 'AYUSH' (Government of India 2003, 2010; Chandra 2011). Since then governmental recognition has further expanded from the original four non-biomedical systems ('ISM&H') to seven officially recognised 'systems', with Sowa Rigpa ('Tibetan medicine') being added in 2010. The acronym AYUSH (*ayush* meaning 'long life' in Sanskrit) has rapidly become a widely used generic descriptor among policy makers, practitioners and sections of the urban public for all non-allopathic forms of treatment. Of course, the 'AYUSH' traditions only have in common the fact that they are not biomedical and, as far as the MoHFW is concerned, are regulated through State-accredited training institutions that award officially recognised degrees (see Lambert 2012 for a fuller account).

Shortly after the formation of the AYUSH Department, the Government of India launched a major initiative to improve primary health care in several Indian States recognised as having particularly poor health service infrastructures. This National Rural Health Mission (NRHM) mandates the posting of a qualified 'AYUSH' practitioner as well as a qualified MBBS (biomedical) doctor at all primary health care centres covered by the NRHM, meaning that practitioners with an accredited degree from any one of the recognised systems of medicine may now obtain government employment as an 'AYUSH doctor' in primary care (Ministry of Health and Family Welfare, n.d.). This initiative signals governmental recognition and institutionalisation of an expanded range of non-biomedical traditions, albeit homogenised within the generic category of 'AYUSH', in the formal health sector. Unregulated therapeutic traditions not included under the components of AYUSH have also been recognised in government policy for the first time, with 'support for revitalisation of local health traditions' (Planning Commission 2008: 114) declared to be part of AYUSH planning strategy in India's eleventh Five-Year Plan. The characterisation of these uncodified traditions as requiring 'revitalisation' (Planning Commission 2008), though, perpetuates a view of these traditions as residua which are in the process of disappearing that is similar to the assumptions contained in much of the anthropological literature reviewed previously. 'Local health traditions' or 'LHTs' are not defined in the Planning Commission or NRHM policy documents, but the implementation activities specified for the 'LHTs' refer to the retrieval, testing and promotion of medicinal plants (Ministry of Health and Family Welfare, n.d.), implying that the primary content of 'LHTs' is ethnobotanical knowledge. Indeed, a pilot scheme to provide accreditation to 'Local Health Practitioners' run by Indira Gandhi Open University offers training and registration only to practitioners who use exclusively medicinal treatment (Roy 2012).

Conclusions

In this chapter I have taken the category of 'medicine' as an object of inquiry, attempting to trace its historical formation and avoiding theoretical definitions in favour of an inductive approach that treats temporal shifts in the boundaries between 'medicine' and 'religion' as emergent from the ethnographic and historical material. Maintaining a separation between ethnographic object and analytic construct allows us to see these categories as produced by particular actors and agents of governance, and to situate shifts in their content over time in relation to the specific cultural, political and institutional positions these agents occupy. This analytic strategy, rooted in Edwin Ardener's 'Oxford School' (McDonald 2017: 206–7) of social anthropology (elements of which are seen in the recent 'ontological' turn), takes language and naming practices seriously as guides to people's realities (Ardener 1982). My account therefore characterises all interventions that aim to alleviate ill health neutrally as 'therapeutic practices', since the selective use of formulations such as 'healing', 'belief' or 'ritual' smuggle normative assumptions regarding mode of action or efficacy into the analysis of archival and ethnographic data. By not taking the categories of 'religion' or 'medicine' as pre-determined, this analytic strategy has allowed me to identify when and how therapeutic practices in one region of India became medical or non-medical.

India is often portrayed as an exemplar of thriving medical pluralism (e.g. Sujatha and Abraham 2012). The codified traditions have been described as 'medical systems' that are contributing to an expansion in the range of therapeutic forms available elsewhere in the world (see e.g. Banerjee 2009; Bode 2006, 2008 describes the commodification of Ayurvedic preparations and Zimmerman 1992 discusses changes in Ayurveda consequent on its uptake among Westerners). Reciprocally, introduced traditions (initially biomedicine but subsequently homeopathy from the early twentieth century and more recently, acupuncture and acupressure) have expanded the medical diversity found within the subcontinent (Bhardwaj 2010).

These contemporary portrayals mask significant shifts in the content of what is taken to constitute 'medicine' over the past 150 years. In this chapter I have shown that between the mid-nineteenth and the late twentieth centuries, the content of the medical domain as represented in documentary accounts produced by and for the state contracted and then, in the early twenty-first century, expanded again. In policy and official accounts, the term 'medicine' has come to designate solely non-religious forms of treatment and in most ethnographic accounts, biomedicine alone. The shift has been most significant with respect to therapeutic forms that can also be referred to under the rubric of 'cultural aspects', 'folk tradition', 'healing', 'religion', 'ritual' or 'superstition' but in colonial accounts were also classified as 'medical'.

Most recently the types of therapy afforded governmental recognition as 'systems of medicine' have expanded, with a commensurate contraction in what is classified as 'medical' outside the formal sector; only informal 'health' traditions which are exclusively *medicinal* in content are a legitimate focus of government planning. The interface between medicine and religion has thereby shifted progressively towards a redefinition of medicine as exclusively secular, materialist and transmissible through accredited training. Anthropological research and official representations of India's 'medical pluralism' alike have paid relatively little attention to the official and unofficial hierarchies between therapeutic traditions, or to historical shifts in these hierarchies (cf. Attewell, Hardiman, Lambert and Mukharji 2012). Since the 1980s, social science and historical research has mainly focused either on the codified traditions (e.g. Abraham 2009; Sebastia 2012) or on religious therapeutic modalities (e.g. Barrett 2008; Sax 2009), with only a few studies documenting contemporary vernacular therapeutic practices that are not categorisable under 'AYUSH' (Mukharji 2006; Hardiman and Mukharji 2012; Lambert 2013; Attewell 2016). In ceasing to attend to non-codified and subaltern therapeutics, most scholarship on 'Indian medicine' has implicitly endorsed the state's modernist narrative of decline regarding these therapeutic forms. 'Medicine' has come to constitute an appropriate designation only for those 'systems' amenable to naturalistic and rationalist renderings. There has been – in scholarship and official accounts if not in reality – a progressive erasure of vernacular therapeutics.

In this chapter I have attempted to trace the historical formation of the categories of 'religion' and 'medicine' as empirical objects of inquiry that are produced by particular actors and agents of governance, and then to situate shifts in the content of these categories over time in relation to the specific cultural and political positions occupied by these agents. I have avoided theoretical definitions in favour of an inductive approach, treating the shifting boundaries of these categories as emergent from my ethnographic and historical material. By not taking the categories of 'religion' or 'medicine' for granted, this analytic strategy – which draws on interpretative anthropological approaches to the study of classification – has allowed me to identify when and how therapeutic practices in one region of India became divided into medicine and non-medicine.

Bibliography

Abraham, L. (2009) 'Medicine As Culture: Indigenous Medicine in Cosmopolitan Mumbai', *Economic and Political Weekly*, XLIV.16: 68–75.

Adams, A. (1899) *The Western Rajputana States: A Medico-topographical and General Account of Marwar, Sirohi, Jaisalmer*. London: Junior Army and Navy Stores. British Library.

Ardener, E. (1982) 'Social anthropology, language, and reality', in D. Parkin (ed.) *Semantic Anthropology*. ASA Monographs 22. London: Academic Press, pp. 1–14.

Attewell, G. (2005) 'The End of the Line? The Fracturing of Authoritative *Tibbi* Knowledge in Twentieth-century India', *Asian Medicine*, 1.2: 387–419.

Attewell, G. (2007) *Refiguring Unani Tibb: Plural Healing in Late Colonial India*. Hyderabad & New Delhi: Orient Longman.

Attewell, G. (2016) Alignments? X-ray Diversions, Haptics, Credibility – With a 'Bone-Setting' Clinic in Hyderabad City. *Medical Anthropology* 35(1): 5–16.

Attewell, G., Hardiman, D., Lambert, H. and Mukharji, P.B. (2012) 'Agendas', in D. Hardiman and P.B. Mukharji (eds) *Medical Marginality in South Asia: Situating Subaltern Therapeutics*. London; New York: Routledge, pp. 1–5.

Banerjee, M. (2009) *Power, Knowledge, Medicine: Ayurvedic Pharmaceuticals at Home and in the World*. Hyderabad: Orient Blackswan.

Banerji, D. (1973) 'Health Behaviour of Rural Populations: Impact of Rural Health Services', *Economic and Political Weekly*, VIII.51: 2261–8.

Barrett, R. (2008) *Aghor Medicine: Pollution, Death, and Healing in Northern India*. Berkeley, CA: University of California Press.

Beals, A. (1976) 'Strategies of Resort to Curers in South India', in C. Leslie (ed.) *Asian Medical Systems*. Berkeley, CA: University of California Press, pp. 184–200.

Bhardwaj, R. (2010) 'Medical Pluralism in India: The Interface of Complementary and Alternative Therapies with Allopathy', in A. Mishra (ed.) *Health, Illness and Medicine: Ethnographic Readings*. Hyderabad: Orient Blackswan, pp. 30–60.

Bode, M. (2006) 'Taking Traditional Knowledge to the Market: The Commodization of Indian Medicine', *Anthropology and Medicine*, 13.3: 225–36.

Bode, M. (2008) *Taking Traditional Knowledge to the Market: The Modern Image of the Ayurvedic and Unani Industry 1980–2000*. Hyderabad: Orient Blackswan.

Burghart, R. (1985) 'Introduction: Theoretical Approaches in the Anthropology of South Asia', in R. Burghart and A. Cantlie (eds) *Indian Religion*. London: Curzon Press, pp. 1–14.

Carstairs, M. (1955) 'Medicine and Faith in Rural Rajasthan', in B. Paul (ed.) *Health, Culture and Community: Case Studies of Public Reactions to Health Programs*. New York: Russell Sage Foundation, pp. 104–34.

Carstairs, G.M. (1961) 'Patterns of Religious Observance in Three Villages of Rajasthan', in L.P. Vidyarthi (ed.) *Aspects of Religion in Indian Society*. Meerut: Kedarnath Ramnath, pp. 59–113.

Chandra, S. (2011) *Status of Indian Medicine and Folk Healing*. New Delhi: Department of AYUSH, Ministry of Health and Family Welfare, Government of India.

Daniel, E.V. and Pugh, J.F. (1984) 'Introduction', in E.V. Daniel and J.F. Pugh (eds) *South Asian Systems of Healing*. Brill: Leiden, pp. i–x.

Dhoundiyal, B.N. (1964) *Rajasthan District Gazeteers: Bundi*. Jaipur: Government of Rajasthan. National Archive of India.

Djurfeldt, G. and Lindberg, S. (1975) *Pills Against Poverty: A Study of the Introduction of Western Medicine in a Tamil Village*. Lund: Curzon.

Dumont, L. (1970) *Homo Hierarchicus*. Chicago: University of Chicago Press.

Evans-Pritchard, E.E. (1937) *Witchcraft, Oracles and Magic among the Azande*. Oxford: Clarendon Press.

Freed, S.A. and Freed, R.S. (1964) 'Spirit Possession as Illness in a North Indian Village', *Ethnology*, 3: 152–71.

Fuchs, S. (1964) 'Magic Healing Techniques among the Balahis in Central India', in A. Kiev (ed.) *Magic, Faith and Healing: Studies in Primitive Psychiatry Today*. London: Free Press of Glencoe, Collier-Macmillan, pp. 121–38.

Goodbody, C.M. (n.d.) *Medico-topographical report on Tonk State*. Ajmer: Scottish Mission Industries Co. Ltd. National Archive of India.

Government of India (1837) *Foreign, Political* No. 72. National Archive of India.

Government of India (1864) *Foreign, General A*, March 1864, Nos 182–185. National Archive of India.

Government of India (1864) *Foreign, General A*, March 1864. Dr. Lownds' report on the Raj Dispensaries in Rajastha. No.182. National Archive of India.

Government of India (1866) *Dr. Lownds's report on the Rajpootana Dispensaries for the half year ending 31st Dec.1865. Foreign. General A.* Aug.1866. Nos. 20–23. National Archive of India.

Government of India (1866) *From the Agent to the Governor General for the States of Rajpootana, to the Secretary to the Government of India, Foreign Department, with the Governor General, No.655–109G, Mount Aboo, the 14th May 1866*. No.20. National Archive of India.

Government of India (1882) *Annual Report of the Jeypore Medical Institutions*. Maharaja's Public Library, Jaipur.

Government of India (2003) Department of AYUSH, http://indianmedicine.nic.in/, accessed 26 January 2011.

Government of India (2010) *Annual Report to the People on Health*. Ministry of Health and Family Welfare, September 2010, http://www.mohfw.nic.in/showfile.php?lid=121, accessed 18 October 2012.

Government of Rajasthan (1996) *Rajasthan State Gazeteer Vol.IV: Administration and Public Welfare*. Jaipur: Government of Rajasthan Directorate, District Gazeteers. National Archive of India.

Hardiman, D. (2009) 'Indian Medical Indigeneity: From Nationalist Assertion to the Global Market', *Social History*, 34.3: 263–83.

Hardiman, D. and Mukharji, P.B. (2012; eds) *Medical Marginality in South Asia: Situating Subaltern Therapeutics*. London; New York: Routledge.

Hendley, T.H. (1895) *A medico-topographical account of Jeypore*. Calcutta: Calcutta Central Press Company. National Archive of India.

Hendley, T.H. (1900) *General medical history of Rajputana*. Calcutta: Office of the Superintendant of Government Printing. National Archive of India.

Irvine, R.H. (1941) *Some account of the General and Medical topography of Ajmeer*. Calcutta: W. Thacker & Co., St. Andrew's Library. National Archive of India.

Jaggi, O.P. (1973) *History of Science and Technology in India, Vol. III: Folk Medicine*. Atma Ram.

Jansen, E. (2011) '"It Is Like Playing with Fire" – The Politics of Registering Naturopaths in South India', Paper presentation, EASA Conference on *Medical Pluralism: Techniques, Politics, Institutions*, Rome, September 2011.

Jeffery, R. (1988) *The Politics of Health in India*. Berkeley, CA: University of California Press.

Khan, S. (2006) 'Systems of Medicine and Nationalist Discourse in India: Towards "New Horizons" in Medical Anthropology and History', *Social Science and Medicine*, 62: 2786–97.

Khare, R.S. (1963) 'Folk Medicine in a North Indian Village', *Human Organization*, 22: 36–40.

Kleinman A. (1980) *Patients and Healers in the Context of Culture: An Exploration of the Borderland between Anthropology, Medicine, and Psychiatry*. Berkeley, CA: University of California Press.

Lambert, H. (1989) 'Medical Knowledge in Rural Rajasthan: Popular Constructions of Illness and Therapeutic Practice'. DPhil thesis, University of Oxford.

Lambert, H. (1992) 'The Cultural Logic of Indian Medicine: Prognosis and Etiology in Rajasthani Popular Therapeutics', *Social Science and Medicine*, 34.10: 1069–76.

Lambert, H. (1995) 'Of Bonesetters and Barber-surgeons: Therapeutic Traditions and the Spread of Allopathic Medicine in Rajasthan', in N.K. Singhi (ed.) *Folk, Faith and Feudalism*. Jaipur: Rawat Publishers, pp. 92–111.

Lambert, H. (1996) 'Popular Therapeutics and Medical Preferences in Rural North India', *The Lancet*, 348: 1706–9.

Lambert, H. (1997) 'Plural traditions? Folk therapeutics and "English" medicine in Rajasthan', in A. Cunningham and B. Andrews (eds) *Western Medicine as Contested Knowledge*. Manchester: Manchester University Press, pp. 191–211.

Lambert, H. (2012a) 'Wrestling with Tradition: Towards a Subaltern Therapeutics of Bonesetting and Vessel Treatment in North India', in D. Hardiman and P.B. Mukharji (eds) *Medical Marginality in South Asia: Situating Subaltern Therapeutics*. London; New York: Routledge, pp. 109–25.

Lambert, H. (2012b) Medical Pluralism and Medical Marginality: Bone Doctors and the Selective Legitimation of Therapeutic Expertise in India, *Social Science & Medicine*, 74: 1029–36.

Lambert, H. (2015) 'Medicine', in K. von Stuckrad and R. Segal (eds) *Vocabulary for the Study of Religion*. Leiden: Brill.

Lambert, H. (2013) 'The Management of Sickness in an Indian Medical Vernacular', in I. Vargas-O'Bryan and X. Zhong (eds) *Disease, Religion and Healing in Asia: Collaborations and Collisions*. London; New York: Routledge, pp. 9–21.

Langford, J. (2002) *Fluent Bodies: Ayurvedic Remedies for Postcolonial Imbalance*. New Delhi: Oxford University Press.

Leslie, C. (ed.) (1976) *Asian Medical Systems: A Comparative Study*. Berkeley, CA: University of California Press.

Leslie, C. (1980) 'Medical Pluralism in World Perspective', *Social Science and Medicine*, 14b.4: 190–6.

Leslie, C. and Young, A. (eds) (1992) *Paths to Asian Medical Knowledge*. Berkeley, CA: University of California Press.

Madan, T.N. (1969) 'Who Chooses Modern Medicine and Why', *Economic and Political Weekly*, IV.37: 1475–84.

Madan, T.N. (1972) 'Doctors in a North Indian City: Recruitment, Role Perception and Role Performance', in S. Saberwal (ed.) *Beyond the Village: Sociological Explorations*. Simla: Indian Institute of Advanced Study, pp. 79–105.

Mandelbaum, D. (1970) *Society in India. Vol. II: Change and continuity*. Berkeley and Los Angeles, CA: University of California Press.

Marriott, M. (1955) 'Little Communities in an Indigenous Civilization', in M. Marriott and A. Beals (eds) *Village India: Studies in the Little Community*. Chicago: University of Chicago Press, pp. 171–222.

McDonald, M. (2017) The ontological turn meets the certainty of death. *Anthropology & Medicine*, 24(2): 205–20.

Ministry of Health and Family Welfare (n.d.) *National Rural Health Mission (2005–2012) Mission document*, http://mohfw.nic.in/NRHM/Documents/Mission_Document.pdf, accessed 26 January 2011.

Minocha, A.A. (1980) 'Medical Pluralism and Health Services in India,' *Social Science and Medicine* 14B.4: 217–23.

Mukharji, P.B. (2006) 'Going Beyond Elite Medical Traditions: The Case of Chandshi', *Asian Medicine: Tradition and Modernity*, 2.2: 277–91.

Opler, M. (1958) 'Spirit Possession in a Rural Area of Northern India', in W. Lessa and E. Vogt (eds) *Reader in Comparative Religion. Part XI: Portraits of Religious Systems*. Illinois: Row, Peterson & Co., pp. 553–66.

Opler, M.E. (1963) 'The Cultural Definition of Illness in Village India', *Human Organization*, 22: 32–5.

Pank, P.D. (1900) *A Medico-topographical Account of Ajmere, Rajputana. With Additional Notes by Lt.Col. D. Ffrench-Mullen, M.D.IMS, Civil Surgeon, Ajmere*. Calcutta: Office of the Superintendent of Government Printing. British Library

Planning Commission, Government of India (2008) *Eleventh Five Year Plan (2007–12) in Social Sector*, Vol. II. New Delhi: Oxford University Press.

Rajputana Political Agency (1857) Report from Dr. Ebden, Agency Surgeon, on the Raja's Dispensaries in Rajputana with Tabular figs. For the year 1st July 1856–1st July 1857. Foreign. Political. No. 349. National Archive of India.

Rivers, W.H.R. (1924) *Medicine, Magic and Religion*. London; New York: Routledge.

Roy, D. (2012) 'The IGNOU (Indira Gandhi National Open University) Method for Certification of Traditional Folk Practitioners and Practices', paper presented at workshop, *Integrating Traditional South Asian Medicine into Modern Health Care Systems*, Jawarharlal Nehru University, Delhi, October 2012.

Sax, W. (2009) *God of Justice: Ritual Healing and Social Justice in the Central Himalayas*. Oxford: Oxford University Press.

Sebastia, B. (2012) 'Competing for Medical Space: Traditional Practitioners in the Transmission and Promotion of Siddha Medicine', in V. Sujatha and L. Abraham (eds) *Medical Pluralism in Contemporary India*. Hyderabad: Orient Blackswan, pp. 165–85.

Shore, R. (1909) *Medico-topographical Account of Mewar*. Calcutta: Office of the Superintendent of Government Printing. British Library.

Sujatha, V. and Abraham L. (2012) 'Introduction' in V. Sujatha and L. Abraham (eds) *Medical Pluralism in Contemporary India*. Hyderabad: Orient Blackswan, pp. 1–34.

Woolbert, H.R. (1905) *Medico-topographical Account of the Merwara regiment*. Calcutta: Office of the Superintendent of Government Printing. British Library

Zimmerman, F. (1982) *The Jungle and the Aroma of Meats: An Ecological Theme in Hindu Medicine*. Berkeley, CA: University of California Press.

Zimmerman, F. (1992) 'Gentle purge: The flower power of Ayurveda', in C. Leslie and A. Young (eds) *Paths to Asian Medical Knowledge*. Berkeley, CA: University of California Press, pp. 209–23.

6

Sound medicine: towards a nomadology of medical *mantras* in seventeenth to twentieth-century Bengal

Projit Bihari Mukharji

Background

On 14th June 2014, a leading Bengali daily, *Anandabajar Patrika*, published a report headlined '*Bodhuke Sarate Arbi Mantra Ojhar*' (Ojha uses Arabic Mantra to Cure Housewife). The report went on to describe the case of a young Bengali Hindu housewife in a village in the West Bengali district of Nadia. According to the biomedical doctor at the state hospital, she was suffering from 'puerperal psychosis'. Her neighbours, however, believed her to be possessed. To the utter consternation of the journalist, at the instance of the latter, a local *Ojha* using 'Arabic mantras' was treating her and there was no way to compel the family to do otherwise. The bio-medical doctors and the district administration both agreed with the journalist that she should be treated by a biomedical doctor rather than the *Ojha*, but pleaded helplessness in the face of the family's decision. The journalist lamented that, 'even in this era of globalisation, far away Bengali villages remain stuck in ways of thinking that belong to the Middle Ages (*modhyo jugiyo dhyan dharonaye pode*)' (Haldar 2014; Lambert, Chapter 5 in this volume). There are many aspects of this incident that bear unpacking. Why, for instance, are *mantras* reminiscent of the Middle Ages? Is globalisation really so incompatible with *mantric* therapies? But these are not the questions I will unpack in this chapter.

The questions I want to pose here are slightly different. *Ojhas*, to begin with, are those who treat snake-bites. There is a long and hallowed tradition in precolonial Bengali literature that tells of the prowess of the *Ojha*. But why is he dealing with a case of possession that has nothing to do with snakes? Moreover, *mantras* in scholarly literature are almost entirely discussed within a Sanskrit or Sanskrit-derived milieu. What then might 'Arabic *mantras*' be? In fact, we are told in the same report that the *Ojha* was actually a Muslim. What then is the relationship between Islam, snake-bites and *mantras*? It is these questions that I want to explore in this chapter.

These explorations shall take us away from the domain of elite medical traditions and into the realm of subaltern therapeutics. Elsewhere I have explored this domain of subaltern therapeutics and argued that its elusive archival traces and fluid characteristics demand a distinctive mode of engagement with the past, viz. a nomadology (Mukharji 2013). In this chapter I hope to further deploy and develop this approach.

Before saying more about my intellectual project, however, it would be useful to briefly situate my study within its proper historical context.[1] The Bengal region, along with much of the fertile Gangetic plains, had formed its own discrete administrative unit during the British colonial era and had even housed the capital of the British Raj, viz. Calcutta, for well over a century until 1911. It was the heartland of British colonial power throughout the long nineteenth century and was therefore exposed to the full force of colonial modernity. The iconic institutions of that colonial modernity in the form of schools, colleges, administrative offices and Western medicine usually arrived first in Calcutta before anywhere else in British India. This deep and intimate engagement with colonial modernity has shaped much in contemporary Bengali culture.

Prior to the advent of colonialism, the region had had a chequered past as an independent kingdom. Textual sources antedating the Common Era refer to a number of separate polities in present-day Bengal. These included the *janapadas* (states) of Anga, Vanga, Pundra, Suhma, Brahma, Rarh, Gauda and Tamralipta in western Bengal. Farther east were states such as Samatata and Harikela. The Gupta Empire absorbed much of Bengal by the fourth century. But many of the Bengali kingdoms asserted their independence once more with the decline of the Guptas towards the end of the sixth century. In this period, King Shashanka (600–625 CE) of Gauda emerged as a powerful monarch. Not only did Shashanka unite much of Bengal, he also made a bid for power in the Gangetic valley lying west of

Bengal. For some time at least, his arms certainly extended to parts of northern India. Shashanka's wars however, also served to consolidate his enemies and Gauda was ravaged after his death.

From the chaos that followed the demise of Shashanka emerged the Pala dynasty. Founded by Gopala, elected to put an end to the post-Shashanka chaos, the Palas unified most of Bengal and created a mighty empire in northern India. From the middle of the eighth century to the late twelfth century, this Buddhist dynasty held sway over most of Bengal. Under them contacts were strengthened with other parts of the Buddhist world. Contacts with Tibet were particularly significant.

Despite the prominence, importance and seeming stability of the Palas in Bengali history, some parts of Bengal continued outside their rule. The Buddhist Deva dynasty, for instance, held power in the southern kingdom of Samatata (eighth to ninth centuries). Further east, the Chandras held power in Harikela (tenth to eleventh centuries). In the eleventh century there also emerged the independent Varman dynasty in south-eastern Bengal.

The Pala ascendancy was finally ended by the rise of the Sena dynasty. The Senas, who are thought to have hailed from the Karnataka region of southern India, ruled roughly from 1097 and 1223. The Sena kings worshipped Hindu deities and they almost certainly withdrew the support that Buddhism had received from the state under the Palas. Yet, to what extent the change in the king's faith led to a change in religious life more generally is relatively unknown. It is highly likely that the Senas continued to preside over a religiously mixed subject population made up of Hindu and Buddhist elements.

By the opening decades of the thirteenth century, new Muslim armies from the northwest began to press into Bengal. In 1206, Muhammad Bakhtiyar Khalji founded the first Sultanate in Bengal. Even though the Sultanate steadily grew after this, vast swaths in the east remained under Sena rule until the 1280s. The status of the Sultanate of Bengal kept varying in its first century of existence, occasionally coming under the rule of the Delhi Sultans and on other occasions being independent. Relative stability was only established by the emergence of the Illyas Shahi dynasty. Under this dynasty, including a brief interlude under a Hindu usurper, Bengal remained an independent polity between 1342 and 1487. In 1487,

Abyssinians who had been enslaved by the Illyas Shahi monarchs, removed the last ruler of the Illyas Shahi dynasty. What followed was a brief period of African kings marked by a series of revolts and usurpations. Eventually, the last of the Abyssinian Sultans, Shamsuddin Muzaffar Shah, was removed and the throne claimed by Alauddin Hussain Shah.

Alauddin Hussain Shah's rule (1494–1538) was one of the most significant in Bengal's cultural history. Though Aluaddin was of Arab descent, he had come to Bengal as a young boy and grew up there. He had been a minister to the ousted Abyssinian Sultan Muzaffar Shah. Under his rule Alauddin promoted the Bengali language, sponsored large-scale Bengali translations of Sanskrit classics and sought to unify Bengal culturally. Alauddin also extended the borders of his kingdom beyond Bengal into modern-day Assam and Odisha. It was also during Alauddin's rule that the first Portuguese mission arrived in Bengal.

Unfortunately, the strong foundation laid by Alauddin did not last long in the hands of his heirs and by the end of the sixteenth century Bengal was once again assailed by Mughal troops pressing in through the Gangetic valley. Power in Bengal then passed briefly into the hands of Afghan warriors, who were being pushed north by the incoming Mughals. But these dynasties were too new and too weak to resist the onslaught of the Mughals. While the central authority in Bengal collapsed quickly in the face of superior Mughal armies, a loose confederacy of powerful landlords and warlords continued, however, to resist Mughal occupation under the remnants of the Afghan aristocracy. Finally, in 1576, Daud Karrani, the last Afghan Sultan, was killed in battle with the Mughals.

Interestingly, through much of this period and well into the Mughal era, large swaths of land in the eastern parts of Bengal, particularly the Chittagong region, remained part of the Arakanese Kingdom of northern Burma with its capital at the city of Mrauk-U. The Arakanese royalty in turn employed, and occasionally even inter-married with, the Portuguese robber-barons, such as Filipe de Brito and Sebastian Gonsalves Tibao, who had established their power in the Bay of Bengal and often acted as mercenaries.[2]

Bengal's existence as a Mughal province was tumultuous. It became a happy hunting ground for rebel princes of the blood. First, Shah Jahan and then one of his sons, Shah Shuja, sought to make their bids for the Mughal throne from Bengal. Whilst Mughal systems of government and culture made a deep impact in Bengal, its political integration with upper India remained tenuous. By the dawn of the eighteenth century, after just over a century of tempestuous Mughal rule, as the Mughal Emperors in Delhi began losing authority, the provincial governors of Bengal assumed de facto monarchic powers as Nawabs. Though the formal ties with Delhi were not repudiated, the office of the Nawab became hereditary and the Mughal Emperor's authority over them declined precipitously.

It was the last of these hereditary governor-monarchs, Nawab Siraj-ud-Daula, who was treacherously defeated by the English East India Company in 1757. What enabled the English victory was a secret alliance with some of the Nawab's foremost generals who, as per earlier agreement with the English, rebelled on the battlefield and joined the enemies. In return, the English briefly propped up one of these rebels as the next Nawab, but from then on real power progressively passed out of the hands of the Nawab and into those of the English. By the end of the eighteenth century, the English were the unquestioned rulers of Bengal.

From then until the British departure in 1947, the British ruled over Bengal. At the moment of decolonisation however, the decision was taken to partition the large and populous region of Bengal between the new dominions of India and Pakistan. The Hindu-majority west went to India and the Muslim-majority east to Pakistan. Subsequently, the eastern part, whose language, culture and even the form of Islam they practised was remarkably distinctive from the rest of Pakistan, emerged through a bloody civil war as an independent state called Bangladesh in 1971.

I would emphasise three aspects within this potted history of Bengal. First, there are at least three distinctive religious traditions which had left their marks on precolonial Bengal, viz. Buddhism, Hinduism and Islam. The relatively long Buddhist rule and the short Hindu rule prior to the establishment of Muslim Sultanates also meant that the Buddhist contribution to the cultural life of the people did not get as thoroughly assimilated into Hinduism as it did in many other parts of India. Second, the region was also deeply influenced by Western forms of Christianity. The presence of the Portuguese pirates-turned-warlords and the early and deep intimacy with the British both left their mark on the region. Finally, though Bengal has usually been seen as a part of South Asia, its historical location is more complicated. Its episodic political integration with the rest of South Asia, its geographic connections to Tibet, the Bay of Bengal and Burma, and its links through a diverse array of ruling houses to the wider worlds of Portugal, Ethiopia and Arabia, made it a veritable melting pot of many distinctive cultural influences.

Ecologically too, as an overwhelmingly riparian and rice-growing region, it shares much with Southeast Asia and is certainly distinctive from the relatively drier Gangetic valley of northern India. Medically, this riparian ecology translated into three major consequences. First was the prevalence of malarial fevers that proliferated due to the increased ease with which mosquitoes reproduced in the waterlogged paddy fields. Second was the higher volume of water-borne diarrhoeal diseases, such as dysentery and cholera. Finally, the wetlands were home to many different types of snakes, and snake-bites formed a large medical problem. Of course, none of these medical consequences were determined exclusively by the climatic conditions. Political and social interventions mattered. Historically strong states in the region, for instance, attended to the dredging of canals, improving irrigation and ensuring the people's relative prosperity, all of which could significantly curtail the ill-health resulting from mosquitoes, poor sanitation and snake-bites. But it cannot be denied that the wetter climate of Bengal contributed towards making these problems much more acute in Bengal than they were in upper India.

Literature

Until recently, the history of medicine in South Asia had been dominated by histories of colonial public health (Arnold 1993; Harrison 1994; Mukharji 2009). The histories of neo-traditional medicines had largely been left to Indologists and Classicists who studied ancient Sanskrit texts (Filliozat and Chanana 1964; Zimmermann 1999). These Indological studies, though hugely informative in their own right, were frequently textualist in orientation and neglected the local contexts within which such texts had been produced. The neglect of local context also meant that their historical relevance was assumed to be equal for all parts of the subcontinent. Regional differences were either neglected or seriously downplayed.

The overwhelming majority of such studies, based as they were on Sanskrit texts, were devoted to the study of Ayurveda. Other South Asian traditions, though codified and textually grounded like Ayurveda, such as Unani Tibb, Siddha and Sowa Rigpa, drew much less scholarly attention. Of the few exceptions to this general trend were Scharffe (1999) and Daniel's (1984) works on Siddha, and the older work of Siddiqi (1959) on Unani.

Another trend that marked some, though certainly not all, of the works of Indological scholarship was an attempt to read ancient texts in the light of current medical science. Authors thus tried to distinguish the 'medical' from the 'magical' or identify how accurately ancient knowledge resembled modern Western notions of anatomy, physiology and disease aetiology (Sinha 1981; Zysk 1986, 1993, 1998).

From the late 1970s, mainly through the efforts of anthropologist Leslie (1977, 1992), there also began to emerge a stream of anthropological literature interested in what might broadly be called the 'modernisation' of Ayurveda. Most of this scholarship, despite being mainly ethnographic, often contained a historical aspect that stretched back to colonial times. Besides Leslie himself, the works of Gupta (1977) and Obeyesekere (1992) are worth mentioning in this regard.

This anthropological literature has continued to blossom, producing in its wake not only a plethora of fine studies of the contemporary lives of Ayurveda, but indeed going further and charting the contemporary conditions of other similarly so-called 'traditional' medicines as well. Langford's (2002) study of Ayurveda, for instance, has opened up entirely new areas of research into Ayurveda's contemporary life by studying contemporary Ayurvedic colleges, textbooks and private practices. Cohen's (2006) brilliant work on Alzheimer's disease has similarly relocated the medical within a thick cultural fabric. More recently, Bode's (2008) wonderfully nuanced account of the medical market in India for non-biomedical products has sought to get beyond the disciplinary divide between Ayurveda and Unani and look at them side by side. Pordie's (2008) work on Sowa Rigpa, on the other hand, has not only documented the hugely complex story of 'Tibetan Medicine' in all its diversity, but in fact has given us a new vocabulary to speak of the altered, modernised and globalised lives of these 'traditions'. Of these, I find his notion of neo-traditional medicine eminently useful in distinguishing classical traditions from their recent avatars. Sheehan and Hussain (2002) have similarly documented the fascinating plurality of neo-traditional Unani Tibb.

This blossoming tradition of anthropological works on neo-traditional medicines is, however, quite distinct from another equally rich body of anthropological works that looked beyond the codified traditions of neo-traditional therapies. Here older anthropological themes of shamanism and possession, for instance, have continued to yield fascinating new insights into health and healing in South Asia. Amongst the better-known and more influential works in this tradition are those of Flueckiger (2006), Sax (2009), Desjarlais (2011) and others.

Historical works devoted to traditional or neo-traditional medicine were initially slow to emerge. The pioneering early works of Hume (1977) and Panikkar (1992) were not immediately followed up with work of equal quality and analytic rigour. The true flourishing of historical works on the subject began more than a decade after Panikkar's work. Sivaramakrishnan's (2006) brilliant work on Ayurveda in colonial Punjab was not only methodologically rigorous but also helped mainstream histories of neo-traditional medicines amongst historians. Berger (2013) on north India has since followed up her work, as has my own work on Bengal (Mukharji 2016). An edited volume by Wujastyk and Smith (2008), on the other hand, has explored Ayurveda's more recent history of globalisation and Alter's (2010) fascinating work has documented the modern history of yoga. A similarly rich seam of work has also appeared on neo-traditional Unani medicine. In this regard Attewell's (2007) and Alavi's (2010) works are particularly worthy of mention (see also Datoo 2020). Both these, however, unfortunately omitted the Bengal region from their studies. The only study on the history of Islamicate medicine in Bengal, therefore, remains a short article of mine (Mukharji 2011). In the case of Siddha medicine too there have been some excellent historical works that have explored its neo-traditional form (Weiss 2009).

Recently, Slouber (2017) has identified a distinctive Garudi medical tradition that relied significantly upon therapeutic *mantras*.

Despite this diverse and rich body of scholarship, or rather one might say precisely because of it, certain major gaps have developed. Lambert (2013, Chapter 5 in this volume) for instance, has pointed out that there is a preponderance of spiritual therapies amongst those who study non-textual traditions of healing. Thus, massaging and bone-setting traditions, which are often prominent within the domain of 'subaltern therapeutics', are frequently ignored in the extant body of scholarship. Interestingly, the case is just the reverse when it comes to studying the textualised and more elite traditions of healing. Here the 'spiritual' and the 'magical' have often been either neglected or mentioned only in passing.

Mantric therapies have suffered particularly in this context. Zysk's chapter (1991: 123–43) in Alper's edited volume, *Understanding Mantras* was, until the recent publication of Slouber's (2017) work, the best-known work on the use of *mantras* in Indic medical traditions. Zysk's study is, however, limited in two explicit ways. First, Zysk looks exclusively at what he calls 'Ancient Indian Medicine'. Leaving aside the politically fraught question of exactly what territory might be considered 'Ancient India' (and where, one wonders, would 'Ancient Pakistan' be?), we can at least agree that this framing immediately excludes from its ambit anything that is not 'ancient'. Again, leaving aside hair-splitting about exactly how old is 'ancient', we can easily agree that in Zysk's view at least anything written in the second millennium, i.e., after the 10th CE, would not be 'ancient'. A second, and even more problematic framing, comes from Zysk's (1991: 133) comment that, 'With the development of [A]yurveda around the Christian era, a quite different approach to medicine began to emerge in India. A more rational or 'scientific' attitude had all but replaced the magico-religious medical doctrines of the *Atharvaveda*; and with these revolutionary ideas, mantras assumed a subordinate, if not anomalous, place in the medical treatments prescribed in the early [A]yurvedic literature'.

Zysk was neither the first nor the last to depict a largely homogeneous and perfectly 'rational' 'Ancient Indian Medicine'. Anticipating many of the core arguments of Zysk, Ray (1970: 90) argued, for instance, that 'the age of Ayurveda', influenced by Buddhism, was one when 'liberal and rational ideas' along with 'freedom from mysticism, restrictions and rigidities of rites and ceremonies' had 'prepared a congenial atmosphere for the growth of a rational system of medicine'. Medicine in this era, Ray asserted, 'emerged out of empirico-magical medicine of the Vedic Age and developed... into an empirico-rational system of lore and practices' (1970: 91). In the same vein, the famous Indian Marxist, Chattopadhyaya (1977: 314–15), wrote that 'though fully acknowledging the importance of the *Atharvaveda* for Indian medical science... the *Caraka-samhita* seems to remind us... that, in spite of the humble beginnings of medicine as magico-religious therapeutics, it has already taken a momentous step forward, i.e. to the system of rational therapeutics...'. It was these frameworks developed by scholars such as Ray and Chattopadhyaya that Zysk came to deploy. Afterwards, other Indian scholars, such as Sharma (1990: 166), still continued to assert that Ayurvedic medicine in the post-Vedic era 'no longer was magico-religious but [became] empirico-rational'. Zysk is, therefore, only the best-known international exemplar of an approach that has long cast its shadow over the history of South Asian medicines.

At its inception this framework was an anticolonial one. It sought to challenge the imperialist denunciations of non-Western and specifically Indic knowledge traditions by claiming for it the same authority as was enjoyed by modern science. Later, authors such as Chattopadhyaya, used the framework to advance a teleological Marxist view of historical progress that viewed religion as little more than a devious ploy to maintain the power of caste elites. Ironically in recent times, however, such anachronistic claims about the rationality (and by implication modernity) of 'ancient India' has become a central plank of the Hindu right. Subrahmaniam (2000, 2017) has called this peculiarly anachronistic search for rational and modern science in ancient India 'archaic modernity'. She points out that this archaic modernity in effect authorises two simultaneous moves. On the one hand, it domesticates science into a deep historical narrative of Hindu nationalism. On the other hand, it also forecloses the possibility of an epistemic critique of contemporary science by papering over all differences and rendering distinctive epistemic frameworks perfectly compatible. Thus, it blends majoritarian Hindu nationalism with a complete embrace of contemporary mainstream science and technology.

It is this archaic modernity that frames extant discussions of *mantric* therapies. By creating a set of ahistorical binary filters, such as extrinsic/intrinsic, scientific/superstitious, magical/empirical etc., scholars such as Ray, Chattopadhyaya and Zysk create a fully rationalised ancient tradition that maps entirely onto a narrow, one might say superficial, understanding of mainstream biomedicine. *Mantric* therapies are extrinsic to this antiquity and hence labelled as fossilised remnants of an earlier, more magical and backward therapeutics. Any 'new' *mantric* therapies that may have developed after the golden age of classical rationality that cannot be identified as a fossil, are simply stigmata of historical retrogression.

Such judgements, which can be passed even before an actual investigation has been undertaken, are a particularly strong example of what Fabian (2014) has called the 'denial of coevalness'. Though Fabian was writing about ethnographic writing where certain ideas, institutions and people were dubbed 'primitive' and thereby excluded from the temporal frame of the modern present to which the author himself or herself belonged, the framework of archaic modernity goes a step further and renders *mantras* anomalous even before studying them.

The denial of coevalness, Chakrabarty (2013) points out, has serious political consequences. He argues that modern capitalist societies necessitate the imagination of individualised bodies that are universally the same. Just as such societies also require a disenchanted world where production can be fully rationalised. Bodies that are amenable to religious and spiritual forces introduce an element of indeterminacy into rationalised production systems. A world animated by spiritual entities and responsive to *mantric* therapies would make both the bodies of potential workers and the system of production reliant on such bodies relatively unpredictable. The disenchanting historicism through which religio-moral imaginations of the body are suppressed and supplanted are, according to Chakrabarty (2007), in concert with capitalist modernity.

Besides these, more subtle political resonances, the disenchanting historicism of archaic modernity that frames the scholarship on *mantras* also have more immediate and obvious political consequences. As Subramaniam has argued (2017), the images of a rational antiquity that is perfectly in-sync with contemporary deployments of mainstream science and technology are explicitly and conspicuously peddled by right-wing Hindu nationalists. This, in turn, has allowed both non-Hindu minorities as well as lower castes and heterodox Hindus, who do not putatively identify with a narrow Sanskrit canon or its rationalised reading, to be viewed with derision and suspicion. The historiographic elisions of *mantric* therapies in general, and non-Hindu *mantras* in particular, have thus played squarely into the corner of right-wing Hindu formations.

Whereas the quest for an archaic modernity has largely written *mantric* therapies out of the histories of medicine, they have had a very different fate within the histories of religion. Until the 1990s, most of the scholarship on *mantras* within the histories of religion avoided dealing with *mantras* as a whole. Instead, scholars slotted them into clearly delineated 'traditions' and studied them strictly within the remit of their respective 'traditions'.

The notion of 'tradition' functioned within this scholarship in a way similar to how the notion of 'context' functioned in social historical scholarship. That is to say that it authorised certain seemingly objective limits to the 'field' against which the 'figure' of the particular set of *mantras* was to be understood. In effect these seemingly objective 'traditions' were textual corpuses identified by scholars as constituting a homogeneous group. Thus Alper's (1991) pioneering volume, which included Zysk's essay on *mantras* in Ayurveda, also carried essays on *mantras* in the Mimamsa tradition, *mantras* in the Vedic tradition, a comparison of Vedic and Tantric *mantras* etc. (Staal; Taber; Wheelock). Other authors (Alper; Coward; Rocher) narrowed their field of vision even further and discussed *mantras* within the context of a single text or author's oeuvre.

Just as the social historian's 'context', notwithstanding their claims, is actually constructed by the historian through her research, so too is the classicists' 'tradition'. Depending on what features one looks for and how one reads inter-textual cues, two scholars might locate the same text within two distinctive 'traditions'. Thus, whereas earlier authors had often spoken of a generalised 'Tantric tradition' of *mantra* use, Slouber's (2017: 39) fascinating recent work has, for instance, identified a distinctive 'Garudam tradition of Tantric medicine' dealing with snakebites and with roots going back to the 'Vedic age and early classical India'.

Whereas these explorations of *mantras* within specific 'traditions' searched for doctrinally coherent textual corpuses, Staal began to advance a radical and controversial alternative approach. Drawing widely on structuralism, neo-Darwinian insights and much else, Staal proposed that *mantras* were a very special type of sound that pre-dated the emergence of human language. Staal (1985, 1996) argued that *mantras* were akin to birdsong and should be treated as sonic fossils dating possibly from the days of the pre-human hominids.

Staal's arguments proved controversial and did not attract too many supporters amongst the classicist circles. Yet, his suggestions had opened up a way of comparing *mantras* beyond and between corpuscular 'traditions' and lonely, individual texts. Thus, even though his evolutionary framework did not catch on, his ideas have contributed to the emerging, new field of study called 'material religion' (The Editors 2005). Keane (1997, 2004), one of the founding figures of 'material religion', for instance, has repeatedly cited the work of Staal. Keane points out that those studying 'material religion' aim to move away from the belief-centric view of religion and focus instead on material practices. This includes attention to specific types of language use. The emphasis on belief, scholars of material religion have argued, reflects both an essentially Protestant Christian view of religion as well as privileging of more scholarly engagements with religion. A focus on material practices aims to redress these problems with the belief-centric approach and open up instead a way of studying and comparing religion without relating it exclusively to doctrinal and textual positions (Keane 2008).

The turn to material religion has structural similarities with the emergent histories of subaltern therapeutics. Both approaches, respectively within the histories of religion and medicine, aspire to decentre earlier approaches that privileged rationalised 'theories' and the doctrinal coherence of their objects.[3] More immediately, both approaches have opened up new grounds and reasons to look at *mantric* therapies. The sources I am going to introduce in the following section, by their very existence, will open up the history of *mantric* therapeutics in the post-classical, especially early modern and modern, eras. They will also illuminate the ways in which the pursuit of doctrinal coherence might actually obscure the significant transaction of therapies beyond and between discrete traditions, whether religious or medical.

Sources

There are three bodies of sources that I shall introduce in this chapter and, to the best of my knowledge, all three have been largely ignored not only by historians of South Asian medicines, but also to a large extent by historians of South Asian religions.

Finding information about the social and cultural aspects of precolonial life in Bengal has always been a problem for historians. The archival record is extremely patchy in every respect. The Sena Kings, for instance, were scholars and poets in their own right and thus left a substantial literary archive. They also often dealt with ethical issues and matters of social and caste organisation, so these too are somewhat accessible. After the fall of the Senas, however, the Sultanate records are extremely uneven. What little exists is often directed towards political and religious ends. Medical manuscripts, while certainly present, have neither been systematically preserved nor studied. In any case, medical manuscripts per se are unlikely to illuminate exactly how they were used. Given all these absences, social and cultural historians of Bengal have long depended upon the handful of Mughal chronicles, such as the *Baharistan-i-Ghaybi* and the older, poetic *Mangal-kabyas* that preached devotion to particular local deities through epic narratives, to reconstruct social and cultural histories of the region (Raychaudhuri 1953; Ostor 1984; Curley 2008).

Through the efforts of Sahityabisharad (1917), Sen (1924), and Sharif (1969) amongst others, however, from the late nineteenth and through the early twentieth century, there emerged a large treasure trove of previously ignored or unknown Bengali works from the precolonial period. Most of these, though not all, were the works of Bengali Muslim authors and written in verse. The subject matters covered in these works varied widely, ranging from esoteric texts about mystical religious practices to poetic adaptations of Perso-Arabic and Sanskrit works. There were also a significant number of original works in this corpus. Ahmed Sharif published the majority of these works either as independent texts or as collections of extracts. Some of these have, sadly, since gone out of print, but the collected extracts remain fairly easy to access. Yet, unfortunately, this entire corpus remains woefully understudied.

Whilst these texts are not about *mantric* therapies per se, many of them give us excellent descriptions of how *mantric* therapies were used in practice. Being Islamicate, they are also overtly outside, though of course not unconnected with, the discrete Vedic tradition about which Zysk and others have written. These texts give us, therefore, a rare glimpse into the social world of precolonial Bengal and help us understand how lay people, rather than scholars and theologians, understood *mantras*.

A second corpus of texts is a cache of manuscripts dating from the eighteenth and very early nineteenth centuries. These were collected, like the former corpus, during the early decades of the twentieth century and are now housed in the archives of the Visva Bharati University in Santiniketan, India. The university itself had been set up by the poet and Nobel-laureate, Rabindranath Tagore, and sought to implement his romantic vision, which included a valorisation of everyday rural life and its culture. The manuscripts were collected from the villages around the university and include a wide variety of texts ranging from old personal letters to collections of songs and some medical manuscripts. The majority of the manuscripts are in Bengali and a good many of them were written by authors who hailed from relatively humble backgrounds.

The medical manuscripts in this cache are, therefore, not the elite Sanskrit manuscripts which Indologists work on. Instead, they are ready-to-hand aids that actual rural physicians, most of whom did not know Sanskrit, used in their everyday practice. They often include a motley assemblage of useful prescriptions, *mantras*, and second-hand quotations from medical classics that passed into a sort of medical common sense.

These manuscripts and the medical world that engendered them are a world apart from the erudite Sanskrit manuscripts kept in royal libraries in Gwalior or Kathmandu. They were never collected by colonial scholars and deposited in elite European repositories in Vienna, Paris or London, and no Indologist will aspire to reconstruct from them any Ayurvedic Ur-text. They are, in short, both in terms of content and provenance, certainly non-classical and perhaps even, on occasion, subaltern texts which existed in the somewhat ambiguous space between orality and literacy.

Though little is yet known about exactly how people actually used these texts in practice, there are enough signs to suggest that these texts did not really stand alone and independent of the world of orality. Both the terms of their lexicon, as well as the occasionally truncated lines of hymns and *mantras* in them, suggest that the books remained connected to an oral/aural milieu outside the text as such.

This implication in a local oral milieu however, presents some challenges to deciphering them. Often the truncated references can no longer be completed. More frequently still, words and spellings have become redundant and difficult to discern. Finally, the cheap locally produced papers on which most of these texts were written are themselves in extremely poor condition and therefore difficult to read.

Happily for our purposes, however, Panchanan Mandal, one of the early archivists at Santiniketan and a man of the greatest erudition when it came to the textual culture of early modern Bengal, published a number of lengthy catalogues in the mid-twentieth century of the manuscripts in the University's collections (Mandal 1951). Not only did Mandal provide an immensely helpful annotated catalogue, but he also included a good number of texts either in full or in extensive extracts. These catalogues, though out of print, can still be reasonably easily accessed through libraries in South Asia and the West.

Amongst Mandal's catalogues are several reprinted manuscripts that deal with medical matters. The majority of such manuscripts, moreover, contain some *mantric* therapies. I will use these reprinted copies to provide a sense of *mantric* therapies.

Curiously, like the poetic and literary texts of the previous corpus, these manuscripts have unfortunately fallen through the scholarly cracks and remained entirely unstudied. It is one of the unfortunate ironies of the way South Asian scholarship, particularly in Bengal, is organised. Whilst modern historians who work on Bengali vernacular material very seldom look to manuscripts, relying instead on printed books and colonial records, classicists seldom show any interest in non-Sanskrit (or, more rarely, Perso-Arabic) manuscripts.

Finally, the last corpus of sources I shall use is a number of printed texts dating roughly from the 1860s to the 1930s that were exclusively compilations of *mantric* therapies. The printing press, though known in precolonial South Asia, had never caught on. Bengali printing was started under direct British efforts in the late eighteenth century. By the 1820s Bengalis had taken up printing and a slew of early texts and newspapers began to appear. It was only from the 1860s, however, that a combination of social and technological factors led to an explosive growth of print culture.

From the 1860s on not only did the number of books printed rise exponentially, but their variety, quality, taste and market all begun to diversify significantly. Historians of Bengali print usually refer to a genre of low-brow publications known as *Bot-tola* literature (Ghosh 2006). While recent work has challenged earlier understandings of a clear-cut and absolute divide between the high-brow world of nineteenth-century progressivism, social reform and Victorian prudishness, and this low-brow world of *Bot-tola,* it is clear that there were significant differences in prices, styles and content between the two strata of Bengali publications (Bhadra 2011).

One of the most popular themes of *Bot-tola* literature was medicine and health. Yet, this world remains very poorly studied. Whatever studies exist look at *Bot-tola* prints as a kind of limiting case to other, better-established medical histories (Mukharji 2009). One of the problems with studying the *Bot-tola* corpus in detail is that only a fraction of what was printed has been preserved. Within that too, predictably, religious or literary works – however racy or low-brow – have tended to be better-preserved than broadly medical works. Neither private collectors nor colonial and postcolonial repositories have retained much of this corpus of printed works.

Notwithstanding the enormous archival losses and the poor state of preservation, I have managed to see quite a few cheaply printed, pamphlet-size works devoted entirely to *mantric* therapies. Some of these, I have seen either at the British Library's old India Office Collection of vernacular Bengali books or at the National Library in Kolkata. But there are also a handful of books that I have managed to buy from old bookstalls in Kolkata and Dhaka that do not appear in any library catalogue.

The earliest of these printed books is a mere 12 pages in length and published, according to the British Library's catalogue, around 1863. It is about six inches by four inches in size. Most of the works up to the Great War are of approximately similar size. After that, their size begins to grow and they also begin to include ritual diagrams and magic squares. I have seen recent editions of such works which run into more than a thousand pages. Interestingly, many of the books printed the *mantras* in red, rather than the usual black ink. This might have started as a mimicry of manuscript practices, but remains in vogue for this kind of literature.

Used together, these three collections of sources, I am confident, will challenge the notion that *mantric* therapies were an 'anomalous' remnant of a classical Vedic antiquity and thus force us to rethink the histories of South Asian medicine.

Intervention

The seventeenth-century poet, Dona Gaji Choudhury, described the equivocal attitude towards *mantric* therapies. In his epic poem, *Saiful Muluk Badiujjamal*, he wrote:

> Some say someone malicious must have uttered *tona* (black magic)
> Some say uttering *mantras* will destroy it all. (Sharif n.d.: 336)

A century later, Nawazish Khan, one of the most accomplished Bengali poets of the eighteenth century, wrote in his *Gule Bakawali* about the power of *mantras:*

> If the *mantras* are pure, all can be achieved
> [Just as] if the ministers are pure, the king keeps his kingdom
> Every single *mantra* destroys sins
> *Mantras* from a guru shows God
> Heaven [may be reached] by *mantras,* Hell [may be reached] by *mantras*,
> By mantras all can be achieved. (Sharif n.d.: 371, 381)

Clearly both authors seemed to believe in the power of *mantras* to do both good and evil. Their role in therapeutics too was clearly established. The foremost Bengali poet of the seventeenth century, Alaol, in his justly famous *Padmabati* (1651) thus described three types of virtuous physicians, viz. *Ojha, Baidya* and *Garudi* (Sharif n.d.: 304). Though the exact boundaries between these three are somewhat vague, particularly in this period, still the *Ojha* and the *Garudi* would certainly have used *mantric* therapies as part of their repertoires.

It is with this preliminary recognition of the widespread faith in the power of *mantric* therapies that we can turn to an examination of the actual *mantric* therapeutic texts we have. The *mantras* we find in both manuscript sources, and later printed texts, come in a variety of lengths. Some are only a single line, whilst others go on for several lines. A single manuscript usually included multiple *mantras* of varying lengths. One manuscript dating from the middle of the eighteenth century, for instance, contained five separate *mantras*. One of these was only a single line, a couple were three lines long, the fourth four lines long and finally, the last one, was of eight lines (Mandal 1963: 365). Some *mantras* in other manuscripts were longer still. There is nothing to suggest that these *mantras* were categorised differently due to their length. Yet, recent ethnographers working with contemporary physicians who use *mantras* have reported the existence of distinct names for *mantras* of different lengths. *Mantras* of a single syllable are called *pinda*, those with two syllables are called *kartari*, and those of between three and nine syllables were known as *bijak*. Similarly, *mantras* of between ten and twenty syllables were called *mantrak* and those longer than twenty syllables were known as *mala* (Samanta and Kabiraj 2002: 9). Notwithstanding these categorisations by some contemporary physicians, there is no evidence to suggest that such names were widely used in the eighteenth or nineteenth centuries. In fact, the manuscript evidence seems to suggest the contrary.

The length is not the only variable and heterogeneous element of these *mantras*. Both the linguistic composition and the sources of power they invoked were equally diverse. One of the early *mantric* therapies is in a two-page manuscript dating from around the 1790s. Written by an unknown Brahmin called Ramlochan, it contains some devotional hymns, riddles and a *mantra* to counteract black magic (*tona*). The *mantra* itself is written in the Bengali script but the language is a slightly garbled Hindustani along with some words that do not seem to have any intelligible meaning. Consider for instance the following lines: '*Kala ghora, nil paon turuk chalta chalta kahan jao/ Asmanme jaon, patalme jaon, tetalme jaon*' (Black horse, blue legs, trots along, where does it trot/It goes to heaven, it goes to hell, it goes to *Tetal*). Amongst the various deities invoked in the *mantra* were Ishwar, Asman Jogi, Kamakhya Devi and Ramji (Mandal 1958: 57).

Another manuscript from the same period contained a few scattered astrological formulae alongside a few *mantric* therapies. One of these was for stomach aches. The *mantra* once again was written in the Bengali script but was linguistically a mix of Bengali and Hindustani. It invoked the authority of the epic heroes Bhim, Arjun and Ram (Mandal 1958: 110). Similarly, another interesting and slightly earlier manuscript dating from the middle of the eighteenth century contains eight, fairly lengthy, *mantras* directed at poisons and snake-bites. Once again, whilst the script is clearly Bengali, the language is a curious mix of Bengali, Hindustani and what appears to be gibberish (Mandal 1958: 251).

One manuscript from the middle of the eighteenth century that contained a *mantra* for a chronically swollen spleen ('*piley*', from Sanskrit *pliha*), invoked the Hindu deity, Narayan, and an anonymous 'mother' (goddess?), alongside Allah and the local Islamic saint, Khwaja Khijir (Khizr/Khidr), in the same line. The relevant line went thus: '*Sri Sri Narayan Ma jol jol Khaj Khidirer jol Allahar bol*' (Sri Sri Narayan, Mother, water, water, Khwaja Khizr's water, Allah's strength) (Mandal 1963: 356). Simultaneous invocations of seemingly 'Hindu' and 'Muslim' sources of divine power are not at all rare in these *mantras*. Another one in a separate manuscript calls upon Allah, Muhammad and the snake-goddess, Manasha, simultaneously (Mandal 1963: 166). Yet another in the same manuscript invoked Khuda Talha (Allah), alongside the heroes of the Ramayan, viz. Ram and Lakshman (Mandal 1963: 168).

The range of divine powers found side-by-side in a single manuscript of a couple of pages is often quite remarkable. The same manuscript that invoked Khwaja Khijir, for instance, contained five further *mantras*. Two of these remaining *mantras* were also for splenic afflictions, whilst the rest were for snake-bites. Amongst the deities invoked in these *mantras* were Ram, Saraswati, Radha, Krishna, Sita, the goddess of Kamakhya and a relatively obscure figure, Hadi Jhi Chandi. Hadis are a low and untouchable caste, and Hadi Jhi Chandi literally means Chandi, the daughter of a Hadi. Despite her obscurity outside Bengal and for that matter even in more elite and urbane circles in Bengal, she is quite readily recognised by Bengali villagers as a powerful deity linked to the goddess Kali at Kamakhya in Assam (Roy 1999: 21–2). Hadi Jhi Chandi, along with the goddess of Kamakhya, is in fact one of the most frequently called upon figures in Bengali *mantric* therapies. There are several other manuscripts with *mantras* that invoke them (Mandal 1963: 366, 369, 371–3). Another relatively obscure figure who is constantly invoked is Neto Dhopani or Nitya the

Washerwoman. This is a minor character from the Bengali *Mangal-kabyo* tradition, who was said to be able to 'kill' and 'revive' her truant son at will, thus allowing her to pursue her work as a washerwoman. She was also one of the most intimate devotees of the snake-goddess Manasha. But in the *mantras* she seems to have emerged almost as an independent source of power (Mandal 1963: 167; McDaniel 2004: 150–2).

Other divinities cited were even more obscure. Amongst them, in more than a couple of *mantras*, were Sahadeb Thakur or Kumar Sahadeb and Narsingh (Mandal 1963: 168, 176, 356). Narsingh might be a Hindustani reference to one of the ten avatars of Vishnu, i.e. Nrisimha, while Kumar Sahadeb might be the fifth, and arguably most obscure, of the five Pandava brothers in the epic Mahabharata. Neither of these figures, however, have any significant independent cults. So their invocation – provided the names do actually refer to these and not to some more localised figures – is still difficult to explain.[4]

Finally, it is worth noting the kind of afflictions that these *mantric* therapies were being used for. Zysk has argued that there were five main occasions upon which *mantras* were medically deployed in classical South Asia, viz. the treatment of swellings and wounds, treatment of poisons, treatment of fevers, treatment of mental disorders and finally the collection and preparation of certain medicines (Zysk 1991: 126). Many of these emphases were retained into the modern period, but there were also some additional applications which extended the older usages. One mid-eighteenth-century manuscript contains *mantra* for different types of wounds, viz. *gha*, including burns (*pora gha*) (Mandal 1958: 249). Another slightly earlier manuscript contains a *mantra* for body-aches (Mandal 1958: 252). A single-page manuscript from 1868 contains a *mantra* for a condition called '*harish*' and was used by a practising physician called Gopal Kaviraj (Mandal 1958: 256). One of the most comprehensive lists of complaints is found in a single manuscript comprising a number of pages all containing *mantras*. A man called Samar owned the manuscript, possibly in the eighteenth century, but not much else is known about it. Amongst the complaints for which it includes *mantras* are burns (*pora gha*), child's indigestion (*chheler rasambal*), a fever called *balsa* that afflicted children, stomach ache, feeling low/unhappy (*mon-kharap*) etc. (Mandal 1963: 165–74).

The vast majority of *mantras*, however, are consistently for poisons, and especially snake-bites. There are also a significant number of *mantras* that counteract black magic, possession, etc.

It is clear from the perusal of both literary representations of *mantric* therapies by early modern poets, like Dona Gaji Choudhury and Nawazish Khan, as well as the relevant extant manuscript material that *mantric* therapies were flourishing in precolonial Bengal. It is also clear that these *mantras* were not in any way derived from the hallowed Sanskrit canon or the *Atharvaveda.* While it might well have been related to older Vedic material, though that will need to be explored separately, the deities invoked and the language used both bear testimony to non-Vedic roots for such therapies. There is, therefore, little justification for seeing them as a Vedic survival, leave alone seeing them as anachronisms.

The advent of colonial modernity, far from rendering *mantras* obsolete, further contributed to their development in at least two ways. The foremost amongst these was undoubtedly the development of the print market. Print capitalism created a context for enterprising publishers to seek out *mantras* previously ensconced in esoteric networks of practice and rendering them public. Whilst this was an enormous shift in terms of the social context of *mantric* therapies, it ensured wider dissemination of these *mantras* and the constitution of a stable archive.

The anonymous publisher of the *Bangiyo Bishwashyo Montraboli*, which I believe might well be the first such publication, described his pioneering project thus: 'It is true that in the great city of Calcutta myriad books on diverse subjects are today being published. Yet, till now, no erudite gentleman has undertaken to publish the *mantras* used by the Bengali lower castes to combat ghosts (*bhut*), spirits (*pret*), witches (*daini*) and snakes etc. (*sarpadi*). [Hence] I have collected these *mantras* after much effort from a practitioner of *mantras* and chosen to publish it' (Anon. 1863: 11). The publisher was also clear that his publication would offend many practitioners who held that *mantras* should be kept secret and circulated only amongst esoteric circles. He wrote that, 'Those who know *mantras* will be offended by the publication of such secret matters, but what can I do? I am compelled to publish them in the belief that nothing under the sun ought to be secret' (Anon. 1863: 12). Given the lack of circulation figures or details about the actual publisher who, notwithstanding his own dictum on keeping no secrets, chose to keep his own identity a secret, it is difficult to evaluate his comments. Was the publisher really inspired by a conviction to bring esoteric knowledge to the public or was he simply an entrepreneur seeking to dignify his profit motive? Studies of Bengali print culture tell us that from around 1860 there emerged an especially large and diverse market for cheap printed works. A significant section of this market was devoted to medical works (Ghosh 2006). So it is highly possible that the lure of a quick profit played some part in bringing these esoteric *mantras* into the world of print. Yet, in the absence of fuller records, such possibilities are precisely that, viz. possibilities.

A second way in which colonial modernity contributed to the development of *mantric* therapies was by introducing new sources of divine power into the region. An undated collection of Bengali *mantras*, possibly from around the time of the First World War, bears striking witness to this aspect of colonial modernity (Anon. [Sri Dere Babaji] n.d.). Though the entire collection was in Bengali, it included two spells in English that it simply called 'English *mantras*'. One such *mantra* was as follows:

> By the virtue of the holy redemption and torments by the damned I conjure and exercise thee to answer my big demands, being obedient to these sacred ceremonies, for fear of everlasting torment and distress.
>
> Berald—Berauld—Balbin
>
> Gab—Gaber—Agaba (Anon. [Sri Dere Babaji] n.d.: 415).

These spells were further accompanied by a ritual illustration showing how to raise the dead. The spells and the illustration, it turns out, were copied from an 1806 edition of the eighteenth-century English occultist and physician, Sibly's (1807: 1106) *New and Complete Illustration of the Celestial Sciences of Astrology*. Amongst the figures invoked in this 'English *mantra*' were 'Imanuel' and 'Harcot Gambalon'. Needless to say these were utterly new sources of divine power in the region.

Notwithstanding these new inclusions, the printed books also demonstrated remarkable continuity with older manuscript cultures. The range of powers invoked and the complaints engaged with in the *Bongiyo Bishwashyo Montraboli* are certainly reminiscent of manuscripts such as Samar's undated manuscript. The 1863 text invoked figures such as Mahadeb (Shiva), Nrisimha, Manasha, Ram, Gaji Pir, Paigambar (The Prophet Muhammad) and so on. The actual afflictions dealt with by these *mantras* are not always clear, since they are not invariably mentioned. The few afflictions that are expressly referred to include *gorol* (allergic rash), *phik-bedona* (pain due to muscle-spasm), snake-bites, and a possession by a variety of different species of malignant spirits, e.g. *Bhut*, *Sankhchunni*, *Dakini*, etc. Another early printed collection, published in 1907, addresses a range of women's health issues, in addition to the usual anti-venom *mantras*. The *mantras* in this collection are applicable in cases of menstrual pains (*ritubedona*), barrenness in women (*kakbondha*), avoiding miscarriage (*garbharaksha*) and excessive bleeding during menstruation (*raktasrab*) (Datta 1907). Another book published the following year expanded the list of cures even further by diversifying the kinds of poisons his *mantras* could counteract. Besides the usual snake venom, this author spoke of the venom of foxes, dogs, cats, rats, scorpions, house lizards, frogs, fishes, mosquitoes, leeches, honeybees, hornets, and even cases of suicidal self-poisoning (Bidyaratna 1908).

Despite greater diversification and extension of the genre, the basic province of *mantric* therapies remained venoms, wounds, aches and so forth. It was these basic complaints that were repeatedly engaged with in the printed works, just as they have been in the pre-print manuscripts. This trend has continued to grow beyond the colonial era and such printed collections of *mantras* have flourished both in West Bengal and Bangladesh.

Analysis

At the most obvious level, the sources I have discussed above demonstrate that there was a thriving culture of *mantric* therapies that predated the advent of colonialism in Bengal and continued to grow and diversify with the onset of colonial modernity. But how does this body of material fit into any larger narrative of the history of South Asian medicines?

Recently, Slouber (2017) has made a powerful case in favour of taking *mantric* therapies seriously. He has recovered a large body of *mantric* therapies that derive from the *Garuda Tantras* and were mainly, though not exclusively, concerned with the treatment of snake-bites. Slouber is also one of the few scholars to have explicitly demonstrated the problems of Zysk's characterisation of *mantras* in the history of South Asian medicines (Slouber 2012: 16–17). My intervention is along the same lines as Slouber's, but I also go further than him in certain respects.

Whilst I am entirely in agreement with Slouber on the continued importance and relevance of *mantric* therapies, I am not as invested in locating them within a single genealogy deriving from a Garudi corpus. My material is also chronologically later than Slouber's texts. Slouber's analysis is roughly focused on the early medieval period (the fifth to thirteenth centuries), whereas mine is mostly focused on the period between roughly the seventeenth to the early twentieth centuries. Finally, the geographic location of my intervention is narrower. I do not speak of all South Asia, but only of Bengal.

What I believe my material shows is that not only did *mantric* therapeutics remain a strong component of the therapeutic landscape in Bengal throughout the period under study, but also its diverse roots. Whereas too rigorous an etymological analysis will certainly make the word *mantra* seem firmly Indic, as I have tried to show above, in Bengal the word was used loosely to incorporate a range of non-Indic material. Nawazish Khan's *Gul-e-Bakawali*, for instance, drew explicitly upon an Indo-Persianate romance tradition. The invocations of Khwaja Khijir, the Prophet, Allah, etc. are all patently outside any specific Indic textual genealogy. Likewise, when the anonymous author of the *Indrajal* incorporated Sibly's (1807) material by calling them 'English *mantras*', he reached beyond any corpuscular Indic tradition.

To make sense of these practices, therefore, I will suggest that we need to go beyond textual genealogies of discrete traditions and look at the shared cultural logic, which makes such borrowings possible. In fact, going further, I will argue that a strictly historical approach with its emphasis on linear genealogies is somewhat inadequate for narrating the past of Bengali *mantric* therapies. Instead, their tendency constantly to scramble disciplinary, traditional and religious boundaries can only be captured by a nomadology.

Elsewhere, I have argued that the pasts of subaltern therapeutics are ill-suited to historicist writing. Borrowing from Giles Deleuze and Felix Guattari, I had suggested that we needed to access the pasts of subaltern therapeutics through more rhizomorphic narrative styles that would be capable of attending to both 'internal' and 'external' heterogeneities, which defy the essentialising logic of historicism (Mukharji 2013). While I have my doubts about whether *mantric* therapies prior to the nineteenth century can in any way be described as 'subaltern therapeutics', it is certainly true that under colonial modernity *mantras* were marginalised and associated, as we notice in the preface to the *Bangiyo Bishwashyo Montraboli*, with lower caste people. But the past leading up to this marginalised identity under colonial modernity was not a simple, linear one commencing in the *Atharvaveda* and passing through the *Garudi Tantras* and so on. It would have to attend to the multiple rough translations that rendered *mantras* akin to a variety of Islamic and Christian esoteric practices and, thereby, incorporated new pasts and other genealogies into the colonial present of *mantric* therapies. It is this non-linear and anti-essentialist, perhaps even anti-historicist, project that I am calling a nomadology.

What enabled this nomadism of the *mantras* at its core was a shared and widespread belief in the power of intangible agencies, whether benevolent or malevolent, and a simultaneous belief in phonic therapies. Without a deeply held belief in the ability of intangible agencies, or in the plausibility of phonic therapies, none of the nomadism and borrowing could have taken place.

The nomadic and constantly incorporative aspect of these *mantras* is reminiscent of the *Grimoires* of the European tradition (Davies 2010). But, unlike the latter, the *mantras* do not seem as closely tied to writing and textuality. 'Grimoires' properly so-called, were after all textual compendia, whereas the *mantras* we have been looking at were rarely available in sizeable compendia formats prior to the twentieth century. Samar's manuscript is exceptional. Most manuscripts were a page or two in length, suggesting that the encyclopedic format was not germane to the manuscript culture of these *mantras*. What they shared with the Grimoires was their eclectic appetite. Though there too, the range of eclectic borrowings which are obviously trans-sectarian are, I feel, much more significant in the Bengali phonic therapies, than in the European Grimoire tradition.

It would be useful here to elaborate precisely what I mean by 'phonic therapies'. To me they are a set of therapies that engender a certain materialist understanding of uttered sound. What is important in these therapies is, therefore, their phonic materiality, rather than the hermeneutics of their meaning/signification. Many of the words used in Bengali *mantras* are often unintelligible to both the practitioner and the patient. This is but natural when we recognise the frequently polyglot nature of the *mantras* themselves. Yet, their efficacy was not doubted.

Slouber has made a forceful case against the contention that *mantras* often contain nonsensical words. He has argued instead that, 'It is highly unlikely that the words are nonsensical; rather, it is our own ignorance of ancient Indic languages that makes them so' (Slouber 2012: 17). While I do not challenge the fact that some words may seem meaningless to us, but may have held meaning for some users, I feel over-emphasising the transparency of meaning misses something crucial about what *mantras* are and how they work. The anonymous compiler of the Indrajal clarified the point when he introduced Sibly's *mantras*. Explaining the words, 'Worrah, Worrah, Harcot Gambalon' in the last line of one of Sibly's *mantras*, the compiler wrote, 'Readers notice the words at the end of this *mantra*. Just as our *mantras* for *bhuts* and *prets* often contain meaningless (*artha-shunya*) or esoterically meaningful (*gurha-athra-jukta*) words such as Hrim, Phat, Swaha etc., so too can we see the use of the words worrah, worrah, Harcot, Gambalon in the English school [of *mantras*]. From this we can gather that these words are not entirely meaningless ravings (*pralap*)' (Anon. [Sri Dere Babaji] n.d.: 414). This is a fascinating gloss. It shows that meaning and its transparency are not the same thing. In fact, we might even speak of layers of meaning. None of the users might comprehend the meanings of sounds and it may appear meaningless, but that does not foreclose the possibility of there being an esoteric meaning that is unintelligible to all the users.

What is necessary for the *mantra* to work in practice is not its meaning, but its correct utterance. Sometimes further minor rituals and props are prescribed, but essentially its sound has a certain materiality which effects the cure. *Mantras* were not the only form of phonic therapy. As I have described elsewhere, precolonial

Bengal evinced faith in a number of different aural therapies, such as Vaishnav *kirtans*, Sufi *zikr*, Sakta custom of ritualised reading aloud texts such as the *Chandimangal*, etc. (Mukharji 2016). The communication or indeed comprehension of meaning in these therapies was never emphasised. What dominated were the acts of uttering and hearing.

Where I feel *mantric* therapies stand apart from this larger corpus of sonic therapies is that there is a greater emphasis in them on phonics or utterance, rather than on acoustics or hearing.[5] The ritualised reading of *Chandimangal* to be therapeutically effective needs, for instance, to take place within the earshot of the patient. *Kirtans* and *zikr* also therapeutically 'work' on a similar principle. But with *mantras* there are cases where the utterance of the *mantras* at a great distance, i.e. well out of the patient's hearing might still have an effect. Writing on Vedic *mantras*, Ellison Banks Findly (1989: 30) clarifies that in the 'mantric conception of speech the locus of power is in its pronunciation by a religious functionary'. Given the broader historical and religio-cultural pasts that have shaped Bengali *mantra* therapeutics, however, the emphasis on pronunciation might need not have derived exclusively from the Vedic tradition. It might equally have been shaped by *ilm al-tawjid*, the complex, rule-bound tradition of Quranic recitations (McMurray 2021).

It is clearly the underlying general plausibility of sonic, and particularly phonic, therapies that allowed for the kind of nomadic exchanges that are attested to in the *mantras*. This led in turn to a constant exchange of divine sources of power, seemingly 'meaningless' words and even entire *mantras* from one tradition into the other. As a result, the *mantras* as texts, are actually remarkably anti-historical. They borrow rather unsystematically and mess up neat chronologies and discrete sectarian boundaries.

Conclusions

What becomes obvious in trying to write about Bengali *mantric* therapies is the voracious appetite their users had for new sources of extramundane power. This in turn makes any kind of linear history of these *mantric* therapies inchoate. Instead, what emerges is a set of constantly mobile, accretive texts and technologies that radiate outwards. On the one hand, they retain a deep historical investment in such figures as Garuda, Nrisimha and even, on occasion, long-forgotten Buddhist monks from the Pala era.[6] On the other hand, they also voraciously add to their repertoire by drawing upon new sources of divine power such as Allah, the Prophet, Khwaja Khijir, Immanuel and Harcot Gambalon.

As *mantric* therapeutics continue to proliferate in postcolonial South Asia, the task of understanding their role within the medical landscape of the region becomes an even more urgent one. What I have shown in this chapter is that there is a rich and diverse archive into which we can tap in order to begin this task. Following Slouber, I have also emphasised the need to get rid of dated and highly prejudicial scholarly frameworks that have for so long marginalised these *mantric* therapeutics. Going further I have also suggested that, as we move from the Sanskrit texts to vernacular archives and more recent times, we might also need a more radical set of conceptual tools that go beyond the rigidity, essentialism and latent historicism that is written into such words as 'system', 'tradition', and 'history' itself.

Notes

1 The potted history of Bengal that follows is largely taken from the 'History' section of *Banglapedia: National Encyclopedia of Bangladesh* http://en.banglapedia.org/index.php?title=History, accessed 21 February 2017. The *Banglapedia* is a national encyclopedia created by the government of Bangladesh in collaboration with private funders and backed by the UNESCO. Available in print, online and CD-ROM versions the encyclopedia, first published in 2003 and since updated, brings together scholars writing on a diverse array of topics related to the historic Bengal and contemporary Bangladesh. Since its inception, noted economic historian and ex-President of the Asiatic Society of Bangladesh, Professor Sirajul Islam, has served as the Chief Editor.

2 For the history of Mrauk-U, which is not adequately covered in the *Banglapedia*, see Galen (1971).

3 For a summary of the critiques of the 'medical systems' approach to South Asian medical history, see Mukharji (2011).

4 In this regard it is worth noting that Slouber (2012: 90–1) mentions that the key *mantra* for snake-bite, viz. the Vipati mantra, was often associated with Narasimha/Nrisimha in the Tantras.
5 This is a point I feel I had inadequately expressed in my own earlier discussion of these sonic therapies in *Doctoring Traditions* (2016).
6 For Buddhist *mantras* to treat snake-bites, see Singha (1978). See also Mukharji (2020).

Bibliography

Alavi, S. (2010) *Islam and Healing: Loss and Recovery of an Indo-Muslim Medical Tradition, 1600–1900*. London: Palgrave Macmillan.
Alper, H.P. (1991) 'The Cosmos as Siva's Language-Game: 'Mantra' According to Ksemraja's Sivasutravimarsini', in P.A. Harvey (ed.) *Understanding Mantras*. Delhi: Motilal Banarsidass, pp. 249–94.
Alter, J.S. (2010) *Yoga in Modern India: The Body Between Science and Philosophy*. Princeton, NJ: Princeton University Press.
Anon. [Gupta Pracharak] (1863) *Bangiya Biswasya Mantrabali* (Trusted Bengali *Mantras*). Calcutta: Prakrita Jantralaya.
Anon. [Sri Dere Babaji] (n.d.) *Indrajal* (Magic). Calcutta: Basak & Sons.
Arnold, D.J. (1993) *Colonizing the Body: State Medicine and Epidemic Disease in Nineteenth-Century India*. Berkeley, CA: University of California Press.
Attewell, G.N.A. (2007) *Refiguring Unani Tibb: Plural Healing in Late Colonial India*. New Delhi: Orient Longman.
Berger, R. (2013) *Ayurveda Made Modern: Political Histories of Indigenous Medicine in North India, 1900–1955*. Basingstoke: Palgrave Macmillan.
Bhadra, G. (2011) *Nyara Bot-tolaye Jaye Kabar?* (How Many Times does Baldy Walk under the Wood-apple Tree?). Calcutta: Chhatim Books.
Bidyaratna, K. (1908) *Guptamantra* (Secret Mantras). Calcutta: Dakshayani Jantra.
Bode, M. (2008) *Taking Traditional Knowledge to the Market: The Modern Image of the Ayurvedic and Unani Industry, 1980–2000*. Hyderabad: Orient Longman.
Chakrabarty, D. (2007) *Provincializing Europe Postcolonial Thought and Historical Difference*. Princeton: Princeton University Press.
Chakrabarty, D. (2013) 'Community, State and the Body: Epidemics and Popular Culture in Colonial India', in D. Hardiman and P.B. Mukharji (eds) *Medical Marginality in South Asia: Situating Subaltern Therapeutics*. Abingdon: Routledge, pp. 36–58.
Chattopadhyaya, D. (1977) *Science and Society in Ancient India*. Calcutta: K.P. Bagchi & Co.

Cohen, L. (2006) *No Aging in India: Alzheimer's, the Bad Family, and Other Modern Things*. Berkeley, CA: University of California Press.

Coward, H. (1991) 'The Meaning and Power of Mantras in Bhartrhari's Vakyapadiya', in P.A. Harvey (ed.) *Understanding Mantras*. Delhi: Motilal Banarsidass, pp. 165–76.

Curley, D.L. (2008) *Poetry and History: Bengali Maṅgal-Kābya and Social Change in Precolonial Bengal*. New Delhi: Chronicle Books.

Daniel, E.V. (1984) 'The Pulse as an Icon in Siddha Medicine', *Contributions to Indian Studies*, 18: 115–26.

Datoo, S. (2020) 'Advertising Medical Technologies in Urdu Print, c. 1930: Prosthesis and Possibility', *South Asia: Journal of South Asian Studies*, 43.6: 1143–62.

Datta, A. (1907) *Guptamantra* (Secret Mantras). Calcutta: Bharat Prabha Press.

Davies, O. (2010) *Grimoires: A History of Magic Books*. Oxford. Oxford University Press.

Desjarlais, R.R. (2011) *Body and Emotion: The Aesthetics of Illness and Healing in the Nepal Himalayas*. Philadelphia: University of Pennsylvania Press.

Fabian, J. (2014) *Time and the Other: How Anthropology Makes Its Object*. New York: Columbia University Press.

Filliozat, J. and Chanana, D.R. (1964) *The Classical Doctrine of Indian Medicine. Its Origins and Its Greek Parallels*, trans. D.R. Chanana. Delhi: Munshiram Manoharlal.

Findly, E.B. (1989) '*Mántra kaviśastá:* Speech as Performative in the Rgveda', in Harvey P. Alpers (ed.) *Mantra*. Albany: State University of New York Press, pp. 15–47.

Flueckiger, J.B. (2006) *In Amma's Healing Room: Gender and Vernacular Islam in South India*. Bloomington: Indiana University Press.

Galen, S.E.A. van (1971) *Arakan and Bengal: The Rise and Decline of the Mrauk-U Kingdom (Burma) from the Fifteenth to the Seventeenth Century AD*, PhD thesis, University of Leiden.

Ghosh, A. (2006) *Power in Print: Popular Publishing and the Politics of Language and Culture in a Colonial Society, 1778–1905*. New Delhi: Oxford University Press.

Gupta, B. (1977) 'Indigenous Medicine in Nineteenth- and Twentieth-Century Bengal', in C.M. Leslie (ed.) *Asian Medical Systems: A Comparative Study*. Berkeley, CA: University of California Press, pp. 368–82.

Haldar, S. (2014) 'Bodhuke Sarate Arbi Mantra Ojhar' (Ojha uses Arabic Mantra to Cure Housewife), *Ananda Bazar Patrika*, June 18, 2014.

Harrison, M. (1994) *Public Health in British India: Anglo-Indian Preventive Medicine, 1859–1914*. Cambridge; New York: Cambridge University Press.

Hume, J.C. (1977) 'Rival Traditions: Western Medicine and Yunan-i-Tibb in the Punjab, 1849–1889', *Bulletin of the History of Medicine*, 51.2: 214–31.

Karim Shahitya-bisharad, A. (1917) *Goraksha-bijaya: Sheikh Faijulla Marhuma Pranita* (Victory of Goraksha: Authored by the Late Sheikh Faijulla). Kalikātā: Bangīẏa-Sāhitya-Parishat.

Keane, W. (1997) 'Religious Language', *Annual Review of Anthropology*, 26: 47–71.

Keane, W. (2004) 'Language and Religion', in A. Duranti (ed.) *A Companion to Linguistic Anthropology*. Malden, MA: Blackwell Publishing, pp. 431–48.

Keane, W. (2008) 'On the Materiality of Religion', *Material Religion*, 4.2: 230–1.

Lambert, H. (2013) 'Wrestling with Tradition: Towards a Subaltern Therapeutics of Bonesetting and Vessel Treatment in North India', in D. Hardiman and P.B. Mukharji (eds) *Medical Marginality in South Asia: Situating Subaltern Therapeutics*. London: Routledge, pp. 109–25.

Langford, J. (2002) *Fluent Bodies: Ayurvedic Remedies for Postcolonial Imbalance*. Durham, NC; London: Duke University Press.

Leslie, C.M. (1977) 'The Ambiguities of Medical Revivalism in Modern India', in C.M. Leslie *Asian Medical Systems: A Comparative Study*. Berkeley, CA: University of California Press, pp. 356–67.

Leslie, C.M. (1992) 'Interpretations of Illness: Syncretism in Modern Ayurveda', in C.M. Leslie and A. Young (eds) *Paths to Asian Medical Knowledge*. Berkeley, CA: University of California Press, pp. 177–208.

Mandal, P. (1951) *Punthi Paricaya*. Vol. 1. 6 vols. Santiniketan: Vidya Bhavan.

Mandal, P. (1958) *Punthi Paricaya*. Vol. 2. 6 vols. Santiniketan: Vidya Bhavan.

Mandal, P. (1963) *Punthi Paricaya*. Vol. 3. 6 vols. Santiniketan: Vidya Bhavan.

McDaniel, J. (2004) *Offering Flowers, Feeding Skulls: Popular Goddess Worship in West Bengal*. New York: Oxford University Press.

McMurray, P. (2021) 'Qur'an Alphabetics and the Timbre of Recitation', in E.I. Dolan and A.Rehding (eds) *The Oxford Handbook of Timbre*. Oxford: Oxford University Press, pp. 93–120.

Mukharji, P.B. (2009) *Nationalizing the Body: the Medical Market, Print and Daktari Medicine*. London: Anthem Press.

Mukharji, P.B. (2011a) 'Lokman, Chholeman and Manik Pir: Multiple Frames of Institutionalising Islamic Medicine in Modern Bengal', *Social History of Medicine*, 24.3: 720–38.

Mukharji, P.B. (2011b) 'Symptoms of Dis-Ease: New Trends in the Histories of 'Indigenous' South Asian Medicines', *History Compass*, 9.12: 887–99.

Mukharji, P.B. (2013) 'Chandshir Chikitsha: A Nomadology of Subaltern Medicine', in D. Hardiman and P.B. Mukharji (eds) *Medical Marginality*

in South Asia Situating Subaltern Therapeutics. Abingdon: Routledge, pp. 85–108.
Mukharji, P.B. (2016) *Doctoring Traditions: Ayurveda, Small Technologies, and Braided Sciences*. Chicago: University of Chicago Press.
Mukharji, P.B. (2020) 'Rediscovering Living Buddhism in Modern Bengal: Maniklal Singha's *The Mantrayāna of Rārh*', in C.P. Salguero (ed.) *Buddhism and Medicine: An Anthology of Modern and Contemporary Sources*. New York: Columbia University Press, pp. 231–4.
Obeysekere, G. (1992) 'Science, Experimentation, and Clinical Practice in Āyurveda', in C.M. Leslie and A. Young (eds) *Paths to Asian Medical Knowledge*. Berkeley, CA: University of California Press, pp. 160–76.
Ostor, A. (1984) *Culture and Power Legend, Ritual, Bazaar and Rebellion in a Bengali Society*. New Delhi: Sage Publications.
Panikkar, K.N. (1992) 'Indigenous Medicine and Cultural Hegemony: A Study of the Revitalization Movement in Keralam', *Studies in History*, 8.2: 283–308.
Pordié, L. (2008) 'Tibetan Medicine Today: Neo-Traditionalism as an Analytical Lens and a Political Tool', in L. Pordié (ed.) *Tibetan Medicine in the Contemporary World. Global Politics of Medical Knowledge and Practice*. London: Routledge, pp. 3–32.
Ray, P. (1970) 'Medicine – As It Evolved in Ancient and Medieval India', *Indian Journal for the History of Science*, 5.1: 86–100.
Raychaudhuri, T.K. (1953) *Bengal under Akbar and Jehangir: An Introductory Study in Social History*. Calcutta: A. Mukherjee & Co.
Rocher, L. (1991) 'Mantras in the Sivapurana', in H.P. Alper (ed.) *Understanding Mantras*. Delhi: Motilal Banarsidass, pp. 177–203.
Roy, S. (1999) *The Bengalees: Glimpses of History and Culture*. New Delhi: Allied Publishers.
Samanta, R. and Kabiraj, S. (2002) *Saper Mantra O Jharphunk* (Mantras for Snakes and Exorcism). Calcutta: Lok Samskriti Gabeshana Parishad.
Sax, W. S. (2009) *God of Justice: Ritual Healing and Social Justice in the Central Himalayas*. New York: Oxford University Press.
Scharfe, H. (1999) 'The Doctrine of the Three Humors in Traditional Indian Medicine and the Alleged Antiquity of Tamil Siddha Medicine', *Journal of the American Oriental Society*, 119.4: 609–29.
Sen, D.C. (1924) *Eastern Bengal Ballads*. Calcutta: University of Calcutta.
Sharif, A. (1969) *Banglara Sufi Sahitya: Alocana O Nayakhani Grantha Sambalita* (Bengal's Sufi Literature: Discussion and Nine Books Collected). Dhaka: Samay Prakashan.
Sharif, A. (n.d.) *Madhyayugera Sahitye Samaja O Samskritira Rupa* (Society and Culture in Medieval Bengali Literature). Dhaka: Muktadhara.
Sharma, O.P. (1990) 'Development of Medicine in Ancient India', in B.K. Matilal and P. Blimoria (eds) *Sanskrit and Related Studies: Contemporary Researches and Reflections*. Delhi: Sri Satguru Publications, pp. 165–76.

Sheehan, H.E. and Hussain, S.J. (2002) 'Unani Tibb: History, Theory, and Contemporary Practice in South Asia', *The Annals of the American Academy of Political and Social Science*, 583.1: 122–35.

Sibly, E. (1807) *A New and Complete Illustration of the Occult Sciences*. London: Champante & Whitrow.

Siddiqi, M.Z. (1959) *Studies in Arabic and Persian Medical Literature*. Calcutta: Calcutta University.

Singha, M. (1978) *Rarher Mantrajan* (The Mantrayana of Rarh). Bankura: The New Minerva Press.

Sinha, A. (1981) 'Physiological Concepts in Ancient and Medieval India', *Advances in Physiological Sciences*, 21: 61–76.

Sivaramakrishnan, K. (2006) *Old Potions, New Bottles: Recasting Indigenous Medicine in Colonial Punjab (1850–1945)*. Hyderabad: Orient Longman.

Slouber, M. (2012) *Garuda Medicine: A History of Snakebite and Religious Healing in South Asia*, PhD thesis, University of California, Berkeley.

Slouber, M. (2017) *Early Tantric Medicine: Snakebite, Mantras, and Healing in the Garuda Tantras*. Oxford: Oxford University Press.

Staal, F. (1985) 'Mantras and Bird Songs', *Journal of the American Oriental Society*, 105.3: 549–58.

Staal, F. (1991) 'Vedic Mantras', in H.P. Alper (ed.) *Understanding Mantras*. Delhi: Motilal Banarsidass, pp. 48–95.

Staal, F. (1996) *Ritual and Mantras Rules without Meaning*. Delhi: Motilal Banarsidass.

Subramaniam, B. (2000) 'Archaic Modernities: Science, Secularism, and Religion in Modern India', *Social Text*, 18.3: 67–86.

Subramaniam, B. (2017) *Ghost Stories for Darwin: The Science of Variation and the Politics of Diversity*. Champaign: University of Illinois Press.

Taber, J. (1991) 'Are Mantras Speech Acts? The Mimamsa Point of View', in H.P. Alper (ed.) *Understanding Mantras*. Delhi: Motilal Banarsidass, pp. 144–65.

The Editors (2005) 'Editorial Statement', *Material Religion*, 1.1: 4–9. https://doi.org/10.2752/174322005778054474, accessed 14 May 2022.

Weiss, R.S. (2009) *Recipes for Immortality: Medicine, Religion, and Community in South India*. Oxford: Oxford University Press.

Wheelock, W.T. (1991) 'The Mantra in Vedic and Tantric Ritual', in H.P. Alper (ed.) *Understanding Mantras*. Delhi: Motilal Banarsidass, pp. 96–122.

Wujastyk, D. and Smith, F.M. (2008) *Modern and Global Ayurveda: Pluralism and Paradigms*. Albany: State University of New York Press.

Zimmermann, F. (1999) *The Jungle and the Aroma of Meats: An Ecological Theme in Hindu Medicine*. Delhi: Motilal Banarsidass.

Zysk, K.G. (1986) 'The Evolution of Anatomical Knowledge in Ancient India, with Special Reference to Cross-Cultural Influences', *Journal of the American Oriental Society*, 106.4: 687–705.

Zysk, K.G. (1991) 'Mantra in Ayurveda: A Study in Magico-Religious Speech in Ancient Indian Medicine', in H.P. Alper (ed.) *Understanding Mantras*. Delhi: Motilal Banarsidass, pp. 123–43.

Zysk, K.G. (1993) 'The Science of Respiration and the Doctrine of the Bodily Winds in Ancient India', *Journal of the American Oriental Society*, 113: 198–213.

Zysk, K.G. (1998) *Asceticism and Healing in Ancient India: Medicine in the Buddhist Monastery*. Delhi: Motilal Banarsidass.

Part III

Himalayas, Southeast Asia

7

Sowa Rigpa, Tibetan medicine, Tibetan healing

Geoffrey Samuel

Background

Like many things about contemporary Tibet and the wider Himalayan region, the history and identity of Tibetan healing practices are contested. There is nevertheless a clearly identifiable medical tradition,[1] which I refer to here as Sowa Rigpa (*gSo ba rig pa*), one of several names that have been used for it in recent years (see below).[2] Medical practice appears to go back at least to the seventh or eighth century CE. The basic structure of Sowa Rigpa as we know it today was codified in a text known as the *rGyud bzhi* ('Four Tantras'), now generally regarded as the work of g.Yu thog Yon tan mgon po in the twelfth century. This text is closely associated with Tibetan Buddhism and was regarded by some, though not all, Tibetan doctors and scholars as the actual word of the Buddha. The medical tradition described in the *rGyud bzhi* has been employed for many centuries both by Tibetans and by other populations throughout those regions of the Himalayas where Tibetan Buddhism is practised. In terms of contemporary political boundaries, these regions include the Tibetan regions of the Chinese People's Republic (the Tibet Autonomous Region, and large parts of Qinghai, Sichuan, Gansu and Yunnan provinces), large parts of northern Nepal, several parts of the Republic of India (Ladakh, Sikkim, areas within West Bengal), and the independent Buddhist kingdom of Bhutan.

The practice of Sowa Rigpa is by no means uniform throughout this vast region today, and undoubtedly was not so in the past either. In some areas, such as Ladakh (Pordié 2007, 2015; Blaikie 2013a, 2013b; Pordié and Kloos 2021) or Spiti (Besch 2009), lineages of family practitioners have long been established at village level, passing on their knowledge from father to child, and accessible to much of the local population. In other areas, such as pre-modern Bhutan, doctors were much rarer and patronised mainly by a small number of elite families. The Lhasa government instituted a medical college on lCags po ri (Chakpori) hill in Lhasa in the seventeenth century (Meyer 2003; Hofer and Larsen 2014; Van Vleet 2015), and a series of further monastic medical colleges (*sman pa grwa tshang*) developed over the following centuries, particularly in Northeast Tibet (Amdo) and Mongolia (cf. Van Vleet 2015). These led to a tradition of monk-doctors. In the early twentieth century, after the 13th Dalai Lama visited India and saw something of public health provision under the Raj, a new medical and astrological college, the Mentsikang (*sMan rtsis khang*), was set up in Lhasa. After 1959, doctors from this college set up a similar institution in Dharamsala, known in English as the Men-Tsee-Khang (Kloos 2008, 2010, 2013; Prost 2003, 2008). The curricula of both these colleges, and most of the other contemporary teaching institutions which have grown up in recent years in Chinese-controlled Tibet, India and Bhutan, have been partially reconstructed under biomedical influence.

Sowa Rigpa is often referred to as 'Tibetan medicine' (*Bod sman* in Tibetan). However, 'Tibetan medicine' tends to imply claims of authority over this tradition by Tibetans (as opposed to Ladakhis, Bhutanese and others), so scholars have employed several alternative terms. Sowa Rigpa (literally the art, science or knowledge of healing) was originally a term for medicine and healing as one of the areas of knowledge traditionally mastered by the Indian scholars from whom the Tibetans derived much of their own scholarly tradition. It is widely accepted among practitioners, and has become increasingly used in recent years both by scholars and by official sources, including the Indian government (e.g. Adams, Schrempf and Craig 2011b).

The *rGyud bzhi* is the central and foundational text of the Sowa Rigpa tradition. In the past, and in some places still today, students of Sowa Rigpa were expected to study and memorise the whole or large parts of this text, which takes the form of a dialogue in verse between two emanations of the Buddha within a visionary, *maṇḍala*-like landscape. The mode of medical practice described within it can best be understood as a syncretic version of material from several Asian medical traditions, with a large dose of Ayurveda and smaller components of Chinese and Greco-Arab medicine, reworked substantially by Tibetan scholars. Like these traditions, it employs compound medicines with herbal, some mineral and (traditionally, at any rate) some animal-derived ingredients. In fact, Tibetan historical texts describe the coming of foreign doctors from the Persian (i.e. Greco-Arabic), Indian and Chinese traditions to Tibet in the seventh and eighth centuries (Beckwith 1979; Yoeli-Tlalim 2012). However, the theoretical structure of the *rGyud bzhi* is essentially based on Ayurveda, with some significant changes, which will be considered later.

The kind of medicine described in the *rGyud bzhi* forms only part of the field of healing in culturally Tibetan societies. In general terms, one can speak of three major areas of healing practice within these societies (see Samuel 2014), as illustrated in Table 7.1.

Table 7.1 The field of Tibetan healing practices

Description	Tibetan names (Wylie)	Conventional English names
Sowa Rigpa: Syncretic variant of Asian medical traditions, reworked in Tibet and canonically specified in the *rGyud bzhi* or 'Four Tantras'. Based on compound medicines with herbal, some mineral and some animal ingredients	*gso ba rig pa, bod sman*	Sowa Rigpa, Tibetan medicine, *amchi* medicine, *gyüshi* medicine
Sophisticated Buddhist ritual procedures for wellbeing and longevity, such as the numerous Tantric longevity practices and the rituals for the empowerment of medicines	*tshe sgrub, tshe dbang, sman sgrub*	*tsedrub, tsewang,* long-life practice, long-life-empowerment; *mendrup*, medicine empowerment
Folk healing rituals, spirit-mediumship and folk dietary practices	No generic name	No generic name

Apart from the Sowa Rigpa remedies based on the *rGyud bzhi* and developed further by later medical practitioners, there is also an important additional category of ritually empowered, mercury-based potions and pills (*rin chen ril bu*, 'precious pills') deriving from mediaeval Tantric alchemy. While there is some mention of these in the *rGyud bzhi*, the processes of manufacture and practice for these pills today are not associated with the *rGyud bzhi*, but with other, more specifically Tantric lineages (cf. Czaja 2013; Gerke 2013).

In the contemporary situation, biomedicine (*rgya sman, phyi sman*) is also a dominant component of the field. Virtually all Tibetan communities today have some access to biomedicine, and it is often more accessible than Sowa Rigpa, especially in urban contexts. Particularly there, biomedicine and Sowa Rigpa exist side by side, in a generally complementary but sometimes uneasy relationship (e.g. Prost 2008; Craig 2011; Hofer 2011; Vargas-O'Bryan 2015). The impact of biomedicine on pre-modern healing practices took place later in Tibet than in many parts of Asia, and is arguably less extensive, but it is scarcely possible to speak about Tibetan healing practices in recent times without a constant awareness of the dominating, and at times hostile, presence of biomedicine.

As many scholars have shown, biomedicine adopts specific forms in the Tibetan context, some of them deriving from the wider contexts of biomedicine within the People's Republic of China (PRC) and the Republic of India (Hofer 2008a; 2008b; 2011, 2012; Kloos 2008, 2010, 2013; Craig 2012; Saxer 2013). While the Tibetan terms for biomedicine ('foreign medicine', 'Indian medicine', 'Chinese medicine') imply an 'outside' status, in practice biomedicine is mostly delivered within Tibetan communities by Tibetan medical and health workers.

Divination also forms a vital component of medical and healing practice. It overlaps with, and in some ways can scarcely be distinguished from, strictly diagnostic procedures, such as the pulse analysis and urine analysis techniques described in the *rGyud bzhi*. Divination also often plays a key role in determining which of the above kinds of healing practice will be brought into play, including the choice between Sowa Rigpa and Tibetan medicine and even which doctors or clinics should be utilised.[3]

The role of divination, and the presence of Tantric alchemy, Buddhist ritual and folk ritual in the above account, point to the mutual involvement in practice between Sowa Rigpa, Buddhism and spirit practices of various kinds. The *rGyud bzhi* itself, while in many respects a secular medical treatise, also deals with spirit-related illness (Samuel 2007). In addition, it supplements the Ayurvedic understanding of illness as produced by the three *doṣa* or pathogenic factors (*nyes pa* in Tibetan[4]) of *vāta*, *pitta* and *kaphā*, conventionally translated as wind, bile and phlegm, with a further, specifically Buddhist, level of explanation for illness in terms of the three root *kleśa* (Tib. *nyon mongs*) of desire, anger and delusion. Thus, *all* illness may be seen as ultimately a result of the fundamental Buddhist issue of ignorance of our true Enlightened nature, which underlies the three *kleśa*.

The extent to which individual practitioners, publicly or privately, are committed to this Buddhist level of explanation, and to seeing Sowa Rigpa as an intrinsically Buddhist tradition, doubtless varied in the past, as it does today. The religious or spiritual dimension of Sowa Rigpa is also a key issue for how Western scholars have approached this Tibetan healing tradition, and will be discussed further in later sections of this chapter.

In contemporary practice, Sowa Rigpa can be presented in more or less 'religious' ways, depending on the context and also on the specific clientele. My initial field research on Tibetan medicine, in 1996, took place at a clinic in a small Indian hill-town, as part of a joint project with Linda Connor and Santi Rozario (Samuel 1999, 2001; Rozario and Samuel 2001). This clinic was the local branch of a network of Tibetan medical clinics administered by the central Men-Tsee-Khang in the North Indian town of Dharamsala, the headquarters of the Tibetan refugee administration, which was about 50 km away. The clinic where we did our research catered mostly to local Tibetans and Indians. Many clients were children from the local Tibetan boarding school, generally wanting medical certificates so that they could go on a visit home to their families elsewhere in India. The local *amchi* conspicuously displayed a stethoscope, and made regular use of a sphygmomanometer to measure the patients' blood pressure. Indeed, that widespread Indian folk syndrome, 'blood pressure' – meaning high blood pressure – was one of the most frequent diagnoses at the clinic, though it does not correspond precisely to any classical Tibetan disease or syndrome. In addition, although the young doctor in charge was a monk, his dress was relatively secular. A red sweater was his main concession to monastic dress (Samuel 1999, 2001).

The relatively matter-of-fact style and mood of the clinic was not much different from that of a biomedical practice in the UK or Australia, though the staff consisted of two people only, the *amchi* and the pharmacist, who also served as receptionist. Patients came through the door, and after a relatively brief encounter were given a prescription or medical certificate, after which they left. It is true that the encounters generally included a Tibetan-style pulse reading, and that the diagnostic categories employed by the *amchi* corresponded for the most part to those in the *rGyud bzhi*. However, the office, desk and equipment looked much more generically biomedical than specifically Tibetan. This was a Tibetan community where there was also a significant presence of biomedicine, both in the form of community nurses and health workers, and of access to biomedical facilities in the Indian town where the community was situated and other nearby centres, and most local Tibetans who used Sowa Rigpa also used biomedical services. Few appeared to have a strong ideological preference for Sowa Rigpa (Samuel 2001).

Visiting the clinic of Dr Yeshi Dhonden, the well-known Tibetan *amchi*, at Dharamsala, also in 1996, I found myself in a quite different symbolic world. Dr Dhonden wore full monastic robes. The atmosphere was pervaded by Buddhist symbolism, with a gentle fragrance of Tibetan temple incense. The walls were adorned with *thang ka*, scroll-paintings of Buddhist deities, and there was not a stethoscope or sphygmomanometer in sight. Dr Yeshi Dhonden had been the personal physician of the 14th Dalai Lama from 1960 to 1980, and was the founder and first director of the Dharamsala Men-Tsee-Khang in the early 1960s. He retired as Director of the Men-Tsee-Khang in 1979 to set up his private practice in Dharamsala. Many of the patients to whom Dr Dhonden catered were Western visitors to Dharamsala, drawn there by their interest in Tibetan religion and culture, and familiar with Dr Yeshi Dhonden through his widely available book, *Health Through Balance* (Dhonden 1986). I have no data on why they chose to use Tibetan medicine, but it would seem likely that some at least were drawn by the mystique of an alternative healing modality, which they assumed to have a strong Buddhist and spiritual orientation. Clearly these two different practitioners were providing the signals and symbols that would be most comfortable, reassuring and attractive to their respective clientele.

This is not an unusual situation, cross-culturally, but it is notable how far the framing of Sowa Rigpa can vary between different contexts. Not only the framing, but the internal understandings of Sowa Rigpa as practised in the urban clinic and hospital context within Tibet and India may be heavily structured by biomedical norms and expectations. Some of this may be little more than window-dressing, as with the unused microwave ovens for sterilising herbal ingredients in the medicine factories discussed by Martin Saxer (2013), presumably there primarily to satisfy visiting government officials. A more complex situation, such as the medicine empowerment (*sman sgrub*) performed in relation to a hospital-based clinical trial of a Tibetan medical formula in Lhasa described by Sienna Craig (2011), may involve a delicate negotiation between Sowa Rigpa and biomedical elements and understandings. Here the trial has to be carried out in a way which will as far as possible satisfy a variety of parties: Craig herself, foreign expert and medical anthropologist; her local colleagues, some of them practitioners of both Sowa Rigpa and biomedicine, others only of biomedicine; the lama who will perform the empowerment; and a variety of government officials. Each of these may frame what is going on in subtly different ways. At the same time, the best interests of the patients also have to be borne in mind (Craig 2011).

Part of the background to this situation is the history of medical training and biomedical syncretism in both Chinese-controlled Tibet (Janes 1995; Garrett 2005–6) and India (Kloos 2008, 2010, 2013). Products of the Tibetan medical training system in China would undergo a more systematically secularised curriculum, but the Men-Tsee-Khang training in India also gave a relatively marginal place to religious or spiritual concerns (cf. Kloos 2013). In other, more rural contexts, particularly outside the PRC, Sowa Rigpa can retain strong elements of more 'traditional' approaches. Consider, for example, Florian Besch's (2009) description of medical practice and its ongoing relationship with Buddhist Tantric healing and the local gods and spirits in Spiti, or Calum Blaikie's (2013a, 2013b) study of the social and spiritual networks still underlying much medicine production in Ladakh.

How important, though, is the Buddhist dimension of Sowa Rigpa? It is probably already evident that there is no simple answer to this question. However, there is plenty of material that bears in varying ways on this issue, and hopefully the reader will have a clearer sense of what is involved by the end of the chapter. The next section provides an overview of the literature on Tibetan medicine in Western languages, with particular reference to the question of the Buddhist dimension of Sowa Rigpa.

Literature

The Western-language literature on Tibetan medicine is by now quite extensive. Jürgen C. Aschoff's 1996 bibliography already included nearly 1700 items, and by now the number must be far higher. While this work is not all of a high scholarly standard (Aschoff included some journalistic and semi-popular literature in his bibliography, and other items date from a period when Western knowledge of Sowa Rigpa was still quite basic), there is undoubtedly a substantial body of research in the area.

This can be divided into three main categories. The first and probably the largest, not discussed here, consists of scientific work on traditional medicinal plants and Tibetan pharmacology, along with research on the possible therapeutic applications of Tibetan medical compounds or (more often) individual ingredients. Two further categories will be discussed in some detail in this section. These are historical and textual works on the Tibetan medical tradition, and research by medical anthropologists on Tibet and other societies where Sowa Rigpa is practised.

I move on to the second category, the textual and historical work. Csoma de Körös (1984) presented a brief summary of the *rGyud bzhi* in 1835, and there was some work on this text in the early twentieth century, mainly in Russian and on the basis of the Mongolian translation (see Emmerick 1975 for references). Claus Vogel (1965) also produced a valuable study of the first five chapters of the Tibetan translation of Vāgbhata's *Aṣṭāṅgahṛdayasa ṃhitā*, one of the most important Ayurvedic treatises on medicine, presenting a verse-by-verse comparison of the Tibetan and Sanskrit texts with translations and detailed notes. Rechung Rinpoche's (1973) *Tibetan Medicine* included a translation of parts of the second and fourth books of the *rGyud bzhi*, along with the hagiography of the elder g.Yu thog pa, a probably legendary ancestor of the twelfth-century compiler of the *Rgyud bzhi* (cf. Yang Ga 2019).

Research and publications on Tibetan medicine really began to take off in Western European languages, however, in the late 1970s and early 1980s. Important early examples include Elisabeth Finckh's (1978, 1985, 1988a, 1988b) writings, particularly her *Grundlagen tibetischer Heilkunde: Nach dem Buche rGyud-bzhi* (translated as *Foundations of Tibetan Medicine: According to the Book rGyud bži*) and the work of Fernand Meyer (1984; see also Meyer 1990, 1992), including his *Gso ba rig pa: Le Système Médical Tibétaine*. Marianne Winder's publications (1981, 1984, 1987) might also be added to this group, along with Terry Clifford's (1984) *Tibetan Buddhist Medicine and Psychiatry: The Diamond Healing*.

Other substantial works, in a more popular style, include Yeshi Dhonden's (1986) *Health Through Balance*, edited and translated by Jeffrey Hopkins, and Tom Dummer's (1988) *Tibetan Medicine and Other Holistic Health Care Systems*. The Library of Tibetan Works and Archives in Dharamsala produced a number of works, including an English-language journal, *Tibetan Medicine*, a series of short books in collaboration with Men-Tsee-Kang doctors, a volume of lectures by the female doctor Lobsang Dolma Khangkar (1986), and a volume by the Ayurvedic scholar Bhagwan Dash (1976). They also produced a translation of the opening sections of the *rGyud bzhi* (Kelsang 1977), while Dash went on to publish seven volumes of an extensive *Encyclopedia of Tibetan Medicine* focused around a reconstructed Sanskrit text of the *rGyud bzhi* (Dash 1994–2001). Other significant authors include T.J. Tsarong (1981, 1986), Dr Lobsang Rabgay (e.g. 1994a, 1994b), and Barry Clark (1995), who provided a complete translation of the first two books of the *rGyud bzhi*.

The most spectacular and impressive achievement of this period was no doubt the massive reproduction of the medical paintings illustrating the 'Blue Beryl' commentary to the *rGyud bzhi* by the sDe srid Sangs rgyas rgya tsho, Regent of Tibet in the early eighteenth century. The volume was edited by Yuri Parfionovitch,

Gyurme Dorje and Fernand Meyer (1992) with an extensive summary of the commentary running in parallel with the paintings.

This is by no means a complete listing,[5] particularly in relation to popular works in English and other European languages, but it indicates the range and type of work produced during this initial period. This shared a number of features. It was generally based closely on the *Rgyud bzhi* as expounded by doctors in the Tibetan diaspora, mostly at the Dharamsala Men-Tsee-Khang. It presented Tibetan medicine as a 'system', and the *rGyud bzhi* as the epitome of that system. The Buddhist nature of the medical tradition was for the most part taken for granted. There was little or no attention to the origins of the *rGyud bzhi,* to its complex textual history, or to its relationship to the remainder of Tibetan medical literature. More will be said about this in the following section on 'Sources'. Nevertheless, as a whole, this work presented a basically sound overview of Sowa Rigpa as presented by the first generation of Tibetan doctors in the diaspora, and it laid the foundations for a real knowledge of Tibetan medicine in the West.

A more critical orientation towards the *rGyud bzhi* was first developed in the work of the late Ronald Emmerick, who demonstrated in his 1977 article, 'Sources of the rGyud bzhi', that substantial parts of the *rGyud bzhi* were closely based on the eleventh century Tibetan translation of Vāgbhata's *Aṣṭāṅgahṛdayasaṃhitā*. Emmerick (1977) also correctly noted that other features connected more with Chinese medicine (see also Emmerick 1975, 1987, 1990, 1991; Hsu 2008). Christopher Beckwith (1979) pointed out that Tibetan historical sources describe a number of doctors from various traditions, including the Greco-Persian (Galenic), Indian and Chinese, as visiting Tibet during the seventh to eighth centuries and founding medical lineages. Ronit Yoeli-Tlalim (2012), who has worked on the medical texts from Dunhuang, noted that while there are traces of 'Galenic' medicine in the later tradition, they are rather limited.

An important article by Samten Karmay, 'Vairocana and the Rgyud-bzhi', first published in 1989, pointed out that Tibetan medical authorities had historically been in disagreement regarding the authorship of the *rGyud bzhi*, with a substantial group arguing that it could not be the literal word of the Buddha. By this stage, it was becoming clear that the *rGyud bzhi* was indeed a compound work synthesising material from a variety of traditions. The work is generally now regarded by Western scholarship as the product of g.Yu thog Yon tan rgyal po 'the Younger' (1126–1202), perhaps in collaboration with one or more of his students, and g.Yu thog pa's eighth-century namesake is seen as probably fictional (cf. Yang Ga 2019). In fact, as argued in the Harvard doctoral thesis of the Tibetan medical scholar Yangga Trarong (Yang Ga 2010), we have a substantial body of other medical writing by the twelfth-century g.Yu thog Yon tan rgyal po, much of which can be viewed as draft material for the *rGyud bzhi.* Yangga Trarong provides a detailed study of the sources of each section of the *rGyud bzhi* demonstrating that, in addition to the material based on the *Aṣṭāṅgahṛdaya-saṃhitā* there is a substantial contribution from Tibetan medical literature predating the translation of Vāgbhata's work.

Karmay's (1989) article was one of the first to explore sources in Tibetan on the history of Tibetan medicine, and subsequent scholars, such as Olaf Czaja (e.g. 2005–6a, 2005–6b, 2007), Janet Gyatso (2004, 2011, 2015), Frances Garrett (2004, 2007, 2013, 2014), Stacey Van Vleet (2010–11, 2013, 2015, 2016), William McGrath (2017) and others gradually built up, on the basis of these and other sources, a fairly detailed picture of the historical evolution of both Tibetan medicine and Tibetan medical scholarship. There is undoubtedly much more to be done, but in reading these more recent works it is clear that there has been a dramatic shift in the level of sophistication of scholarship in this area.

Most of this work has been aimed primarily at other Tibetanists. A major exception has been the writings of Janet Gyatso, already well-known for earlier work on the *gter ma* or visionary traditions within Tibetan Buddhism, who produced an important article in 2004 (reprinted as Gyatso 2011) aimed at a more general audience, and argued for an ongoing tension between the empiricist orientation of Tibetan medicine and the rigid presuppositions of Tibetan tantra. Her 2015 book, *Being Human in a Buddhist World: An Intellectual History of Medicine in Early Modern Tibet*, was likewise aimed at bringing what is in many ways a challenging and radical interpretation of Tibetan medical history to the awareness of the wider world of scholarship on medicine and science. I discuss this work later in this chapter (see 'Analysis').

I move on to the third category, writing by scholars working primarily in the field of medical anthropology. There is by now a substantial body of work in this area, focusing on the contemporary practice of Tibetan medicine and other Tibetan healing modalities in a wide range of communities. Early authors include Alice Kuhn (1988, 1994) writing on Ladakh, Craig Janes (1995, 1999a, 1999b, 2001) and Vincanne Adams (1998, 2001a, 2001b) on Central Tibet, as well as my own early articles on Tibetan medicine in Himachal Pradesh (Samuel 1999, 2001). Since then a whole series of younger scholars have produced substantial and impressive work using primarily ethnographic approaches. They include Resi Hofer (2005, 2008a, 2008b, 2011, 2012), Sienna Craig (2006, 2009, 2011, 2012, 2014), Mona Schrempf (2010, 2015a, 2015b, 2015c), Martin Saxer (2013, 2014), Stephan Kloos (2008, 2010, 2013), Florian Besch (2009), Calum Blaikie (2009, 2013a, 2013b), Barbara Gerke (2010a, 2010b, 2012, 2013, 2014), Audrey Prost (2003, 2006, 2007, 2008), Colin Millard (2002, 2006, 2007, 2013), Laurent Pordié (2007, 2015), Patrizia Bassini (2007, 2013), Susannah Deane (2014, 2015, 2018), Ivette Vargas (2010), Ivette Vargas-O'Bryan (2015), and Jonathan Taee (2017) among others.

While there is undoubtedly a contrast in style and approach between this anthropologically inspired work and that of the textualists, one can also exaggerate the differences. Many of the younger generation of anthropologists who work in Tibetan medicine, as in other areas of Tibetan culture, have also a sound textual and philological grounding, and some of them have written work which might be seen as belonging more to the textual school: Theresia Hofer's 2007 article on the *byang lugs* medical tradition, moving fluidly between ethnographic and textual material, might serve as an example. Equally, many 'textual' scholars have spent time with Tibetan doctors and lamas in Asia, and are willing to employ ethnographic as well as traditional textual approaches: Olaf Czaja's 2011 study of a conference where Tibetan doctors were discussing how to understand cancer in Tibetan terms could be cited here. The two approaches, however, yield different kinds of information, and the strong presence on both sides has contributed to the rich and nuanced picture that we are acquiring of the history and practice of the Sowa Rigpa tradition.

The following listing gives an idea of some of the questions that have been significant in the ethnographic literature on Sowa Rigpa over the last few years:

How is Tibetan medicine delivered in practice? Who by? In what setting?
How are practitioners trained? By whom? What texts are used? What is learned by heart? How is practical experience acquired? If there are family networks, how do they operate? What is the relationship between medical literature and practice?
How are *materia medica* gathered or acquired? How do these practices relate to 'traditional' specifications? What practices of substitution are used when ingredients are not available or too expensive?
How are medicines produced? By whom? In what form? Is production commercial or personal? Is there a Buddhist ritual component, if so how does it work? Are there international networks of production and distribution?
What is the role of official regulation of medical formulae and medical production?
How do patients understand the meaning, efficacy and safety of treatments? Is ritual empowerment of medicines significant for them? How do they understand the relationship between biomedical and Sowa Rigpa treatment? How do they understand the difference between Sowa Rigpa treatment and ritual treatment? Who provides ritual treatment?
Are there popular and folk medicinal practices within the community? Is there local use of herbs by lay people?
How do people without training in Sowa Rigpa understand illness? Do they use Sowa Rigpa categories?
What is the nature of the professional community (or communities) of Sowa Rigpa practitioners? How do they interact with other communities of health and medical practitioners? How do they interact with Government regulation of medical practice?
What are the wider implications, for public health and society more generally, of the practice of Sowa Rigpa within Tibetan and other societies?
Who uses Sowa Rigpa? What is the role of Sowa Rigpa in relation to Tibetan or other ethnic identity?
How have any or all of these issues changed over the recent historical period? How are they changing now?

A detailed survey of this material would go well beyond the bounds of the present chapter, though one significant collective volume will be discussed at some length in the following section. It is worth noting, though, that this ethnographic work covers at least three different, if overlapping, contexts. First, there are studies of medical practice still embedded in regions, mainly in the Indian and Nepalese Himalayas, where much of the logic of traditional medicine practice still prevails, if increasingly challenged by state authorities, biomedical practice and other modernising forces. Studies, such as Besch's (2009) of medicine in Spiti, or Blaikie's (2013a, 2013b) accounts of medicine production in Ladakh might serve as examples. Then there are studies of the practice of medicine in areas such as Chinese-controlled Tibet, where there have been radical processes of transformation and restructuring, and Sowa Rigpa is in the process of ongoing adjustment to a very different kind of health environment. The work of Janes (1995), Adams (2001b) and Hofer (2011) fit into this category. Finally, there are studies where diasporic populations and international flows come to the fore, and Sowa Rigpa is seen as part of global networks of both economic and therapeutic exchange and creation of new meanings. Studies by Kloos (2010, 2013), Saxer (2013) or Craig (2012) are of this kind. But these divisions can be somewhat artificial, since even in remote valleys in the Indian Himalayas, Sowa Rigpa is not insulated these days from a global context. The point is more that one of the most important contributions of the ethnographic material on Tibetan medicine has been precisely to give a detailed and realistic account of the vast range of situations and contexts within which the practice of Sowa Rigpa is now located. The *rGyud bzhi* may still serve in important ways as the foundation and root text of Tibetan medicine, but medical practice goes far beyond anything that might be understood simply by a study of the *rGyud bzhi*.

Sources

In fact, despite the undoubtedly important role of the *rGyud bzhi*, its role in relation to the quite extensive indigenous medical literature in Tibetan has always been more exemplary than exhaustive. Garrett's (2004) PhD dissertation provided a useful summary of the various genres of Tibetan medical writing, outlining nine kinds of text (Garrett 2004: 48–69). Her nine categories are:

Nosology (Disease Classification)
Pharmacy and *materia medica*, including therapeutic prescriptions
Dictionaries of medical terminology, *materia medica*, etc.
Histories of medicine
Biographies of medical figures
Medicine Buddha liturgies
Descriptions of the human body
Documents on medical iconography
The Four Tantras (*rGyud bzhi*) and its commentaries

This is not exhaustive, and individual texts can span more than one category, but it gives a sense of what is in fact a very substantial body of literature. One should, at the same time, bear in mind that Tibetan medical literature, like much of Tibetan religious and other literature, formed in the past part of structures of transmission and distribution different from that of its Western equivalents. Texts were tied up with concepts of lineage and property. They were part of the passing down of medical knowledge through specific lineages of people who had the rights to use those texts through family connection or attachment to a particular teaching lineage. While there were certainly scholars who could and did read comparatively across a body of similar texts, this was not normal practice.

I move on now to a discussion of two specific texts or bodies of texts, the *rGyud bzhi* and the *g.Yu thog snying thig*.

The rGyud bzhi

The formal title of this text is the *Bdud rtsi snying po yan lag brgyad pa gsang ba man ngag gi rgyud ces bya ba* (Eightfold Ambrosial Heart, entitled the Secret Oral Instruction Tantra). The title reflects both the title of the *Aṣṭāṅgahṛdayasaṃhitā* (Summary of the Eightfold Heart), which refers to the classical Ayurvedic division of medicine into eight *aṅga* (limbs or parts), and the Tibetan text's claims to originate in a secret Tantric transmission. It is popularly known simply as the *rGyud bzhi*, the 'Four Tantras' or 'Fourfold Tantra', from the four major sections into which it is divided. As both titles suggest, the *rGyud bzhi* is presented as a 'Tantra', that is an esoteric text which is held to be the actual word of the Buddha, and its overall structure follows the literary conventions of such a text, being framed as an instructional dialogue between Tantric manifestations of the Buddha.

It has consequently been regarded as a sacred and authoritative text, as the literal word of the Buddha in one of his Tantric manifestations, by many Tibetan scholars and medical practitioners. It is not included, however, in the Tantric section of the *bKa' 'gyur*, the canonical collection of the translated words (*bka'*) of the Buddha, as one would expect were it a Tantra transmitted from India, nor, like other Indian medical treatises such as the *Aṣṭāṅgahṛdayasaṃhitā*, is it in the *bsTan 'gyur*, the collection of translated works by Indian scholars. For this and other reasons, some Tibetan scholars argued from soon after the appearance of the *rGyud bzhi* that it was in fact a Tibetan product. This is also the view adopted by almost all Western scholars.[6]

The *rGyud bzhi* owes part of its title and a substantial part of its contents to the *Aṣṭāṅgahṛdayasaṃhitā* (Emmerick 1977; Yang Ga 2010). However, as noted earlier, this is by no means the only source which G.yu thog pa used for the work, assuming that it was indeed he who wrote it. Substantial parts of the text originate from other sources, including Chinese, Greco-Islamic and indigenous contributions (see Hsu 2008; Yang Ga 2010; Yoeli-Tlalim 2012). Thus, Tibetan medicine as practised according to the *rGyud bzhi* is not a simple transposition of Ayurveda from India to Tibet.

A further question concerns the degree to which the *rGyud bzhi* can be seen as definitive of Tibetan healing practices. I have already discussed the wide range of textual material regarding aspects of Sowa Rigpa, dating from both before and after the *rGyud bzhi*. It is also important to appreciate that the *rGyud bzhi* is a verse text, often condensed and even cryptic. Consequently, it is generally approached via a commentary that expands and explains the text, as well as through oral explanation. The text itself has undergone substantial revisions by later scholars. A number of lineages of interpretation developed in the centuries after its appearance, of which the two best-known are the Jang (*Byang*) tradition founded by Byang pa rNam rgyal grags bzang and the Sur (*Zur*) tradition founded by Zur mkhar mNyam nyid rdo rje and continued by, among others, Zur mkhar bLo gros rgyal po (Gerke 1999; Hofer 2007; see also Van Vleet 2015; McGrath 2017).

In the seventeenth century, Sangs rgyas rgya mtsho (1653–1705), the sDe srid (regent) of the Lhasa state at the time of the fifth Dalai Lama (1617–1682) and also a major scholar of medicine, is regarded as having combined elements from these two lineages. In reality, his work was far more extensive than a simple comparison or conflation (Czaja 2007; Van Vleet 2016). He re-edited the text of the *rGyud bzhi* and provided his own extensive commentary, the *Vaiḍūrya sngon po* or 'Blue Beryl' (Sangs rgyas rgya mtsho 1994). While we have other textual versions of the *rGyud bzhi* material, including the *'Bum bzhi* associated with the Bon po medical tradition, and other commentaries, the *rGyud bzhi* today is generally viewed through a perspective created by the sDe srid.[7] He was also responsible for several other important medical texts, including the 'Supplement' or *lhan thabs* to the *rGyud bzhi* (Sangs rgyas rgya mtsho 1978), and an extensive and influential medical history, recently translated as the 'Mirror of Beryl' (*Vaidūrya'i me long*)' (Sangyé Gyatso 2010). He also founded the medical college of lCags po ri, mentioned earlier (cf. Meyer 2003).

The sDe srid was also responsible for commissioning a famous series of paintings illustrating the *rGyud bzhi*, subsequently repainted and copied many times (Parfionovitch, Dorje and Meyer 1992). Much early Western scholarly literature on Sowa Rigpa took the sDe srid's work as representing the *rGyud bzhi* in an unproblematic way, but it is becoming clear that he made a significant and creative contribution to the tradition. At the same, as he himself pointed out, he had limited experience of medical practice (e.g. Sangyé Gyatso 2010: 487–8). Czaja (2007: 363) says of the sDe srid's relationship to the Zur pa and Byang pa school that he 'attempted to smooth out their differences in order to create an intellectually coherent system regarding the understanding of the *rGyud bzhi*'. Czaja, Gyatso and others have argued plausibly that the sDe srid's work on the *rGyud bzhi*, including lCags po ri college and the paintings, needs to be understood in relation to his State-building project in relation to the Lhasa government (Gyatso 2015; Van Vleet 2015, 2016).

The *rGyud bzhi*, generally in combination with the sDe srid's 'Blue Beryl' (*Bai ḍūrya sngon po*) commentary, is often treated as authoritative or definitive of the Sowa Rigpa tradition, and substantial parts of the text are still memorised by Sowa Rigpa practitioners as part of their training. As with other such canonical texts, while memorisation may lead to internalising the diagnostic categories and basic techniques of the body of knowledge in question, it does not really, as and of itself, make you into a doctor, which is more a matter of practical apprenticeship to an established practitioner.

In any case, the *rGyud bzhi*, with or without commentary, hardly provides an adequate basis for practice as a Tibetan doctor today. The *rGyud bzhi*'s disease categories, defined in the third and longest of its four treatises, the *Man ngag rgyud*, are still widely used, but the remedies employed today are generally different and more complex than those prescribed in the *rGyud bzhi*, often containing up to fifty ingredients. Pharmacology has developed considerably since the time of the *rGyud bzhi*, when the process of identifying Tibetan plant varieties and medicinal substances that were effective equivalents for the largely Ayurvedic pharmacopoeia in the *rGyud bzhi* was still at a fairly early stage. Later works such as the *Shel gong shel phreng* of the eighteenth-century medical scholar De'u dmar dge bshes bsTan 'dzin phun tshogs are fundamental to Sowa Rigpa pharmacology, and later works and recipes also provide the basis for the compounding of medicines.

Two specific features of the *rGyud bzhi* are worth pointing out here. The first has already been mentioned. The *rGyud bzhi* incorporates the standard Ayurvedic model of disease as being caused by three pathogenic factors, the three *doṣa* or pathogenic factors (*vāta*, *pitta*, *kaphā*). It, however, adds a further layer of explanation to the essentially materialistic Ayurvedic theory of the *doṣa*, by claiming that the three *nyes pa* are themselves caused by the three basic *nyon mongs* (Sanskrit *kleśa*), mental obscurations or negative emotional factors, greed, hatred and delusion. Thus, what is in the *Aṣṭāṅgahṛdayasaṃhitā* a basically materialist account of illness causation caused by organic factors acquires in the *rGyud bzhi* an underlying level of explanation that links directly with the world of Buddhist philosophy and practice (see also Samuel 2019: 771–2).

There is another important linkage to Buddhist practice. The *rGyud bzhi* also includes substantial references to elements from Buddhist Tantric theory, including the 'subtle body' concepts that form part of both Hindu and Buddhist Tantra (e.g. Samuel and Johnston 2013; Yangönpa 2015; Samuel 2019: 779–82). These encompass a network of 'channels' (Sanskrit *nāḍī*, Tibetan *rtsa*) within the body through which flow the substance known in Tibetan as *rlung*. *Rlung* is conventionally translated as 'wind' or 'air', and corresponds to *vāta*, one of the three *doṣa* of the Ayurvedic system. However, the same Tibetan term is also used to translate Sanskrit *prāṇa* or 'breath', the substance that flows through the Tantric system of *nāḍī*, and these two different concepts, deriving from different bodies of discourse in India, have clearly become conflated in Tibetan writing. A key concept within the Tantric context is that of 'untying the knots' within the (Tantric) channels so that *rlung* (*prāṇa*) can flow freely, and exercises to do with controlling and directing *rlung* through the channels form an important part of Tantric practice. Practitioners of Tantric meditation are thought to be particularly susceptible to *rlung* disorders, which often manifest as what biomedicine might regard as mental or psychiatric disorders, such as depression, anxiety or forms of psychosis. Specific forms of Tantric therapy focus on working with *rlung* (see e.g. Lipman 2010; Samuel 2019).

The *rGyud bzhi* contains a description of the system of *rtsa* within the body, but the term *rtsa* also refers to veins, arteries and other visible and material structures within the body, including the nervous system, and the interpretation of this passage caused major difficulties for later Tibetan medical scholars (see Gyatso 2015: 193–249, especially 200–2). This was particularly so because it became increasingly apparent that the *rlung* channels did not have a visible material existence and could not be identified, for example, in an autopsy. They can perhaps be explained in other ways that are compatible with how they are employed in Tantric practice (Samuel 2019), but it was also quite difficult to reconcile the *rGyud bzhi*'s description of the *rtsa* with the Tantric understandings of the subtle body. Since working with the *rlung* is a central component of Tantric yoga, this was not a trivial matter.

The g.Yu thog snying thig

There is another important linkage between the *rGyud bzhi*, or at any rate the great twelfth-century physician who is generally assumed to have written it, g.Yu thog pa, and the world of Buddhist practice. This is g.Yu thog pa's other great creation, the Tantric practice cycle known as the *g.Yu thog snying thig* (Yuthok Heart Essence) (Ehrhard 2007, Garrett 2009, Samuel 2017).

The term *snying thig* refers to a number of traditions of oral transmission of rDzogs chen, a specific form of the Buddhist teachings, which were codified in textual form from the eleventh century onwards. The conventional understanding of 'discovered' (*gter ma*) texts, such as the *snying thig*, is that they were the result of visionary revelation from Tantric deities. In practice, they appear to result from a complex mix of visionary processes, newly composed material, and material adapted from previous *gter ma* texts (Mayer 2013–14). *Snying thig* traditions in particular are of considerable importance within the wider world of Tibetan Buddhist practice, especially in Eastern Tibet.

The *g.Yu thog snying thig* shares in this general milieu in that it has the overall structure and includes the core components of a *snying thig*. Thus, it includes a set of central practices aimed at the achievement of Buddhahood, and other practices aimed at various this-worldly purposes, as well as accessory rituals and texts, such as the empowerment rituals for passing the practice on to disciples. It is, however, intended specifically for medical practitioners, and many of its rituals and practices are specifically connected with healing and medicine. A short historical text included in the cycle describes the *g.Yu thog snying thig* as claiming to originate in teachings passed on to G.yu thog pa from a *ḍākinī* (female initiatory deity) during a visit he made to India, while implying that it was in fact derived from G.yu thog pa's personal vision (*thugs gter*) (Ehrhard 2007: 163–4; Samuel 2017). However the central texts of the cycle were created, the core of the *g.Yu thog snying thig* does indeed appear to go back to the time of g.Yu thog pa and his immediate disciple Sum ston Ye shes gzungs.

The *g.Yu thog snying thig* lineage has been passed down to the present day but, while it has had some high-profile exponents, such as the late Trogawa Rinpoche, it has become marginal to the practice of most contemporary Tibetan *amchi*. It is not taught directly as part of the Men-Tsee-Kang curriculum in Dharamsala, nor in the equivalent institutions in Tibet, and while *amchi* may take the opportunity to receive the associated empowerment ritual, if available, it seems that few commit themselves to these demanding practices on a regular basis. Yet it is striking that this cycle of practices appears to have been seen, through eight or nine centuries of Tibetan medical history, as an essential complement to the practice of medicine according to the *rGyud bzhi*. The main contemporary use of the *g.Yu thog snying thig* is as a source of the most commonly employed *sman sgrub* (medicine empowerment) ritual. Here, as in other features such as the role of greed, hatred and delusion as underlying the three *nyes pa*, or the significance of medicine-empowerment in the preparation of medicines, we see Tibetan medicine as adopting a specifically Buddhist identity.

Analysis

By this point, some of the reasons why Sowa Rigpa today might be understood and indeed practised in terms which are either more religious or more secular have perhaps become clear. Sowa Rigpa derives in large part from medical traditions, Indian, Chinese and Greco-Arab, that were not framed primarily as spiritual practices, but as practical approaches for the understanding of illness and the bringing about of healing. Yet it incorporated other elements that have a different and more explicitly spiritual orientation. My concern in the remainder of this chapter is with the consequences of this inbuilt ambiguity or tension. I shall discuss two recent works of Western scholarship which might be seen as exemplifying the two contrasting approaches. These are the joint-edited volume, *Medicine, Science and Religion: Explorations on Tibetan Grounds* (Adams, Schrempf and Craig 2011a), and Janet Gyatso's recent work on Tibetan medicine, particularly her 2015 volume, *Being Human in a Buddhist World: An Intellectual History of Medicine in Early Modern Tibet.*

Medicine Between Science and Religion

I begin with the *Medicine Between Science and Religion* collection, which is an edited volume of original contributions on the Sowa Rigpa tradition (Adams, Schrempf and Craig 2011a). It began with a group of papers by scholars who came together at the 11th Seminar of the International Association of Tibetan Studies in Germany in 2006. A number of further invited contributions were included in the final volume, including an epilogue that I contributed myself (Samuel 2011). The three editors, Vincanne Adams, Mona Schrempf and Sienna R. Craig, are all medical anthropologists working on Sowa Rigpa. I will focus here on their joint introduction to the volume (Adams, Schrempf and Craig 2011b) which constitutes a manifesto for a radical shift in our view of Tibetan healing practices, and indeed of healing as a whole. In the following passage, they set out to explain the perspective from which the book is written:

> Most ethnographic analyses of science and medicine in cross-cultural encounters begin with analytical frameworks adopted from biological science or social science methodology, which can presume an objectivist and empirical reporting of encounters without recognizing that the very notions of objectivity and empiricism are themselves already embedded in a specific kind of modernity and scientific discourse [...]. In these accounts, biomedicine (as a normative ideal and, often, a locally specific set of practices) offers the analytical framework for comparison, as if the encounter with the 'other' on medical terrain always presupposes the need for an engagement with the biological sciences that derives first and foremost from a modern, Western viewpoint.
>
> Instead of starting with the supposition that such translations of medicine across cultures must begin with, or emerge from, a biomedical frame, we adopt and apply an approach that begins with *sowa rigpa*. The 'science of healing' – as *sowa rigpa* is most often translated and used to denote the foundations of traditional Tibetan medicine – is our epistemological starting point, our orientation. We chose the terms 'science of healing', from among the various possible translations of these Tibetan words, in order to deliberately complicate the notion of science, as we explain below [...]. Our use of the term *sowa rigpa* signifies more than the classical body of Tibetan medical knowledge, as expounded in the *Gyüshi* or the Four Tantras, to include other forms of Tibetan healing knowledge and practices that have either become marginalized within modern institutions of Tibetan medicine or have been seen as belonging to the domain of 'religion' (2011b: 3–4).

The authors make a number of moves in the above passage, but the key ones are their insistence that biomedicine should not be taken as the primary frame of reference, and that their epistemological starting point treats 'medical' and 'religious' healing practices as essentially on the same level. These moves complement each other. If biomedicine is no longer the sole judge of effective healing, there is no reason to regard Tantric ritual or shamanic healing as some kind of inferior, marginal practice.

Both 'medical' and 'religious' practices may form part of *sowa rigpa*, the 'science of healing', which is here clearly wider than 'Sowa Rigpa' in the sense of, for example, the medical modality approved by the Government of India's Department of AYUSH. The 'science of healing' encompasses spirit-mediums, diviners and Tantric lamas, as much as practitioners of medicine according to the canons of the *rGyud bzhi*.

This is a radical move, and goes well beyond the critique of biomedicine found in most of the classical authors in medical anthropology. For such medical anthropologists as Arthur Kleinman, the problem is not with biomedical science itself, but with the way it is practised. By focusing on the biomedically defined 'disease' as an organic process, and failing to see the need to treat the 'illness', the patient's subjective experience of his or her situation, contemporary biomedical doctors may miss a vital part of the process of healing. Yet the ultimate assessment of efficacy remains that of biomedicine (Kleinman and Sung 1979; Kleinman 1980, 1988; Samuel 2010). For Adams, Schrempf and Craig (2011b), efficacy is a question of how effectively one treats the illness, the patient's holistic experience, not the biomedically defined disease. The demands of effective healing may, and will, cut across any formal distinctions between medical systems and practices.

After this explicit expansion of the field to include practices that might conventionally be labelled as religious, Adams, Schrempf and Craig (2011b: 4) describe their approach as deriving from a '*sowa rigpa* "sensibility"':

> Such a sensibility begins with the processes of looking at medical and social worlds – participating in them, empirically knowing them, and being conscious of their effects on health and well-being.

The perspective that the three editors adopt derives most obviously from a substantial body of earlier work by the senior author, Vincanne Adams, Professor of Medical Anthropology at the University of California, San Francisco (e.g. Adams 2001a,

2002, 2010), but it can also be seen in the writings of the other two authors (e.g. Schrempf 2010; Craig 2011, 2012). One could perhaps question how far their intention is carried through in the subsequent chapters of the book, especially those by authors other than the three editors, and there are unresolved tensions in the introductory chapter itself. One might also ask how far the *sowa rigpa* sensibility sketched in this chapter represents an approach integral to healing in Tibetan society, and how far it derives from the authors' critique of Western and global biomedical practice. The overall intention as outlined in the introduction is, however, clear enough: Tibetan healing practices should be seen as various, and as applied creatively and situationally by a range of healing specialists in order to achieve the most effective result for the patient. Within this process, the boundary between 'medical' and 'religious' aspects is meaningless, and the question of how biomedicine might assess the techniques employed is irrelevant.

Being Human in a Buddhist World

Janet Gyatso is Hershey Professor of Buddhist Studies at Harvard University. Her earlier work was mainly on visionary (*gter ma*, 'Treasure') traditions in Tibet and Buddhism; she has also been a pioneering scholar of gender issues in Tibet and the place of women in Tibetan society. Her work on medicine is relatively recent, and I focus here on two works: her first major article in this area, 'The Authority of Empiricism and the Empricism of Authority' (Gyatso 2004, reprinted as Gyatso 2011), and her recent book, *Being Human in a Buddhist World* (Gyatso 2015). The book is an expansion of the argument in the article, although it also contains a great deal of additional material.

Gyatso's first publication on Tibetan medicine, the short but tightly argued 'Authority of Empiricism' article, came out in 2004. Her move to work on medicine was for some a surprise, but in fact there are continuities between Gyatso's medical work and many of her earlier writings (e.g. Gyatso 1986, 1993, 1999). The ways in which knowledge and experience were constituted and legitimated within various Tibetan traditions had long been key issues in her work. They were also important in her 1998 book, *Apparitions of the Self*, on the important eighteenth-century lama 'Jigs med gling pa. Indeed, Gyatso's book on 'Jigs med gling pa is not really about the career of that very distinguished visionary lama, whose work had such a dominant influence over the non-Gelugpa traditions of Tibet in the nineteenth and twentieth century. Rather, it is a subtle and delicate reading of two short autobiographical texts by 'Jigs med gling pa. Its aim is both to discover the person behind the texts, unpicking the irony and complexity of 'Jigs med gling pa's words, and to explore the whole question of individuality and personal experience within Tibetan society.

Thus, in most of her major writings, Gyatso has used her detailed readings of Tibetan texts to explore general issues, which are more connected with wider work in the humanities – experience, life-writing, the constitution of the self – than with the internal debates of the field of Tibetan Studies. This has been one of the great strengths of her work, and has meant that she is probably much more widely read *outside* Tibetan studies than many of her colleagues. It has also, however, I think made it harder at times for Tibetanists themselves to appreciate what she has been doing and to engage fully with it.

This is true both of the 'Authority of Empiricism' (2004) article, which appeared in a general Asian and African studies journal, not a Tibetanist publication, and of her subsequent writings on Sowa Rigpa, culminating in the 2015 book. Gyatso's interest is less in Tibetan medical writings for their own sake than in what they might tell us about how Tibetans made sense of and understood their experience of the world. Medicine, and specifically the conflicts between Buddhist doctrine and empirical data in the history of Tibetan medical scholarship, provides an illuminating field to examine these issues.

There are other significant aspects to Gyatso's writing on Sowa Rigpa. These relate to what her work might say to the Tibetan community, and particularly to younger Tibetans educated in the diaspora or in the modern Chinese educational system, about the empirical and non-religious aspects of Tibetan thought. In this respect, it links up with a literature on secularism in Tibet which is just starting to get under way (see e.g. Gayley and Willock 2016).

From this point of view, Gyatso's book can be read in part as an assertion that the Tibetans were not perpetually lost in some mystical Buddhist universe. They were as capable of empirical thought as anyone else, and a succession of medical scholars stand as exemplars of their abilities in this area. For most of us who have had some acquaintance with Tibetans, this is hardly a surprise, but it is a useful reminder all the same. It is a message also to the wider world, which often assumes that pre-modern Tibetans lived their lives in some kind of theocratic fantasy-universe.

I turn now to consider some central themes of Gyatso's work, beginning with the 2004 article. After some introductory material on Sowa Rigpa, this article moves to a discussion of the *nyams yig* literature, a body of medical writings from the sixteenth century onwards which as its name implies were indeed based – or in some cases regarded by later authorities as being based – on the author's experience (*nyams*). The growth of the *nyams yig* literature appears to reflect a widespread feeling that doctors should rely more on practical experience and less on what was said in the *rGyud bzhi*. sDe srid Sangs rgyas rgya mtsho, the famous medical scholar and regent for the fifth Dalai Lama, was a particular advocate of the *nyams yig* genre, and Gyatso argues that writings of this kind gradually came to replace the *rGyud bzhi* as the primary sources for medical practice:

> sDe-srid labels his work a 'supplement' to the Four Tantras, but the ineluctable trend is that the nyams-yigs were beginning to supplant the root text. The upshot was that the Four Tantras fell out of use, even if the medical colleges still compelled students to memorize it. At least by the nineteenth century, authors of nyams-yigs could speak directly of the Four Tantras' limitations, as when Kong-sprul describes the many sources to which he had to resort for information that was lacking in the root text, while Mi-pham can distinguish the way he found to read pulse based on his own experience from an array of authoritative precedents in Tibet and China alike (2004: 86).

But what happens when the results of experiential knowledge directly contradict what is in the texts? Gyatso suggests that this was much less of a problem for the medical scholars than for religious scholars:

> In Tibet neither Buddhist nor medical writers considered experience ever to be entirely free of ideational content. Hence their presumption that it is necessary to educate experience in the right way; left uneducated, experience is subject to emotional prejudice and error.

> But while medical writers worried about physicians who practiced only on the basis of their experience, we find far less suspicion of experience as a category as such than we do in Buddhist epistemology and meditation theory. Experience appears to have been unambiguously a good thing in medical learning, even if it could not suffice on its own (2004: 87).

We find, Gyatso argues, 'a greater respect for the realities of the physical world in medicine than in Buddhism' (2004). After all, 'for Buddhist theory what appears to be direct perception in the conventional world will on close analysis prove to be but an illusion' (2004) while '[t]he medical tradition had no interest in arguing that the physical death of a patient is an illusion'. Thus, 'we find medicine in Tibet struggling with classical Buddhist doctrine throughout its history' (2004). That is a key theme for her approach, and the 2004 article is orientated around demonstrating its validity.

Her first key example in the article is the controversy over the various channels within the body described in the *rGyud bzhi*. The *rGyud bzhi*'s account of the channels, which Gyatso summarises here and translates in full in the later book, is as I mentioned earlier famously confused and difficult, conflating what appear to be data from medical anatomy with the well-known channels of Tantric theory. Later doctors clearly struggled to make sense of this account. Gyatso begins with Byang ba bKra shis dpal bzang in the late fifteenth century, and proceeds to Zur mkhar ba Blo gros mtha yas in the sixteenth century and the sDe srid in the seventeenth, ending with the dPal spungs scholar Gling sman bkra shis in the eighteenth century.

She also considers another debate, that about the *rGyud bzhi*'s insistence that the tip of the heart points in different directions in men and women, on which most of the same scholars also commented. It is not very clear what the tip of the heart is meant to be, but it is difficult to find any straightforward interpretation of this statement that is not contradicted by the physical evidence.

Of the five scholars mentioned above, and various others who occur in the narrative of the article and the subsequent book, there is no doubt that the central figures for Gyatso are Zur mkhar ba and the sDe srid. These two were not actual contemporaries – the sDe srid was born some 75 years after Zur mkhar ba's death – but they nevertheless have a complex mutual relationship in Gyatso's work.

As she shows, both the sDe srid and Zur mkhar ba are proponents of a critical and empiricist approach to Sowa Rigpa, but there are significant differences in their positions. The sDe srid's development of Sowa Rigpa as a significant component of the new Lhasa state was heavily dependent on Zur mkhar ba's earlier work, but the sDe srid's attitude to Zur mkhar ba, as expressed in his own writings, is at times quite critical.

The sDe srid, unlike Zur mkhar ba, was not just a medical scholar or even a lama. He was also a major figure in Tibetan politics, and this is part of what Gyatso uses to decode the meaning of the differences between their positions. The centralisation of Tibet under the Fifth Dalai Lama led to an encouragement of medical learning, including empirical study, as in the research that underlay the famous collection of medical paintings produced under the Sde srid's supervision. Tantric ritual and Tantric theory, as in the incarnation status of the Fifth Dalai Lama himself were, however, at the core of the new state. What did this mean for the development of empirical science?

After the debates about the channels and the heart-tip, Gyatso moves – still in the 2004 article – to another critical debate, that on whether the *rGyud bzhi* was Buddha-word, as its form might imply, or a composition by a historical Tibetan author or authors, presumably g.Yu thog pa and his students in the twelfth century. Here Zur mkhar ba and the sDe srid take different positions, with Zur mkhar ba regarding the *rGyud bzhi* as an independent treatise, the sDe srid as Buddha word. Zur mkhar ba appears, however, to be very cautious about his statements in this regard, and is denounced for them in the following century by the sDe srid. This is one of Gyatso's principal arguments for the risks involved in Tibetan doctors making suggestions that contravene scriptural authority. But how real was this tension? In the 2004 article she is cautious in committing herself too far: 'If, then, we find an uneasy tension remaining between the claims of perceptibility and the claims of soteriological transformation [i.e. experience and Buddhist doctrine], the tension may turn out to be mainly in our eyes'. (2004: 93). It is also difficult to know how real the dangers were for those who committed themselves to an overt critique of the official position. As Gyatso (2004: 92) says herself, 'surely the actors at the time didn't know either, even if they felt a risk'.

Being Human in a Buddhist World (2015), which came out 11 years later, is in many ways an expansion of the 2004 article. The three case studies remain at its core, forming Part II, the central part of the book, though the accounts in the original article are re-arranged and considerably expanded, and further chapters added.[8] Both in the book and the article, Gyatso demonstrates convincingly that some Tibetan medical scholars at least did think critically about traditional scholarship in ways based on empirical observation. My impression is that the political argument becomes stronger in the book. Thus, for example, in her discussion of why the sDe srid criticised Zur mkhar ba's assertion that the *rGyud bzhi* was not the word of the Buddha, she tells us that:

> It is all about authority. The foundation of the new state rested on the absolute truth of intentional reincarnation and the accompanying yogic power and apotheosis of the Dalai Lama – all deeply dependent on the magisterial authority of the Buddha's teachings... The Desi moved medicine further into a critical and empiricist direction, but tried simultaneously to keep it domesticated under the sign of Buddhism (2015: 137).

At the same time, she explicitly retains a sense of openness about just what the texts may mean. Neither the sDe srid's position nor that of Zur mkhar ba are easy to read:

> Zurkharwa continuously blurred his own positions. Just when he made his most radical moves that would truly create an epistemic space apart for medicine, he also obscured the effect, precisely, I would say, so as to effect an allegiance to a Buddhist universe on every other front (2015: 138).

Discussion

If Adams, Schrempf and Craig (2011b) stress the otherness of Tibetan healing practices in contrast to biomedical science, and celebrate the religious contribution to the Tibetan 'science of healing', Gyatso's perspective is in many ways the reverse. For her, what is interesting about Tibetan medical scholarship in the *rGyud bzhi* tradition (there is little in her published work about other forms of Tibetan healing) is how close it comes to the empirical approach of Western medical science (i.e. the body of theory and research that underlies biomedicine). Gyatso regards medicine as the area of Tibetan scholarship where empirical research was most evident, and her focus is largely on how medical scholars negotiated the ongoing conflict between textually defined doctrine and their own empirical findings. If Adams and her colleagues celebrate the Buddhist elements of Tibetan healing, Gyatso celebrates the rebels against Buddhist religious dominance. Her heroes are men such as Zur mkhar ba Blo gros rgyal po (1509–79). She views them as empirical scholars who know that, for example, the Tantric channels cannot be physically located in the human body, but who are forced by the religious authorities to conceal or compromise their findings. These men's near-contemporaries in Europe achieved the breakthrough to scientific empiricism and modernity. Tibet's failure to make the same transition has ultimately to be blamed on the dead hand of religious authority.

> There can be no question that we are looking at a knotty set of issues about authority. While we can find examples of commentators overtly correcting the Four Tantras' statements, these tend to be cautious and minor. More commonly, the Four Tantras is upheld, in a display of loyalty that is more important for what it says socially than what it actually means for the practice and theory of medicine, which was evolving. The impulse to show loyalty also has something to do with reticence to dismiss tantric anatomy, even when there was really no way to make its extravagant claims empirically plausible. A twentieth-century commentator's warning probably reflects a long-standing sentiment: 'If [the channels are] explained other than this, that is, if one makes a claim that goes against the theories of the subtle meaning of the tantras that explains the natural condition of the body's channels, then a thesis that invalidates the scriptures would be established. Therefore, it is best to abandon personal arrogance and follow the experts' (Gyatso 2004: 90).

As Gyatso herself admits (2004: 92), there is a speculative aspect to her argument. There are certainly plenty of signs of empirical research within Tibetan medicine, but establishing why this research did not develop into the full-blown empirical approach to knowledge that was taking shape in Europe at the same time is less straightforward. It is difficult to know how real the dangers were for those who committed themselves to an overt critique of the official position. As Gyatso (2004) says, 'surely the actors at the time didn't know either, even if they felt a risk'.

In reality, even Zur mkhar ba adopted a position that respected the Tantric teachings as well as empirical knowledge. Perhaps he was taking the safe option, but perhaps he was also personally committed to the value and efficacy, if not necessarily the precise correspondence to empirical observation, of the Tantric teachings. He was after all a major figure in the lineage of the *G.yu thog snying thig*, the specifically religious teachings held to have been passed down from G.yu thog pa through the Zur mkhar family, and he had received these teachings in a direct line from his famous predecessor in the same medical lineage, Zur mkhar ba Mnyam nyid Rdo rje (Czaja 2005–6: 131). Zur mkhar ba Blo gros rgyal po may have had a critical orientation towards the empirical truth of the Tantric teachings, but we cannot assume that he did not take them seriously as religious teachings, or that they did not play an important role in his own formation as a doctor and medical scholar. What Zur mkhar ba 'really' thought is unknowable. Gyatso is fully aware of such complexities, but the structure of her argument leads her to emphasise the critical scholar in Zur mkhar ba, rather than the spiritually committed medical practitioner.

There is no doubt that Gyatso's book is a major achievement, and that it makes the question of the empirical aspects of Sowa Rigpa into an important issue for scholarship in general. However, there is more to Gyatso's argument than this. In particular, the book proposes a certain relationship between religion – meaning primarily Tantric Buddhism, both as theory and practice – and medicine in Tibet. That relationship is essentially hostile and conflictual. In Gyatso's argument, there is a strong implication that the religious authorities are the villains of the piece, and that it is the dead hand of religious dogma – whether for religious or political reasons – that prevents Sowa Rigpa from reaching its true potential. Gyatso is careful with the parallels to Western history, but underlying her argument in the book – more than in the earlier article – is the parallel with the transition to modern science in Europe, a process which was beginning to get under way at the time of Zur mkhar ba and the Sde srid. There is at least a suggestion that, but for Tantric Buddhism and a state that needed to preserve the authority of Tantric Buddhism to maintain its own legitimacy, the Tibetans might have got much further with achieving their own transition to science, at least in the area of medicine. There are echoes here of the debates years ago, centring on Joseph Needham's *Science and Civilisation in China* (Needham 1954 onwards), about why China failed to develop modern science, and there are suggestions here and there in Gyatso's writings that she sees her own work as engaging with the Tibetan version of this debate, though this never becomes a major theme.

Both *Medicine between Science and Religion* (Adam, Schrempf and Craig 2011b) and *Being Human in a Buddhist World* (Gyatso 2015) are works that take a strong interpretive orientation towards their material. Both are in their different ways major contributions to scholarship on Tibetan medicine, and it would make little sense simply to claim that one of these books is right and the other wrong. What is at issue here is more subtle. I do think, however, that there are questions here that need some serious consideration. If we take Gyatso's overall orientation, for example, and regard Tantric practice as essentially a negative force that obstructed the progress of Tibetan medical science, then what do we make of the vital place that *sman grub*, the Tantric empowerment of medicines, continues to have in most modern Sowa Rigpa practice (e.g. Blaikie 2013b; Craig 2011; Kind 2002)? Or what about the role of *tshe grub* and *tshe dbang*, of long life practice and long life empowerments, in the wider world of Tibetan health? Do we simply treat these as an embarrassing hangover from a pre-scientific world view, or do we accept that they may contribute in some real way to the efficacy of Tibetan practice (cf. Samuel 2013, 2016)?

We do not need, I think, to adopt Tantric theory as a whole to see *sman grub*, *tshe grub*, *tshe dbang* and similar processes as making a vital contribution to healing. Recent re-analyses of what used to be called the 'placebo effect' are making it increasingly clear that ritual and symbolism can indeed have a very strong positive – or for that matter negative – effect on healing the human organism (Samuel 2010, 2014). And, if we are willing to go that far, perhaps we can also concede that men like Zur mkhar ba, who were members of important Tantric lineages as well as major medical scholars, may have had quite a complex and sophisticated understanding of the relationship between empirical science and Tantric practice.

One could, I think, argue that Tantric theory might, at times at least, have assisted rather than obstructed that understanding.

To move to a related point: if g.Yu thog pa, perhaps with his immediate disciples, wrote the *rGyud bzhi* – and most modern scholars would probably concur with Zur mkhar ba on that point – then what do we make of the importance for many Tibetan doctors of g.Yu thog pa's other great contribution to Sowa Rigpa, the *g.Yu thog snying thig*? This lineage of Dzogchen and Tantric practice goes back fairly reliably to g.Yu thog pa's immediate circle, and has been seen throughout much of Tibetan medical history as a vital complement to the *rGyud bzhi*-based system of mostly pharmacological practice. It was also a key property of Zur mkhar ba's own medical lineage. The *g.Yu thog snying thig* has become somewhat sidelined in recent medical training programmes, both in Chinese-controlled Tibet and in the diaspora, but it continues to signal an approach to Sowa Rigpa in which Tantric practice is central, not an uncomfortable and peripheral add-on.

Much here depends on how one reads the texts, and what one reads into them. Gyatso notes in the first chapter of her book how she aims to read with 'a humanistic eye', attuned to 'processes (reaches, retreats, experiments, questions, worries) rather than positions' (2015: 18). She looks for the subtle signs that medical scholars are straining to push further, but are scared that, in her image, they are moving onto thin ice, and that it might crack beneath them. This approach has enabled her to provide an important and insightful approach to Tibetan medicine, but it leaves open the possibility that a different reading might uncover a different Zur mkhar ba and perhaps also a different sDe srid, men less concerned with the political risk of an epistemological breakthrough, and more with the best way of combining Tantric and medical procedures to achieve healing.

Gyatso's work is far richer than my brief remarks can indicate, and goes well beyond the issues raised here into the social and political forces that arguably gave them meaning. It is worth pointing, however, to the implications of Gyatso's overall framing of the Tibetan medical material in contrast to that of *Medicine Between Science and Religion*. Gyatso's central problematic is Tibet's failed transition to scientific modernity, and the dominance of religion and politics over science that dictated that failure. Adams, Schrempf and Craig's central contention is that Tibet, in large part precisely because it failed to make the transition to scientific modernity, retained a fluid and effective set of healing practices, encompassing both 'scientific' and 'religious' elements. Gyatso's framing leads to a focus on the *rGyud bzhi*, the commentarial writing to which it gave birth, and the controversies that took shape within that literature. The framing within *Medicine Between Science and Religion* tends to push in the opposite direction, and to see the *rGyud bzhi* as part of a fluid and situationally determined tradition of medical practice, aimed at efficacious practice in the healing of the patient. To the extent that Gyatso is concerned with efficacy, it is not that of medicine, but that of discourse about medicine as part of the State-building process in seventeenth-century Tibet. She provides a lengthy discussion of the Sde srid's famous set of medical paintings as an integral part of the new political structure that he and his patron the 'Great Fifth' Dalai Lama were creating within Tibet. Her frame and that of *Medicine Between Science and Religion* are not necessarily in direct conflict, but they lead to a very different reading and situating of 'Tibetan medicine' or Sowa Rigpa.

Neither the perspective taken in the introduction to *Medicine Between Science and Religion*, nor that adopted by Gyatso in her book and article, are precisely the same as that of other scholars in the field of Tibetan healing, but they echo concerns characteristic of other scholars in this area and in Tibetan studies more widely.[9] Many Western scholars were attracted to the field by a personal interest in Tibetan Buddhism, and have to negotiate the relationship between Tibetan and Western modes of knowledge within their lives and academic careers. They may also need to negotiate the politics of Tibet under Chinese rule; Gyatso was for several years the President of the International Association of Tibetan Studies (IATS), and was instrumental in maintaining IATS as a location in which Tibetan scholars from around the world could meet and exchange ideas on politically neutral ground.

In such a context, both Adams, Schrempf and Craig's assertion of the primacy of a Tibetan perspective on Tibetan healing (a *sowa rigpa* sensibility), and Gyatso's demonstration of empirical and rational thought within the allegedly Buddhist-dominated culture of Tibet, are likely to arise from complex and multiple sources and concerns. The perspective adopted by Adams, Schrempf and Craig could be seen, among other things, as an attempt to defend

Sowa Rigpa against the biomedical assaults routinely mounted in the West and in Asia against Asian and other 'alternative' medical traditions. This is certainly a concern Adams has expressed in her own earlier work (cf. Adams 2002), and it has also been an issue for other medical anthropologists working on Asian medical and healing traditions. Gyatso's position might be seen as arising mainly from her involvement with Western scholarship on the history of science and the development of scientific modes of thought.[10] It also echoes the concern of some Tibetan scholars to rescue rational and empirical elements in Tibetan culture from Western tendencies to see Tibet exclusively in Buddhist terms. The specific disciplinary locations of Adams, Schrempf and Craig on the one hand (medical anthropology) and Gyatso on the other (religious studies) have also doubtless had an influence on how they framed their projects.

These two 'framings' of the science–religion debate in relation to Tibetan healing are presented as exemplary, rather than exhaustive, of what has happened within this field. Hopefully though, through exploring them, I have helped suggest to the reader both the complexity and richness of the material available on the Tibetan medical tradition, and some of the issues which underlie recent writing in this area.

Notes

1 I use the term 'tradition' with some caution since, as Stephan Kloos (2013) pointed out some years ago, the creation of 'Tibetan medicine' within the Tibetan diasporic context as a self-conscious medical system was itself a political act, and a problematic one at that. 'Tradition' is intended to make fewer claims about unity over time, space and political boundaries than 'system'.
2 Tibetan terms are given in Wylie transcription, except for names and terms which have become familiar in other forms (Lhasa, lama, etc.). Technical terms are italicised; proper names are not.
3 For a more detailed survey, see Samuel (2014a).
4 I avoid the term 'humours' which is problematic both in the Indian and Tibetan contexts. See Tokar (2008); Yonten Gyatso (2005–6).
5 It also omits the very substantial number of publications in Russian, many of which are detailed in Aschoff's (1996) bibliography. The presence of Tibetan medicine in European Russia goes back to the late

nineteenth century, and the Badmaev family, who were key figures, were also eventually to be responsible indirectly for the first European producer of Tibetan pharmaceuticals, Padma AG in Switzerland (see Saxer 2014; van der Walk 2017).

6 The medical lineages associated with the Bon tradition of Tibet, which claims an alternative origin independent of Indian Buddhism, argue that G.yu thog pa adapted the Rgyud bzhi from an earlier Bon medical text, the 'Bum bzhi, which had been handed down for many centuries within the Bon tradition (Millard 2014). Versions of the 'Bum bzhi are still extant, and the relative priority of the 'Bum bzhi and Rgyud bzhi is not entirely certain, but the heavy dependence of both texts (which are verbally for the most part very close to each other) on the Tibetan translation of the *Aṣṭāṅgahṛdayasaṃhitā* implies that they were written after the *Aṣṭāṅgahṛdayasaṃhitā* was translated in the eleventh century.

7 The important new German translation of the *rGyud bzhi* by Florian Ploberger (2013, 2015, 2021), which takes into account a variety of textual and commentarial traditions outside the Sangs rgyas rgya mtsho material, should finally make a more comprehensive view of the *rGyud bzhi* available to Western readers. So far the translation covers the first, third and fourth tantras and the first twenty-seven chapters of the third tantra.

8 The new material consists of two chapters in Part I that serve as an introduction to the sDe srid and the political context of the seventeenth century, and two in Part III, one dealing with gender issues in the *rGyud bzhi* and another on medical ethics.

9 Consider for example some of the studies in the volume edited by Wallace (2003) on Buddhism and science.

10 Cf. Gyatso (2015: x) and references in her book to scholars, such as Shapin (1994) or Hanson (2003).

Bibliography

Adams, V. (1998) 'Suffering the Winds of Lhasa: Politicized Bodies, Human Rights, Cultural Difference, and Humanism in Tibet', *Medical Anthropology Quarterly*, 12.1: 74–102.

Adams, V. (2001a) 'The Sacred in the Scientific: Ambiguous Practices of Science in Tibetan Medicine', *Cultural Anthropology*, 16: 542–75.

Adams, V. (2001b) 'Particularizing Modernity: Tibetan Medical Theorizing of Women's Health in Lhasa, Tibet', in L.H. Connor and G. Samuel (eds) *Healing Powers and Modernity in Asian Societies*. Westport, CT: Bergin and Garvey, pp. 222–46.

Adams, V. (2002) 'Randomized Controlled Crime: Postcolonial Sciences in Alternative Medical Research', *Social Studies of Science*, 32: 659–90.

Adams, V. (2010) 'Encounters with Efficacy', *Asian Medicine*, 6: 1–21.

Adams, V., Schrempf, M. and Craig, S.R. (2011a) *Medicine Between Science and Religion: Explorations on Tibetan Grounds*. New York; Oxford: Berghahn Books.

Adams, V., Schrempf, M. and Craig, S.R. (2011b) 'Introduction: Medicine in Translation between Science and Religion', in V. Adams, M. Schrempf and S.R. Craig (eds) *Medicine Between Science and Religion: Explorations on Tibetan Grounds*. New York; Oxford: Berghahn Books, pp. 1–28.

Adams, V., Schrempf, M. and Craig, S.R. (2011b) *Medicine Between Science and Religion: Explorations on Tibetan Grounds*. New York; Oxford: Berghahn Books.

Aschoff, J.C. (1996) *Annotated Bibliography of Tibetan Medicine (1789–1995)*. Ulm: Fabri Verlag and Dietikon. Switzerland: Garuda.

Bassini, P. (2007) 'Heart Distress and Other Illnesses on the Sino-Tibetan Frontier: Home-Based Tibetan Perspectives from the Qinghai Part of Amdo'. DPhil thesis, University of Oxford.

Bassini, P. (2013) 'The Hierarchy of Food Consumption and Tibetan Experience of Gastric and Gallbladder Disorders in Amdo', *East Asia Science, Technology and Society* (*EASTS*), 7: 453–66.

Beckwith, C.I. (1979) 'The Introduction of Greek Medicine into Tibet in the Seventh and Eighth Centuries', *Journal of the American Oriental Society*, 99: 297–313.

Besch, F. (2009) *Tibetan Medicine Off the Roads: Modernising the Work of the Amchi in Spiti*, PhD thesis, Ethnologie, Ruprecht-Karls-Universität Heidelberg.

Blaikie, C. (2009) 'Critically Endangered? Medicinal Plant Cultivation and the Reconfiguration of Sowa Rigpa in Ladakh', *Asian Medicine: Tradition and Modernity*, 5: 243–72.

Blaikie, C. (2013a) 'Making Medicine: Materia Medica, Pharmacy and the Production of Sowa Rigpa in Ladakh'. PhD thesis, University of Kent.

Blaikie, C. (2013b) 'Currents of Tradition in Sowa Rigpa Pharmacy', *East Asian Science, Technology and Society*, 7: 425–51.

Blezer, H. (2012) 'Light' On the Human Body: The Coarse Physical Body and its Functions in the Aural Transmission from Zhang Zhung on the Six Lamps', *Revue d'Études Tibétaines*, 23: 117–68.

Clark, B. (1995) *The Quintessence Tantras of Tibetan Medicine*. Ithaca, NY: Snow Lion Publications.

Clifford, T. (1984) *Tibetan Buddhist Medicine and Psychiatry: The Diamond Healing*. Wellingborough: Aquarian Press.

Connor, L., Monro, K. and McIntyre, E. (1996) 'Healing Resources in Tibetan Settlements in North India', *Asian Studies Review*, 20.1: 108–18.

Connor, L. (1996) 'Underdetermining the Empirical Ground of Therapy Regimens among Tibetan Refugee Patients', Paper for the International Research Workshop, *Healing Powers and Modernity in Asian Societies*.

Faculty of Arts and Social Science, University of Newcastle, Australia, December 1996.

Connor, L. and Samuel, G. (eds) (2001) *Healing Powers and Modernity in Asian Societies*. Westport, CT: Bergin and Garvey.

Craig, S.R. (2006) 'On the "Science of Healing": Efficacy and the Metamorphosis of Tibetan Medicine'. PhD thesis, Cornell University.

Craig, S.R. and Glover, D.M. (eds) (2009) 'Conservation, Cultivation, and Commodification of Medicinal Plants in the Greater Himalayan-Tibetan Plateau', *Asian Medicine: Tradition and Modernity*, 5: 219–42.

Craig, S.R. (2011) 'From Empowerments to Power Calculations: Notes on Efficacy, Value and Method', in V. Adams, M. Schrempf and S.R. Craig (eds) *Medicine Between Science and Religion: Explorations on Tibetan Grounds*. New York; Oxford: Berghahn Books, pp. 215–44.

Craig, S.R. (2012) *Healing Elements: Efficacy and the Social Ecologies of Tibetan Medicine*. Berkeley, CA: University of California Press.

Craig, S.R. (2014) 'Tibetan Medicine in the World: Local Scenes, Global Transformations', in *Bodies in Balance: The Art of Tibetan Medicine*. Seattle: Washington University Press in association with Rubin Museum of Art, New York, pp. 110–27.

Csoma de Körös, A. (1984) 'Analysis of a Tibetan Medical Work', in J. Terjek (ed.) *Tibetan Studies*, being a reprint of the articles contributed to the Journal of the Asiatic Society of Bengal and Asiatic Researches. Budapest: Akademiai Kiadö, pp. 47–65.

Czaja, O. (2005–6b) 'A Hitherto Unknown "Medical History" of mTsho smad mkhan chen (b.16th cent.)', *Tibet Journal*, 30.4 and 31.1: 153–72.

Czaja, O. (2005–6a) 'Zurkharwa Lodro Gyalpo (1509–1579) on the Controversy of the Indian Origin of the rGyud bzhi', *Tibet Journal*, 30.4 and 31.1: 131–52.

Czaja, O. (2007) 'The Making of the Blue Beryl: Some Remarks on the Textual Sources of the Famous Commentary of Sangye Gyatsho (1653–1705)', in M. Schrempf (ed.) *Soundings in Tibetan Medicine. Proceedings of the Tenth Seminar of the International Association of Tibetan Studies, 2003*. Vol. 10. Leiden: Brill, pp. 345–72.

Czaja, O. (2013) 'On the History of Refining Mercury in Tibetan Medicine', *Asian Medicine*, 8.1: 75–105.

Dash, V.B. (1976) *Tibetan Medicine with Special Reference to Yoga Śataka*. Dharamsala: Library of Tibetan Works and Archives.

Dash, V.B. (1994–2001) *Encyclopaedia of Tibetan Medicine: Being the Tibetan Text of the Rgyud Bźi and Sanskrit Restoration of the Amṛta Hṛdaya Aṣṭāṅga Guhyopadeśa Tantra and Expository Translation in English*. Delhi: Sri Satguru Publications.

Deane, S. (2014) 'From Sadness to Madness: Tibetan Perspectives on the Causation and Treatment of Psychiatric Illness', *Religions*, 5.2: 444–58.

Deane, S. (2015) 'Sowa Rigpa, Spirits and Biomedicine: Lay Tibetan Perspectives on Mental Illness and its Healing in a Medically-pluralistic Context in Darjeeling, Northeast India'. PhD thesis, Cardiff University.

Deane, S. (2018) *Tibetan Medicine, Buddhism and Psychiatry: Mental health and healing in a Tibetan Exile Community*. Durham, NC: Carolina Academic Press.

Debreczeny, K. and Tuttle, G. (eds) (2010) *The Tenth Karmapa and Tibet's Turbulent Seventeenth Century*. Serindia: Chicago.

Deumar Tenzin Phuntsog (De'u dmar bstan 'dzin phun tshogs) (1970) *Dri med shel gong dang dri med shel phreng dang lag len gces bsdus*. Series: Smanrtsis shesrig spendzod. Reprint, Leh Ladakh: S. W. Tashigangpa. First published 1897 by Lcags po ri par khang, Chagpori Printing Press.

Dhonden, Y. (1986) *Health through Balance: An Introduction to Tibetan medicine*, edited and translated by J. Hopkins. Ithaca, NY: Snow Lion Publications.

Dummer, T. (1988) *Tibetan Medicine and Other Holistic Health Care Systems*. London: Routledge.

Ehrhard, F.-P. (2007) 'A Short History of the *g.Yu thog snying thig*', in K. Klaus and J. Hartmann (eds) *Indica et Tibetica: Festschrift für Michael Hahn*. Zum 65. Geburtstag von Freunden und Schulern Uberreicht. Wien: Arbeitskreis fur Tibetische und Buddhistische Studien Universitat Wien, pp. 151–70.

Emmerick, R.E. (1975) 'A Chapter from the Rgyud-bzhi', *Asia Major*, XIX.2: 141–62.

Emmerick, R.E. (1977) 'Sources of the rGyud-bzhi (Supplement, Deutscher Orientalistentag vom 28. Sept. bis 4. Okt. 1975 in Freiburg i. Br.)', *Zeitschrift der Deutschen Morgenländischen Gesellschaft* (Wiesbaden), III.2: 1135–42.

Emmerick, R.E. (1987) 'Epilepsy according to the *Rgyud*-bzi', in G.J. Meulenbeld and D. Wujastyk (eds) *Studies on Indian Medical History: Papers Presented at the International Workshop on the Study of Indian Medicine held at the Wellcome Institute for the History of Medicine, 2–4 September 1985*. Groningen: Egbert Forsten.

Emmerick, R.E. (1990) 'rGas-pa gso-ba', in T. Skorupski (ed.) *Indo-Tibetan Studies: Papers in Honour and Appreciation of Professor David L. Snellgrove's Contribution to Indo-Tibetan Studies*. Tring, Herts.: The Institute of Buddhist Studies, pp. 89–99.

Emmerick, R.E. (1991) 'Some remarks on Tibetan sphygmology', in G.J. Meulenbeld (ed.) *Medical literature from India, Sri Lanka and Tibet*, Vol.8, Panels of the Seventh World Sanskrit Conference, Kern Institute, Leiden August 23–29, 1987. Leiden: E.J. Brill.

Finckh, E. (1978) *Grundlagen tibetischer Heilkunde, Band 1*. Uelzen: Medizinische Literarische Verlagsgesellschaft.

Finckh, E. (1985) *Grundlagen tibetischer Heilkunde, Band 2*. Uelzen: Medizinische Literarische Verlagsgesellschaft.

Finckh, E. (1988a) *Studies in Tibetan Medicine*, Vol. I. Ithaca, NY: Snow Lion Publications.

Finckh, E. (1988b) *Foundations of Tibetan Medicine*, Vol. II, Shaftesbury: Element Books.

Garrett, F. (2004) 'Narratives of Embryology: Becoming Human in Tibetan Literature'. PhD thesis, University of Virginia.

Garrett, F. (2005–6) 'Hybrid Methodologies in the Lhasa Mentsikhang: A Summary of Resources for Teaching about Tibetan Medicine', *Tibet Journal*, 30.4 & 31.1: 55–64.

Garrett, F. (2007) 'Buddhism and the Historicizing of Medicine in Thirteenth Century Tibet', *Asian Medicine: Tradition and Modernity*, 2.2: 204–24.

Garrett, F. (2009) 'The Alchemy of Accomplishing Medicine (Sman Sgrub): Situating the Yuthok Heart Essence (*G.yu thog snying thig*) in Literature and History', *Journal of Indian Philosophy*, 37.3: 207–30.

Garrett, F. (2013) 'Mercury, Mad Dogs, and Smallpox: Medicine in the Si tu Paṇ chen Tradition', *Journal of the International Association of Tibetan Studies*, 7: 277–301.

Garrett, F. (2014) 'The Making of Medical History, Twelfth to Seventeenth Century', in *Bodies in Balance: The Art of Tibetan* Medicine. Seattle and London: Washington University Press in association with Rubin Museum of Art, New York, pp. 178–97.

Gayley, H. and Willock, N. (2016) 'Introduction. Theorizing the Secular in Tibetan Cultural Worlds', *Himalaya*, 36.1, Article 8.

Gerke, B. (1999) 'On the History of the Two Tibetan Medical Schools, Janglug and Zurlug', *AyurVijnana*, 6: 17–25.

Gerke, B. (2010a) 'Correlating Biomedical and Tibetan Medical Terms in amchi Medical Practice', in V. Adams, M. Schrempf and S. Craig (eds) *Medicine between Science and Religion: Explorations on Tibetan Grounds*. London: Berghahn Books, pp. 127–52.

Gerke, B. (2010b) 'Tibetan Treatment Choices in the Context of Medical Pluralism in the Darjeeling Hills', in S. Craig, M. Cuomo, F. Garrett and M. Schrempf (eds) *Studies of Medical Pluralism in Tibetan History and Society*. PIATS 2006: Proceedings of the 11th Seminar of the International Association of Tibetan Studies, Königswinter. Andiast: International Institute for Tibetan and Buddhist Studies, pp. 337–76.

Gerke, B. (2012) *Long Lives and Untimely Deaths: Life-Span Concepts and Longevity Practices among Tibetans in the Darjeeling Hills, India*. Leiden: Brill.

Gerke, B. (2013) 'The Social Life of Tsotel: Processing Mercury in Contemporary Tibetan Medicine', *Asian Medicine*, 8: 120–52.

Gerke, B. (2014) 'The Art of Tibetan Medical Practice', in Pa-sangs-yon-tan and T. Hofer (eds) *Bodies in Balance: The Art of Tibetan Medicine*. Seattle: Washington University Press in association with Rubin Museum of Art, New York, pp. 16–31.

Gyatso, J. (1986) 'Signs, Memory and History: A Tantric Buddhist Theory of Scriptural Transmission', *Journal of the International Association of Buddhist Studies*, 9: 7–36.

Gyatso, J. (1993) 'The Logic of Legitimation in the Tibetan Treasure Tradition', *History of Religions*, 33: 97–134.

Gyatso, J. (1998) *Apparitions of the Self: The Secret Autobiographies of a Tibetan Visionary*. Princeton, NJ: Princeton University Press.
Gyatso, J. (1999) 'Healing Burns with Fire: The Facilitations of Experience in Tibetan Buddhism', *Journal of the American Academy of Religion*, 67: 113–47.
Gyatso, J. (2004) 'The Authority of Empiricism and the Empiricism of Authority: Medicine and Buddhism in Tibet on the Eve of Modernity', *Comparative Studies of South Asia, Africa and the Middle East*, 24: 83–96.
Gyatso, J. (2011) 'Experience, Empiricism and the Fortunes of Authority: Tibetan Medicine and Buddhism on the Eve of Modernity', in S. Pollock (ed.) *Forms of Knowledge in Early Modern Asia: Explorations in the Intellectual History of India and Tibet, 1500–1800*. Durham, NC: Duke University Press, pp. 311–35.
Gyatso, J. (2015) *Being Human in a Buddhist World: An Intellectual History of Medicine in Early Modern Tibet*. New York: Columbia University Press.
Hanson, M. (2003) 'The "Golden Mirror" in the Imperial Court of the Qianlong Emperor, 1739–1742', *Early Science and Medicine*, 8: 111–47.
Hofer, T. (2005) 'Tibetan Medicine in Ngamring'. MPhil thesis, Institute of Ethnology, Cultural and Social Anthropology, University of Vienna.
Hofer, T. (2007) 'Preliminary Investigations into New Oral and Textual Sources on Byang Lugs: The 'Northern School' of Tibetan Medicine', in M. Schrempf (ed.) *Soundings in Tibetan Medicine. Proceedings of the Tenth Seminar of the International Association of Tibetan Studies, 2003*. Volume 10. Leiden: Brill, pp. 373–410.
Hofer, T. (2008a) 'Socio-Economic Dimensions of Tibetan Medicine in the Tibet Autonomous Region, China, Part One', *Asian Medicine: Tradition and Modernity*, 4.1: 174–200.
Hofer, T. (2008b) 'Socio-Economic Dimensions of Tibetan Medicine in the Tibet Autonomous Region, China, Part Two', *Asian Medicine: Tradition and Modernity*, 4.2: 492–514.
Hofer, T. (2011) 'Tibetan Medicine on the Margins: Twentieth Century Transformations and the Traditions of Sowa Rigpa in Central Tibet'. PhD thesis, University College London.
Hofer, T. (2012) *The Inheritance of Change: Transmission and Practice of Tibetan Medicine in Ngamring*. Vienna: Wiener Studien zur Tibetologie und Buddhismuskunde.
Hofer, T. and Larsen, K. (2014) 'Pillars of Tibetan Medicine: The Chagpori and the Mentsikhang Institutes in Lhasa', in *Bodies in Balance: The Art of Tibetan Medicine*. Seattle; London: Washington University Press in association with Rubin Museum of Art, New York, pp. 257–67.
Hsu, E. (2008) 'A Hybrid Body Technique: Does the Pulse Diagnostic cun guan chi Method Have Chinese-Tibetan Origins?', *Gesnerus*, 65: 5–29.
Janes, C.R. (1995) 'The Transformations of Tibetan Medicine', *Medical Anthropology Quarterly*, N.S.9: 6–39.

Janes, C.R. (1999a) 'The Health Transition, Global Modernity and the Crisis of Traditional Medicine: The Tibetan Case', *Social Science and Medicine*, 48: 1803–20.

Janes, C.R. (1999b) 'Imagined Lives, Suffering and the Work of Culture: The Embodied Discourses of Conflict in Modern Tibet', *Medical Anthropology Quarterly*, 13: 391–412.

Janes, C.R. (2001) 'Tibetan Medicine at the Crossroads: Radical Modernity and the Social Organization of Traditional Medicine in the Tibet Autonomous Region, China', in L. Connor and G. Samuel (eds) *Healing Powers and Modernity in Asian Societies*. Westport, CT: Bergin and Garvey, pp. 197–221.

Karmay, S.G. (1989) 'Vairocana and the Rgyud-bzhi', *Tibetan Medicine*, 12: 19–31, reprinted (1998) as 'The Four Medical Treatises and Their Critics' in S.G. Karmay (ed.) *The Arrow and the Spindle*. Kathmandu: Mandala Book Point, pp. 228–37.

Kelsang, J. (1977) *The Ambrosia Heart Tantra: The Secret Oral Teaching on the Eight Branches of the Science of Healing*, translated by Jhamapa Kelsang and annotated by Y. Dönden. Dharamsala: Library of Tibetan Works and Archives.

Khangkar, L.D. (1986) *Lectures on Tibetan Medicine by Lady Dr. Lobsang Dolma Khangkar*, (ed.) K. Dhondup. Dharamsala: Library of Tibetan Works and Archives.

Kind, M. (2002) *Mendrub: A Bonpo Ritual for the Benefit of all Living Beings and the Empowerment of Medicine Performed in Tsho, Dolpo*. Kathmandu: WWF Nepal.

Kleinman, A. and Sung, L.H. (1979) 'Why Do Indigenous Practitioners Successfully Heal?' *Social Science and Medicine*, 13b: 7–26.

Kleinman, A. (1980) *Patients and Healers in the Context of Culture: An Exploration of the Borderland between Anthropology, Medicine, and Psychiatry*. Berkeley; Los Angeles: University of California Press.

Kleinman, A. (1988) *The Illness Narratives: Suffering, Healing and the Human Condition*. New York: Basic Books.

Kloos, S. (2008) 'History of Tibetan Medical Institute', *Tibet Journal*, 33: 15–49.

Kloos, S. (2010) 'Tibetan Medicine in Exile: The Ethics, Politics, and Science of Cultural Survival'. PhD thesis, University of California, San Francisco and University of California, Berkeley.

Kloos, S. (2013) 'How Tibetan Medicine in Exile Became a "Medical System"', *East Asian Science, Technology and Society*, 7: 381–95.

Kuhn, A.S. (1994) 'Ladakh: A Pluralistic Medical System under Acculturation and domination', in D. Sich and W. Gottschalk (eds) *Acculturation and Domination in Traditional Asian Medical Systems*. Stuttgart: Franz Steiner, pp. 61–73.

Kuhn, A.S. (1988) *Heiler und ihre Patienten auf dem Dach der Welt: Ladakh aus ethnomedizinischer Sicht*. Frankfurt: Peter Lang (Medizin in Entwicklungsländern 25).

Lipman, K. (2010) *Secret Teachings of Padmasambhava: Essential Instructions on Mastering the Energies of Life*. Boston; London: Shambhala.

Mayer, R. (2013–14) 'gTer ston and Tradent: Innovation and Conservation within Tibetan Treasure Literature', *Journal of the International Association of Buddhist Studies*, 36–37: 227–42.

McGrath, W.A. (2017) 'Buddhism and Medicine in Tibet: Origins, Ethics, and Tradition'. PhD thesis, University of Virginia.

Meyer, F. (1984) *Gso-ba rig-pa, le système médical tibétain*. 2^d^ ed. Paris: Editions du Centre National de la Recherche Scientifique.

Meyer, F. (1990) 'Théorie et pratique de l'examen des pouls dans un chapitre du rGyud-bzhi. in Tadeusz Skorupski (ed.) *Indo-Tibetan Studies: Papers in Honour and Appreciation of Professor David L. Snellgrove's Contribution to Indo-Tibetan Studies*. Tring, Herts.: The Institute of Buddhist Studies, pp. 209–56.

Meyer, F. (1992) 'Introduction: The Medical Paintings of Tibet', in Y. Parfionovich, G. Dorje and F. Meyer (eds) *Tibetan Medical Paintings: Illustrations to the "Blue Beryl" Treatise of Sangye Gyamtso (1653–1705)*, London: Serindia Publications; New York: Harry N. Abrams, Inc. Publishers, pp. 2–13.

Meyer, F. (2003) 'The Golden Century of Tibetan Medicine', in F. Pommaret (ed.) *Lhasa in the Seventeenth Century: The Capital of the Dalai Lamas*, trans. H. Solverson. Leiden; Boston: Brill, pp. 99–117.

Millard, C. (2002) 'Learning Processes in a Tibetan Medical School'. PhD thesis, University of Edinburgh.

Millard, C. (2006) '*sMan* and *Glud*: Standard Tibetan Medicine and Ritual Medicine in a Bon Medical School in Nepal', *The Tibet Journal, Special Edition on Tibetan Medicine*, 30.4.1: 3–30.

Millard, C. (2007) 'Tibetan Medicine and the Classification and Treatment of Psychiatric Disorders', in M. Schrempf (ed.) *Soundings in Tibetan Medicine: Anthropological and Historical Perspectives*, Proceedings of the 10th Seminar of the International Association of Tibetan Studies 2003. Leiden: Brill, pp. 247–83.

Millard, C. (2010) *Bon Medicine*, www.bodyhealthreligion.org.uk/BAHAR/bon-medical-tradition.html, accessed 5 March 2018.

Millard, C. (2013) 'Bon Medical Practitioners in Contemporary Tibet: The Continuity of a Tradition', *East Asian Science, Technology and Society*, 7: 353–79.

Needham, J. (1954) *Science and Civilisation in China*. Vol.1. London: Cambridge University Press.

Parfionovitch, Y., Dorje, G. and Meyer, F. (eds) (1992) *Tibetan Medical Paintings: Illustrations to the 'Blue Beryl' Treatise of Sangs rgyas Rgya mtsho (1653–1705)*. 2 vols. London: Serindia.

Pei Shengji, Huai Huyin and Yang Lixin (2009) 'Medicinal Plants and Their Conservation in China with Reference to the Chinese Himalayan Region', *Asian Medicine: Tradition and Modernity*, 5: 273–90.

Ploberger, F. (2013) *Wurzeltantra und Tantra der Erklärungen der tibetischen Medizin.* 2. Auflage. Schiedlberg: Bacopa.
Ploberger, F. (2015) *Das letzte Tantra aus die vier Tantra der tibetischen Medizin.* Schiedlberg: Bacopa.
Ploberger, F. (2021) *Das Tantra der mündlichen Überlieferung der vier Tantras der Tibetischen Medizin, 1. Teil.* Schiedlberg: Bacopa.
Pordié, L. (2007) 'Buddhism in the Everyday Medical Practice of the Ladakhi "Amchi"', *Indian Anthropologist*, 37: 93–116.
Pordié, Laurent (ed.) (2008) *Tibetan Medicine in the Contemporary World: Global Politics of Medical Knowledge and Practice.* London; New York: Routledge.
Pordié, L. (2015) 'Genealogy and Ambivalence of a Therapeutic Heterodoxy. Islam and Tibetan Medicine in North-western India', *Modern Asian Studies*, 49: 1772–807.
Pordié, L. and Kloos, S. (eds) (2021) *Healing at the Periphery: Ethnographies of Tibetan Medicine in India.* Durham, NC: Duke University Press.
Prost, A.G. (2003) 'Exile, Social Change and Medicine among Tibetans in Dharamsala, Himachal Pradesh, India'. PhD thesis, University College, London.
Prost, A.G. (2006) 'Causation as Strategy: Interpreting Humours among Tibetan Refugees', *Anthropology and Medicine*, 13.2: 119–30.
Prost, A.G. (2007) 'Sa cha 'di ma 'phrod na ... Displacement and Traditional Tibetan Medicine among Tibetan Refugees In India', in M. Schrempf (ed.) *Soundings in Tibetan Medicine: Anthropological and Historical Perspectives*, Proceedings of the 10th Seminar of the International Association of Tibetan Studies (IATS) Oxford 2003. Leiden: Brill Academic Publishers, pp. 45–64.
Prost, A. (2008) *Precious Pills: Medicine and Social Change among Tibetan Refugees in India.* Oxford: Berghahn.
Rapgay, L. (1994a) 'Pulse Analysis in Tibetan Medicine', *Tibetan Medicine*, 3 (revised edition): 47–54.
Rapgay, L. (1994b) 'Urine Analysis in Tibetan Medicine', *Tibetan Medicine*, 3 (revised edition): 55–62.
Rechung Rinpoche, Ven. (1973) *Tibetan Medicine. Illustrated in Original texts*, presented and translated by the Ven. Rechung Rinpoche Jampal Kunzang. London: Wellcome Trust.
Rossi D. and Oliphant of Rossie, C.J. (eds) *Sharro: Festschrift for Chögyal Namkhai Norbu.* Switzerland: Garuda Verlag.
Rozario, S. and Samuel, G. (2002) 'Tibetan and Indian ideas of Birth Pollution', in S. Rozario and G. Samuel (eds) *The Daughters of Hāritī: Childbirth and Female Healers in South and Southeast* Asia. London; New York: Routledge, pp. 182–208.
Samuel, G. (1999) 'Religion, Health and Suffering among Contemporary Tibetans', in J.R. Hinnells and R. Porter (eds) *Religion, Health and* Suffering. London; New York: Kegan Paul International, pp. 85–110.

Samuel, G. (2001) 'Tibetan Medicine in Contemporary India: Theory and Practice', in L.H. Connor and G. Samuel (eds) *Healing Powers and Modernity in Asian Societies: Traditional Medicine, Shamanism and Science*, Westport: CT: Bergin and Garvey (Greenwood Publishing), pp. 247–68.

Samuel, G. (2007) 'Spirit Causation and Illness in Tibetan Medicine', in M. Schrempf (ed.) *Soundings in Tibetan Medicine. Historical and Anthropological Perspectives. Proceedings of the Tenth Seminar of the International Association of Tibetan Studies, Oxford 2003*. Leiden: Brill, pp. 213–24.

Samuel, G. (2010) 'Healing, Efficacy and the Spirits', *Journal of Ritual Studies*, 24: 7–20.

Samuel, G. (2011) 'Epilogue: Towards a *Sowa Rigpa* Sensibility', in V. Adams, M. Schrempf and S.R. Craig (eds) *Medicine Between Science and Religion: Explorations on Tibetan Grounds*. New York; Oxford: Berghahn Books, pp. 319–31.

Samuel, G. (2013) 'Panentheism and the Longevity Practices of Tibetan Buddhism', in L. Biernacki and P. Clayton (eds) *Panentheism Across the World's Traditions*. New York: Oxford University Press, pp. 83–99.

Samuel, G. (2014) 'Healing in Tibetan Buddhism', in M. Poceski (ed.) *The Wiley Blackwell Companion to East and Inner Asian Buddhism*. Oxford: Blackwell Publishing, pp. 278–96.

Samuel, G. (2016) 'Tibetan Longevity Meditation', in H. Eifring (ed.) *Asian Traditions of Meditation*. Honolulu: University of Hawai'i Press, pp. 145–64.

Samuel, G. (2017) 'The g.Yu Thog sNying thig and the Spiritual Dimension of Tibetan Medicine', in D. Rossi and C. Jamyang Oliphant of Rossie (eds) *Sharro: Festschrift for Chögyal Namkhai Norbu*. Switzerland: Garuda Verlag, pp. 214–25.

Samuel, G. (2019) 'Unbalanced Flows in the Subtle Body: Tibetan Understandings of Psychiatric Illness and How to Deal With It', *Journal of Religion and Health*, 58: 770–94.

Samuel, G. and Johnston, J. (eds) (2013) *Religion and the Subtle Body in Asia and the West: Between Mind and Body*. London; New York: Routledge.

Sangs rgyas rgya mtsho, sDe srid (1978) *Lamaist Medical Practice: Being the Text of the* Man ngag yon tan rgyud kyi lhan thabs zug r'u'i tsha gdu' sel ba'i katpu ra dus min 'chi zhags gcod pa'i ral gri, reproduced from a print from the 1733 sDe-dGe blocks by O-rgyan rnam-rgyal, Smanrtsis Shesrig Spendzod vol. 86. Leh: T.S. Tashigangpa.

Sangs rgyas rgya mtsho, sDe srid (1994) *Gso ba rig pa'i bstan bcos sman bla'i dgongs rgyan rgyud bzhi'i gsal byed ba'i ḍurya sngon po 'i mallika zhes bya ba*. Dharamsala: Men-Tsee-Khang.

Sangyé Gyatso, D. (2010) *Mirror of Beryl: A Historical Introduction to Tibetan Medicine*, trans. G. Kilty. Boston: Wisdom Publications in Association with the Institution of Tibetan Classics.

Saxer, M. (2013) *Manufacturing Tibetan Medicine: The Creation of an Industry and the Moral Economy of Tibetanness*. New York; Oxford: Berghahn Books.

Saxer, M. (2014) 'The Journeys of Tibetan Medicine', in *Bodies in Balance: The Art of Tibetan* Medicine. Seattle and London: Washington University Press in association with Rubin Museum of Art, New York, pp. 246–56.

Schrempf, M. (ed.) *Soundings in Tibetan Medicine: Anthropological and Historical Perspectives*, Proceedings of the 10th Seminar of the International Association of Tibetan Studies 2003. Leiden: Brill.

Schrempf, M. (2010) 'Between *Mantra* and Syringe: Healing and Health-Seeking Behaviour in Contemporary Amdo', in V. Adams, M. Schrempf and S.R. Craig (eds) *Medicine Between Science and Religion: Explorations on Tibetan Grounds*. New York; Oxford: Berghahn Books, pp. 157–83.

Schrempf, M. (2015a) 'Becoming a Female Ritual Healer in Eastern Bhutan', *Revue d'Etudes Tibétaines*, 34: 189–213.

Schrempf, M. (2015b) 'Fighting Illness with Gesar – A Healing Ritual from Eastern Bhutan', in C. Ramble and U. Rösler (eds) *Tibetan and Himalayan Healing – An Anthology for Anthony Aris*. Oxford: Oxford University, pp. 621–30.

Schrempf, M. (2015c) 'Contested Issues of Efficacy and Safety between Transnational Formulation Regimes of Tibetan Medicine in China and Europe', *Asian Medicine: Tradition and Modernity*, 10: 273–315.

Shapin, S. (1994) *A Social History of Truth: Civility and Science in Seventeenth-Century England*. Chicago: University of Chicago Press.

Sich D. and Gottschalk, W. (eds) *Acculturation and Domination in Traditional Asian Medical Systems*. Stuttgart: Franz Steiner.

Skorupski, T. (ed.) (1990) *Indo-Tibetan Studies: Papers in Honour and Appreciation of Professor David L. Snellgrove's Contribution to Indo-Tibetan Studies*. Tring, Herts.: The Institute of Buddhist Studies.

Taee, J. (2017) *The Patient Multiple: An Ethnography of Health Care and Decision-Making in Bhutan*. New York: Berghahn.

Tokar, E. (2008) 'An Ancient Medicine in a New World: A Tibetan Medicine Doctor's Reflections From "Inside"', in L. Pordié (ed.), *Tibetan Medicine in the Contemporary World: Global Politics of Tibetan Medicine and Practice*. London; New York: Routledge.

Tsarong, T.J. (1981) *Fundamentals of Tibetan Medicine according to the rGyud-bzhi*. Dharamsala: Tibetan Medical Centre.

Tsarong, T.J. (1986) *Handbook of Traditional Tibetan Drugs*. Kalimpong: Tibetan Medical Publications.

Van der Walk, J. (2017) *Alternative Pharmaceuticals: The Technoscientific Becomings of Tibetan Medicines In-Between India and Switzerland*, PhD thesis, University of Kent.

Van Vleet, S. (2010–11) 'Children's Healthcare and Astrology in the Nurturing of a Central Tibetan Nation-State, 1916–24', *Asian Medicine*, 6: 348–86.

Van Vleet, S. (2013) 'An Introduction to *Music to Delight all the Sages*, The Medical History of Drakkar Taso Trulku Chökyi Wangchuk (1775–1837)', *Bulletin of Tibetology*, 48.2: 55–79.

Van Vleet, S. (2015) *Medicine, Monasteries, and Empire: Tibetan Buddhism and the Politics of Learning in Qing China*, PhD thesis, Columbia University.

Van Vleet, S. (2016) 'Medicine as Impartial Knowledge: The Fifth Dalai Lama, the Tsarong School, and Debates of Tibetan Medical Orthodoxy', in K. Debreczeny and G. Tuttle (eds) *The Tenth Karmapa and Tibet's Turbulent Seventeenth Century*. Chicago: Serindia, pp. 263–91.

Vargas, l. (2010) 'Legitimising Demon Diseases in Tibetan Medicine: The Conjoining of Religion, Medicine, and Ecology', in S. Craig, M. Cuomo, F. Garrett and M. Schrempf (eds) *Studies of Medical Pluralism 1n Tibetan History and* Society. PlATS 2006: Proceedings of the 11th Seminar of the International Association of Tibetan Studies, Königswinter. Andiast: International institute for Tibetan and Buddhist Studies, pp. 379–404.

Vargas-O'Bryan, I.M. (2015) 'Balancing Tradition Alongside a Progressively Scientific Tibetan Medical System', in I. Vargas-O'Bryan and Zhou Xun (eds) *Disease, Religion and Healing in Asia: Collaborations and Collisions*. New York; London: Routledge, pp. 122–45.

Vogel, C. (1965) *Vagbhata's Astangahrdayasamhita. The first five chapters of its Tibetan version. Edited and rendered into English along with the original Sanskrit.* Accompanied by a literary introduction and a running commentary on the Tibetan Translating-Technique. (Abhandlungen für die Kunde des Morgenlandes 37, 2). Wiesbaden: Deutsche Morgenländische Gesellschaft, in Kommission Franz Steiner.

Wallace, B.A. (2003) (ed.) *Buddhism and Science: Breaking New Ground*. New York: Columbia University Press.

Winder, M. (1981) 'Tibetan Medicine Compared with Ancient and Mediaeval Western Medicine', *Bulletin of Tibetology*, N.S.1: 5–22.

Winder, M. (1984) 'Tibetan Medicine, Its Humours and Elements', *Bulletin of Tibetology*, 1: 11–25.

Winder, M. (1987) 'Vaiḍūrya', in G.J. Meulenbeld and D. Wujastyk (eds) *Studies on Indian Medical History: Papers Presented at the International Workshop on the Study of Indian Medicine held at the Wellcome Institute for the History of Medicine, 2–4 September 1985*. Groningen: E. Forsten, pp. 85–94.

Yang Ga (2010) *The Sources for the Writing of the "Rgyud bzhi": Tibetan Medical Classic*, PhD thesis, Harvard University.

Yang Ga (2019) 'A Preliminary Study on the Biography of Yutok Yönten Gönpo the Elder: Reflections on the Origins of Tibetan Medicine', in W.A. McGrath (ed.) *Knowledge and Context in Tibetan Medicine.* Leiden and Boston: Brill, pp. 59–84.
Yangönpa, G. (2015) *Secret Map of the Body: Visions of the Human Energy Structure.* Translated and annotated by E. Guarisco. Merigar, Arcidosso: Shang Shung Publications.
Yoeli-Tlalim, R. (2012) 'Re-visiting "Galen in Tibet"', *Medical History*, 56.3: 355–65.
Yonten Gyatso (2005–6) 'Nyes pa: A Brief Review of Its English Translation', *Tibet Journal*, 30.4 and 31.1: 109–18.

8

Homeopathy and Islam in Malaysia: encounters of religion and complementary medical traditions in a modern Asian multi-ethnic society

Constantin Canavas

Background

The starting point of the present study is the hypothesis that coexisting ethnic groups, including migrants, transfer and eventually preserve differing, culturally connoted medical practices and health concepts. The external perception of these concepts and practices, whether by medical anthropology or by the established biomedical system, is based on several rather vaguely defined terms: traditional, alternative, complementary, etc. In spite of the terminological problems, the term 'traditional, alternative or complementary medicine' (TACM) will be used in the present study to refer to concepts and practices beyond the limits of the established, more or less centrally administered biomedical system, as far as they are interwoven with social movements or ethnic groups. In this context the central administration may be colonial or that of an independent state, whose relations and politics towards the actors of TACM are subjected to priorities and conditions that are parts of specific historical processes (Jütte 1996a: 11–16). Anthropologists would probably emphasise terms like 'healing practices in local communities' to avoid the ideological and political bias of TACM. Since the present study traces, among other issues, the relations between such practices and the official Malaysian administration, the TACM term renders these relations more visible and recognisable in the general network of medical services and healing practices.

The common expectation of TACM practices, beyond the 'Western' borders implies local traditions and practices 'outside' the modern, 'Western', biomedical horizon. In the present study the focus is on cross-over phenomena, i.e. when Western and non-Western TACM traditions meet, interact, etc.

Terminology, narratives and forms of description of TACM involve epistemological problems whose tackling has a long scholarly tradition, especially in the case of cultural frames beyond typical 'Western' Eurocentric discourses. A special category of difficulties should be expected when European alternative medical traditions beyond the allopathic biomedical model are appropriated and re-interpreted in a new cultural context – eventually with a new specific religious bias. In the present study homeopathy will be considered as reclaimed in a Malay Muslim context. What is the semantic and cultural para-text of the term 'homeopathy' itself – as used in epistemological discourses in the Malaysian context, or when referred to in the present study? Internalistic definitions would comply somehow with some aspects of the theoretical background proposed by several European physicians, and, in one way or the other, would refer to the works and the impact of Samuel Hahnemann (1755–1843) – beginning symbolically with his self-healing experiment and his initial publication in 1796. It is certainly true, that the European historical frame was substantial for the development and strengthening of public perception of homeopathy – at least in Europe (Jütte 1996a: 179–221). The focus of the present study is, however, directed far beyond the direct influence of European traditions; it encompasses regions in Southeast Asia, where European colonial heritage crosses the paths of medical practices transmitted by several ethnic groups and coloured by various religions.

The first goal of the present study is to identify and extract evidence on the *types of relationship* (e.g. dominance, coexistence, mutual influence, syncretism, fusion) among different TACM concepts and practices inside and across the borders of ethnic or religion-based groups in the case of Malaysia. Examining homeopathy in the Malaysian context, the main focus of the study, will serve as a critical view of such categorisations. The provenance of the data considered include a few accessible primary references, as well as studies on TACM practice in Malaysia published after 1940.

In order to describe adequately the social background of the TACM practices, and to assess their specific weight in the multi-ethnic nation of Malaysia, it is crucial to obtain a clear picture of the ethno-political structure and the significance of the related statistical data regarding the ethnic groups in the historical framework of this Southeast Asian country.

There exist long debates and several perceptions and misperceptions of the terms Malay and Malaysian. The term Melayu/Malay was already used by Ptolemy as a geographical name (Μαλέου κῶλον) in the second century CE, possibly derived from the Sanskrit *malaykolam* referring to some part of the Malay Peninsula. The earliest reference in Chinese sources goes back to a mission to the Chinese court in 644 CE. The modern use of the term in European languages began in the sixteenth and early seventeenth centuries with varying linguistic, ethnic or geographical meaning (Reid 2010: 81; Milner 2011: 18).

The present state of Malaysia was established on 16 September 1963. It was the result of joining together the Federation of Malaya, which became independent in 1957, with the British colonies of Sarawak, Sabah, Labuan (on the island of Borneo) and Singapore, which left (rather was 'expelled' from) Malaysia in 1965 and became independent (Somers Heidhues 2000: 12). Today the Federation of Malaysia comprises eleven Peninsular states and the territories, Kuala Lumpur and Putrajaya in West Malaysia, as well as the two states, Sarawak and Sabah, and the territory of Labuan, in east Malaysia on the island of Borneo.

Malaysian citizens are officially registered according to their adherence to one of the officially recognised ethnic groups: the box *bangsa* (race, ethnic group, people) figures in all official and unofficial forms (Ma 2012: 29); even the ways that names are registered in Malaysian passports differ accordingly. The options in the racial/ethnic classification are Malay (*bangsa Melayu*), Chinese, Indian, Orang Asli (lit. 'original people'), and the indigenous East Malaysians of Sabah and Sarawak.[1] The criteria of the classification are primarily related to the parental lineage. Of particular significance for the present study on encounters between homeopathy and Islam in Malaysia are the controversies related to the definition of 'Malayness'. The differentiation between Malay and non-Malay inhabitants was first introduced by the

British colonial administration in order to distinguish the Sultans' subjects from Indian or Chinese immigrants (Schreiber 2017: 184). The 'Malayness' issue is a major controversy in Southeast Asia with a plethora of essays, books (e.g. McAmis 2002; Reid 2010; Hoffstaedter 2011; Milner 2011; Dannaud 2013) and political debates dedicated to it. According to the Malaysian constitution 'a Malay is a person who professes the religion of Islam, habitually speaks the Malay language and conforms to Malay customs (*adat*)' (Hoffstaedter 2011: 17). 'Malayness' is in many cases understood as the goal or the outcome of a process of 'Malayisation'. This process can be seen as initiated by an individual, or it can be referred to a whole group as a target, e.g. in the perspective of Malay activists referring to Orang Asli people (Milner 2011: 199). However, it can also be regarded as an exclusion discourse in which the peculiarities of a major ethnic group – not only in Malaysia, but also in the whole of Southeast Asia – namely the Chinese – are not represented.[2] Significant for the present study is the simplifying but seducing narrative in which Malay is identified with Muslim.

The ambition of preserving Malay hegemony in the new independent state as claimed by several (Malay) political actors became the reason for 'expelling' Singapore from the federation on August 9, 1965. Singapore's population consisted at that time mainly of ethnic Chinese and Indians with a percentage of 83%, and its government promoted multiculturalism, thus challenging the legitimacy of the claim of Malay electoral and political supremacy (Means 2009: 81).

The Malaysian population has increased: at the time of the Independence (1957) the population of Malaya was c. 10 million, consisting of 47% ethnic Malays, 42% ethnic Chinese and ca. 11% Indians and others (Bianco 1969: 298–301). During the years following the creation of Malaya the population (embracing the integrated eastern territories) increased to 22 million (1999), to reach 28.3 million in 2010. As mentioned above, the population composition regarding the major ethnic groups has been a major political concern since the British colonial administration. This officially registered categorisation may reflect privileged treatment by the state, e.g. regarding engagement in the public sector or the support of economic initiatives, both cases foreseen by the constitutional change of 1969, which privileges ethnic Malays. The official

Malaysian statistics of 2010 report 63.1% Malays, 24.6% Chinese, 7.3% Indians, 0.7% 'others' (presumably Europeans and Eurasians), and (presumably) 4.3% indigenous groups/aborigines (Orang Asli) (Department of Statistics, Malaysia 2011: 5). Recent writers have suggested that the figures may be slightly different, e.g. 60% for Malays, 25% for Chinese, 10% for Indians and 5% for indigenous groups/aborigines (Dannaud: 2013).[3]

Malays would collectively call themselves *bumiputras* (sons of the soil) – a term which would be deliberately applied to include indigenous groups too (e.g. in official documents). This practice is the explanation for contested, apparently inconsistent or contradictory statistics – e.g. in the 63.1% Malays stated in the official Malaysian statistics of 2010 many East Malaysian inhabitants are included as Malays. The background of this controversy is the fact that these statistics were and are still used (and abused) as a political instrument of exclusion and inclusion – especially in the multilevel rivalry between Malays and Chinese (dichotomy *bumiputra* vs. *non-bumiputra*). Typical examples are the 'affirmative-action policies' of the Malaysian governments issued explicitly in favour of the *bumiputra* since 1969 (Liow 2009: 103–5).

The spectrum of religions, as well as their correlation with specific ethnic groups, is significant for the scope of the present study. Practically all Malays are Sunni Muslims, or at least considered as such; they follow the *Shāfiʿī* school of Islamic law. Besides, there exist significant *ṣūfī* traditions of Islamic mysticism, as well as numerous forms of historical experiences and current trends of what anthropologists would call *popular Islam* (Weintraub 2011). For the discussion on traditional medical practices beyond theological confines, local expressions of popular culture in conjunction with Islam become of particular interest.

The majority of ethnic Chinese Malaysians follow Buddhist, and to a lesser extent, Daoist practices (Dannaud 2013). Ethnic Indians are considered in their majority to follow Hinduism. From the perspective of the Malaysian administration this statistical fact deprives Indian Muslims from 'Malayness' and excludes them from privileges officially reserved for (Malay) Muslims. Indigenous groups are included as *bumiputras* and, in a political frame of dealing with ethnic groups, they are often considered close to or together with the group of Malay Muslims.

Islam has the status of the official religion of the federal state; at the same time, freedom of religion is constitutionally guaranteed. Officially Malaysia is not an Islamic state but Islamic symbols are omnipresent, and several adherents of political Islam would claim that Malaysia is *de facto* an Islamic state. The correlation of Muslim confession with political representation and power varies regionally, and fluctuated through Malaysian history (Reid 1993). Both ethnicity and adherence to a specific religion are officially documented, e.g. in the Malaysian passport. The Malaysian Census (Department of Statistics, Malaysia 2011: 9) reports 61.3% Muslims, 19.8% Buddhists, 9.2% Christians, 6.3% Hindus and 1.3% belonging to Confucianism, Daoism and 'other traditional Chinese religion', while 2.1% are categorised as following 'other or no religion'.[4]

The decisive steps of a policy characterised by assimilating Islamic values in the administration and correlating legally Muslim status with Malay ethnicity were undertaken early in the history of Malaysia; they became fashioned during the era of Mahathir Mohamad, leader of the United Malays National Organisation (UMNO) and Prime Minister from 1981 to 2003 (Means 2009: 121–49). Mahathir openly contested the description of Malaysia as a secular state stressing the concept of an administration in *accordance with Islam* (Liow 2009: xii). It is remarkable that the Islamic Party of Malaysia (Persatuan Aislam Se-Malaysia, popularly known as Partai Islam, PAS) was formed out of UMNO as a radical reaction to UMNO's moderate Islamisation policy. Being in opposition to the UMNO government, PAS reclaims Malaysia as an explicitly *Islamic state* (Jelonek 2004). Even if not so radical as the PAS claims, Mahathir followed a policy of synchronising an Islamic discourse with the Malay ethnic perception (i.e. equating Malay with Muslim). In this political framework, quotas on ethnic basis (Malays vs. non-Malays) were gradually introduced in industrial activities, education, and public administration – a policy which practically stressed the privileges of the Malay Muslims.

It should be remarked that cultural distinctions in Malaysia do not generally coincide with religious beliefs or group limits in political representation. Thus, the current political parties in Sarawak represent Muslim *bumiputra*, non-Muslim *bumiputra* and Chinese. Nevertheless, in the context of 'Islamic revival and pious social and political movements' during the three decades, 1980–2010, the discourse on the role of Islam in Malaysian society has become a major issue in the political rivalry between Malays who assign themselves with the *bumiputra* quality, and the Chinese ethnic community who – from the perspective of Malays – are situated outside the *bumiputra* confinement (Daniels 2013: 1 ff.).

TACM methods are practised in Malaysia both independently and as a parallel or additional concept to the official biomedical health care system (Talib 2006: 447). These practices generally have a strong ethnic bias. Traditional Chinese Medicine – mainly based on the use of herbs, acupressure and acupuncture – is commonly practiced in the Chinese ethnic group. Ayurveda (literally 'Knowledge of Life'), Unani and Siddha medical practices are mainly associated with Indians (Chen 1975: 176; Chen 1981: 130; Ariff and Beng: 2006). A large spectre of native (indigenous) medical practices can be traced among Malays and indigenous ethnic groups – a fact that shifts ethno-medicine into the *bumiputra* confinement. Typical actors are the female birth attendants, *bidan kampung*, and the healer, *bomoh*, who is often involved in ritual performances (Winstedt 1951; Chen 1975: 172; Chen 1981: 128 ff.; Bach 1991: 13–14, 74). These medical practitioners are well known in Malaysian society, even beyond the vague confines of persons who would seek their services. Finally, the vaguely confined field of popular Islamic medicine (including practices sometimes called 'Medicine of the Prophet') should be mentioned (Kehl-Bodrogi: 2012); this is practised by Muslims especially in rural areas.

Notwithstanding the above schematic and oversimplifying description, cross-over in medical practices, i.e. seeking for treatment beyond ethnic or religious confinements, has been repeatedly reported (Edman and Koon 2000: 103). This phenomenon consists in integrating healing rituals, herbal therapy, massage, acupuncture, etc. in several traditional practices – including cases of mental illnesses. The result could be regarded as a form of medical syncretism, with medical actors (patients, healers, etc.) transgressing formal ethnic or religious limits.

One of these transgression movements has brought the practice of certain Malaysian physicians into the field and terminology of homeopathy. Is this encounter with terminology and practice (already known in the 'Western' medical tradition) a form of appropriation or integration of 'Western' ACM practices? Or is it an independent development on the basis of affinity among medical concepts beyond cultural confinements?

Literature

Any attempt to clarify this double question in a historical perspective should rely on interpreting historical data on medical patterns, practices and discourses in the area of present-day Malaysia, at least since independence. Unfortunately, the evidence in the form of reports and studies, both in the setting as well as in the questioning of the scarce field studies, is biased by the stance and the historically determined ideological assumptions which influence the perspective of each study. The question about TACM practices was motivated by different interests in several periods. Especially the relationship between religion (e.g. Islam) and medical practices was not always an issue of interest, as we will comment on below. The status and practice of homeopathy were often beyond the scope of the research – or they were masked by the ideological bias which did not include homeopathy in medical traditions connoted by ethnicity in the Malaysian state. Therefore, the evidence provided by the research reports yields a picture composed by the specific perspective of the authors, the historical conjuncture that induced the specific perspective, and the stage of development of the TACM practices in the national framework of Malaysia and Singapore.

A lot of the studies concerned with TACM practices in Malaysia published since the 1940s can be categorised chronologically into seven groups.

The first group comprises studies of history and anthropology from the late colonial period (1940–1950s). During this time the colonial focus of the (scarce) studies was directed on the 'primitive' medical practices of the rural Malay population. The leading scholar figure of that period is Richard Winstedt with his seminal treatise *The Malay Magician being Shaman, Shaiva and Sufi* (Winstedt 1951). The viewing angle of Winstedt is determined by his model of a religion-inspired healing syncretism. He regarded the Malay healer as a primitive animistic magician subdued to

Islamic and Hindu influences. Winstedt described the status of the Malay magician basically in a parallel to Islamic ritual by quoting from *Ninety-Nine Laws of Perak*, an Islamic treatise compiled in the eighteenth century by a family of descendants of the Prophet Muhammad and edited in 1908 in Kuala Lumpur: 'The *muezzin* is king in the mosque and the magician is king in the house of the sick, in the rice-field and on the mine' (Winstedt 1951: 72). In order to frame a theological basis of the Hindu–Islamic syncretism, Winstedt elaborated the model of a tolerant Malay Islam that can absorb 'foreign' elements which are active in the healing performance of the magician: 'Tolerant Islam allowed the Malay to retain the nature-spirits of the animist and even the gods of the Hindu under the orthodox designation of infidel genies or *jinn*' (Winstedt 1951: 97). In classical colonial style he does not forget to exalt British colonial medical measures in dealing with the 'primitive' population – e.g. regarding measures against tropical diseases like beri-beri, malaria, etc. (Winstedt 1948).

During the next period (1970–1980s) studies of medical anthropology emerge as a reaction to the colonial ideological bias. The authors of the decolonisation period are concerned with the role TACM practices can play inside the framework of a national health system in the independent state of Malaysia. A major author of that period is Paul C.Y. Chen (1972; 1975; 1979; 1981), who has played an important role in the formation of discourses concerning Malaysian health policies. He was Professor of Preventive Medicine in the University of Malaya and Professor of Community Medicine in the International Medical University, Kuala Lumpur. His administrative influence is related to his engagement in the World Health Organization (WHO) in Southeast Asia, e.g. as Head of WHO Programmes in Papua New Guinea.[5] In his publications he focuses on the actors of various TACM practices in Malaysia, as well as on the public perception of these practices in relation to the modern scientific medical system. He summarises his observations in a model of medical pluralism, according to which modern scientific medicine 'is not replacing traditional medicine but is rather being added on to largely vigorous and continuing systems of traditional beliefs and practices' (Chen 1975: 171). In a quasi-structural approach of medical anthropology he extends the spectrum of native (Malay) medical culture, traditional Chinese medicine and traditional Indian

(Ayurveda, Siddha, Unani) practice by considering also the medical practices of indigenous groups (without elaborating on the question of isolation or contact possibilities between them and the major ethnic groups in Malaysia). On the descriptive level he distinguishes between insular East Malaysians, including Iban as the major group in Sarawak and Kadazan in Sabah, and Orang Asli on the Peninsula. A prevalent common feature, according to his comparison, is the medicine-man (or woman): *bomoh* among the Malays, *manang* among the Iban, the female *bobolian* among the Kadazan, *halaa'* among the Orang Asli, *sin-she* (standard Mandarin: *xiānshēng* 先生) in the Chinese tradition. Chen considers the coexistence of several traditional medical cultures beside the scientific medicine as a challenge for the latter, but also as an opportunity for the state – especially in medical fields with strongly cultural connotation and social entanglement, such as the beginning of life, mental illnesses, or drug addiction.

An important aspect of Chen's studies is the way they enable a diachronic comparison of the TACM practices in Malaysia between the beginning of the 1970s and the 1980s. From his assessments it can be deduced that the 'differential use' of traditional and modern medical services, i.e. the parallel, selective or consecutive use of (shifting into) various medical systems by the same patient (a form of medical pluralism) according to the perception of the specific case, is present and dominant in this decade. Especially the traditional Chinese medicine has obtained more public attention during this period regarding 'modernised' methods and the presence of local training institutions. Chen mentions also homeopathy among the traditional Indian medical systems; however, he provides no comment and no references to other studies. It is also remarkable that he refers neither to any relations between traditional Malay medical practice and popular or scriptural Islam, nor to the so-called medicine of the Prophet.

Special studies of that period on Indian medicine or on 'the Malay healer' have been published by Colley (1978) and Werner (1986), respectively. Other scholars of this period investigated practices among the ethnic groups beyond the schematic borders of Malay–Chinese–Indians by using interview and methods of the medical anthropology, e.g. on black magic and illness in a Malaysian Chinese community. The evidence provided supports the hypothesis of public perception of medical systems and traditional medical practices that 'cross the borders of ethnic communities' (Mo 1984: 155). Other anthropologists have investigated practices affecting the health of Malaysian Orang Asli (Foong-San 1972). A common vision in these studies is the idea that TACM can become an instrument (or shooting target) in ethnocentric tendencies which can effectively support the national medical system – 'particularly when the existing system of health care seems to be inadequate'. A typical field for such TACM engagement is the environment around giving birth, where registration of *traditional* midwives (*bidan kampung*) becomes a suggested instrument for TACM intervention. A similar practice is reported from Indonesia (Bandel 2004: 43). Evidence of repercussions from these studies in later decades can be found in Bach's (1991) dissertation on Malay medical practices in Singapore in the 1980s which will be discussed below.

In the 2000s, comparative epidemiological studies with public health perspectives were published on the basis of ethnic differentiation. The studies of this (third) group focused on the prevalence of certain diseases (e.g. cancer) and on the perception of alternative cure practices regarding these diseases among certain populations. Comparison of mental illness beliefs across ethnic groups, as well as differential behaviour of the patients regarding the various TACM options, were central issues. Statistical analysis of data based on questionnaires about the use of traditional and complementary medicine in Malaysia substituted cultural connotation and ethnological explanation models. Homeopathy was not an object of study (Edman and Koon 2000; Hamidah *et al.* 2009; Siti *et al.* 2009). An increased emphasis on Islamic religious beliefs replacing spiritual assertions in the Malay perception of illness causation was documented by Edman and Koon (2000: 107).

A fourth group comprises studies with a special focus on the relations between TACM and Islam in Malaysia and Singapore. The studies adopted explicitly the perspective of medical anthropology and were published in the 1990s. The work of the German anthropologist Bach (1991) focuses on the relations between state ideology, religions and medical practices in Singapore. Following approaches of medical anthropology, Bach compares patterns of behaviour in dealing with illness and healing options in the different ethnic groups. Regarding the behaviour of Muslims, she underlines the influence of the various *tareqat* (*ṣūfī* groups with several traditions of performing healing rituals). At the time of her PhD research (1990) no institutionalised network of TACM practices existed in Singapore (1991: 160). Nonetheless, she reports upon homeopathic activities and upon her interviews with healers and patients in homeopathic clinics in Singapore. Common statements of homeopathy practitioners interviewed by her evoke vague claims of homeopathy basics to be found in the *sunna* (Islamic tradition) and the Qur'an, e.g. the absence of aggressive interventions in the body, or the parallelism of a soft medicine for peaceful people (Malays). Commenting on homeopathic literature published in Singapore she mentions general allusions to Islam in the introductory parts, but no further references, conceptual or not, in the main corpus of these texts. Another remark on the interviews with homeopathy practitioners regards the syncretism of Malay popular medicine (e.g. performances against evil magic forces), popular performances linked with practising the 'medicine of the Prophet' (e.g. reciting certain verses from the Qur'an), and homeopathy curing practices (1991: 172–5).

A similar focus characterises the work of Eppenich (1998), some years later in Peninsular Malaysia. He underlines explanations provided by the Malaysian homeopaths he interviewed regarding the stronger affinity of homeopathy with Islamic medicine than with traditional Malay medicine. Homeopathic medicaments are not poisonous, and the treatment itself refrains from threatening the patient, like the *halāl* ingredients in Islamic food and the confidential relationships between a Muslim spiritual master (healer of the soul) and the faithful Muslim (patient). These claims evoke the impression of constructing affinities *a posteriori*, a criticism formulated by Eppenich himself. However, they provide evidence about the self-perception of a generation of healers who position the homeopathic practice in the newly strengthened imaginary of Malay Islam. In fact, Eppenich documents the development of a new generation of Malaysian homeopaths (such as Nic Omar, born in 1950), who have left as dissidents from the 'old' Malaysian associations of homeopathy, have founded new ones, while introducing new syncretic elements (from Chinese or Ayurveda medicine) into the 'classical' homeopathy under social and political conditions marked by the new dynamics of political Islam.

Since 2005 onwards there is a revival of the scholar and the administration interest for TACM methods and practitioners in Malaysia (Talib 2006). The main goal of the renewed interest is the integration of TACM into the national health care system (Merican 2002), a trend that is also depicted in the activities of the health authorities, as will be discussed below in relation to the sources. This revitalisation of the scholar and institutional interest for TACM was induced by WHO reports on the spreading of the use of TACM in industrialised countries, but also on the potential of TACM forms for installing a functioning public health system in developing countries. The considerations of these studies (the fifth group of the categorisation) are inspired by the hypothesis that integration of traditional alternative or complementary medical concepts into a modern national public health system (mostly based on 'Western' allopathic bio-medical concepts) may improve the societal acceptance and efficiency of national medical services (including cost reduction).

Since 2010, new critical views under the influence of post-colonial studies have been applied in reconstructing the history and documenting the present of TACM practices in Malaysia. A representative study of this (sixth) group was published by Leow (2014) under the programmatic title 'Healing the nation' in which he described TACM discourses and practices as parts of political strategies focusing on the activities of the physician-politicians Mahathir Mohamad and Burhanuddin Al-Helmy.

A special group of studies that refer to TACM practices in Malaysia is characterised by specific motives of focusing on the relationship between biomedical demands and traditional medical as well as religious discourses. In her dissertation on organ transplantation experiences and discourses in Malaysia, Schreiber (2017) analyses the relationship between the modern biomedical system and the perception of organ donation through the various ethnic and religious groups. The relevance of Schreiber's treatise for the present study results from her evidence-based comments on the complex relationships between culture, ethnicity and religion in a medical context in present-day Malaysia. The religiously coloured discourses, in the case of organ donation and transplantation (especially in an Islamic context), can be read as a parallel to the issue of homeopathy when focusing upon the ambitions of the actors, e.g. Muslim scholars or physicians referring to an Islamic imaginary to localise global narratives in the Malay communities. Schreiber follows Lee and Ackerman (1997) in describing the Malaysian society by a plural religious framing in which Islamic, Buddhist and Daoist groups are internally so diverse that the behaviour patterns of persons belonging officially to these religious communities can't be generally explained or anticipated merely by their adherence to the specific community (Schreiber 2017: 46). In dealing with individual choices and with legitimising discourses regarding traditional medicine she prefers the concept of – Malay or Chinese – lifeworld (*Lebenswelt*); acting in such a lifeworld is not necessarily free of conflicts with religious normative obligations allegedly shared by the community members.

Sources

The overview of the literature implies the necessity of reconstructing a historical hermeneutical framework that enables a better understanding of the emergence, the further development, and the present status of homeopathy as a TACM practice in Malaysia. Information regarding the official status of homeopathy in the present-day medical system of Malaysia is provided in English and Malay versions by the Traditional & Complementary Medicine Division (T&CMD) of the Ministry of Health of Malaysia, which was founded in 2004, following the launching of the National Policy on Traditional and Complementary Medicine and the establishing of the Malaysian Homeopathic Medical Council (MHMC) by the Minister of Health in 2001. MHMC was appointed by the Ministry of Health as the umbrella body for all homeopathic practitioners (http://tcm.moh.gov.my/en/index.php/background). The T&CMD annual reports provide the reader with figures on traditional and complementary medicine programmes offered at institutions of higher and university education since the 2000s, courses (sessions) of Continuous Professional Development (CPD) offered by government hospitals in the fields of T&CMD, as well as with numbers of T&CMD practitioners voluntarily registered since 2008.

Several organisations of homeopathy practitioners (e.g. Majlis Perubatan Homeopathy Malaysia, MPHM) have installed online platforms documenting the history of homeopathy in Malaysia and the interaction with governmental initiatives and institutions (e.g. Persatuan Perubatan Homeopathy Bumiputera Malaysia [PPHBM], Persatuan Perubatan Homeopathy Malaysia [PPHM], Persatuan Perubatan Homeopathy Sarawak [PPHS], Persatuan Homeopati Dan Biokimia Malaysia [PHDBM] and Bahagian Perubatan Tradisional & Komplentari [TCM – The Faculty of Traditional and Complementary Medicine]). Even if such documentation is subject to the perspective and interests of the specific organisation, they enable a rough overview of crucial intersections of national policy and private initiatives in the field of education and practice of homeopathy in Malaysia. The following events could be considered representative for the institutionalisation of homeopathy in Malaysia, as well as for the creation of documents and files on this development:

> 2002: First workshop on formulating standards and criteria for homeopathic education and training. This workshop was held at Kota Bahru, Kelantan, with the collaboration of the Ministry of Health, the National Accreditation Board (Ministry of Health), representatives of selected local universities, and MHMC. Further workshops followed in 2003, 2006 and later.
>
> 2003: First National Seminar on Homeopathy, co-sponsored by MHMC and the Ministry of Health.
>
> 2007: Standards and criteria for homeopathic practices were approved by the Malaysian Qualifying Agency (MQA), Ministry of Higher Education. This approval included the degree program for a Bachelor in Homeopathic Medical Science (BHMS). The first degree-course in homeopathy (BHMS) was offered to the public in 2010 by the Cyberjaya University College for Medical Sciences (CUCMS).
>
> 2011: The Guideline for the Registration of Homeopathic Products was approved by The National Pharmaceutical Control Bureau, Ministry of Health. On 15–17 July 2011 an International Conference on Homeopathy was held at the Putra World Trade Centre, Kuala Lumpur, in a collaboration between the Traditional and Complementary Medicine Division (T&CMD), Ministry of Health, and MHMC under the theme 'Is Homeopathy Evidence-based Medicine?'.

The legal framework for practising homeopathy in Malaysia was reconstrued by the Traditional and Complementary Medicine Act 775 (2016), which established the TCM Council to regulate TCM services and the registration of TCM practitioners in Malaysia. A crucial issue is the recognised practice area in which only registered practitioners are authorised to operate. According to Section 20 (1) 'no person shall practise in any practice area which is not recognised as a practice area'. One of these recognised practice areas is homeopathy. In fact, the registration practice existed already before the TCM Act of 2016 on a voluntary basis according to the Traditional and Complementary Medicine Act 756 (Institute for Public Health 2015: 9). As an example, the new registrations in 2011 were 181 for Traditional Malay Medicine (11%), 1985 for Traditional Chinese Medicine, one for Traditional Indian Medicine, 136 for Complementary Medicine, 71 for Homeopathy and 257 for Islamic Medical Practice (data retrieved from the 2011 Annual Report of the T&CMD, Ministry of Health of Malaysia, p. 88). These figures should not be misunderstood as corresponding to the total offer or to the specific demand for each area. One reason is related to the registration practice, which varied considerably over the years in the various TACM areas. Another reason is the dynamic of medical pluralism in the behaviour and choices of patients across the various TACM areas – an issue of medical anthropology that has been mentioned in the literature quoted above. The governmental statistics of 2012 report an actual total of 13,202 registered practitioners: 3,722 in Traditional Malay Medicine, 6,151 in Traditional Chinese Medicine, 363 in Traditional Indian Medicine, 1,500 in Complementary Medicine, 868 in Homeopathy and 600 in Islamic Medicine. In fact, homeopathy as a category of the T&CMD reports is often 'squeezed' between traditional ethnic Malay medicine, Islamic medicine and other complementary practices. The distinction is mainly based on the data provided by the associations of the Traditional and Complementary Medicine areas as recognised by the authorities. In the past, the practice of homeopathy in Malaysia was strongly associated with Indian traditions (especially Ayurveda), as documented in the short references by Chen (1972, 1975, 1979, 1981). Perhaps the Indian background of the medical studies of the charismatic founding figure of homeopathy in Malaysia, Burhanuddin Al-Helmy (1911–1969), has also contributed to this discourse.[6] Indeed, Ayurveda has often been evoked as a reference for several traditional medical practices understood as alternative or complementary to biomedical methods in the Malaysian regional framework (see, for instance, the comparative study on Ayurveda and Malay traditional medicine by Wan and Wan 2018). In recent years, the representation of homeopathy seems to be dominated by the Registered Homeopathic Medical Practitioners Association of Malaysia (MRHP) founded by Nic Omar in 1984. Nic Omar belongs to the second generation of homeopathy practitioners in Malaysia, the founding figure of the first generation being Burhanuddin Al-Helmy, whose history is described below. Further societies are the Bumiputra Society of Homoeopathy Medical Association (PPHBM) established by Mohamad Hj. Yaakob and headquartered in Johor Bahru, and the Malaysian Homoeopathic Practitioners Association (PPPHM) based in Alor Star, Kedah.

In the meantime, further groups and organisations are engaged in the practice of homeopathy in Malaysia. They offer websites, and they provide information on current trends and demands in the field of homeopathy in Malaysia, e.g. announcements of the Malaysian Government about recruiting homeopathic medical officers. Representative examples are the sites supported by Dr. Nisanth Nambison, President of the Malaysian Homeopathic Medical Council (MPHM) under the TCM Division, Ministry of Health, Malaysia.[7]

A particular problem regarding access to primary sources on homeopathy in Malaysia relates to the biography and the publishing of the works of Burhanuddin Al-Helmy. There are (vague) references about possible practising of homeopathy before the setting up of the first homeopathy association (1937) and the opening of homeopathic clinics in 1939 by Burhanuddin – mostly allusions in some of his speeches. Burhanuddin was a major political activist. Interestingly, his joining the KMM (Kesatuan Melayu Muda), a Malay nationalist anti-British, anti-Sultanate movement, probably took place in his Homeopathy Clinic in 1939 (Omar 2005: 295). A lot of his political writings have been documented. Unfortunately, this is not the case regarding his works on homeopathy in Malaysia. Except for some speeches, these works (essays he allegedly wrote while in prison in 1950) remained unknown to the broader public.[8] They were compiled and published (posthumously) by the HBI Homeopathy Center in Kota Bharu, Terengganu, in 2011 from photocopies made by Dali Muin, a disciple and friend of Burhanuddin – under the title *Pengantar Falsafah Perubatan Homeopathy* (Introduction to the Philosophy of Medical Homeopathy), however, they are still difficult to access (Leow 2014: n. 16).[9] Considering the importance of Burhanuddin Al-Helmy as *the* iconic figure of Malaysian homeopathy and his ideological, political and Islamic theological commitments, it seems reasonable that his speeches and writings have been extensively (even if mostly rather vaguely and superficially) discussed. In a synopsis of Burhanuddin's work published under the title *Pengantar Falsafah Perubatan Homeopati*,[10] attributed to Dali Muin himself and dated on January 1981, Islam is stressed as the basis of Burhanuddin's thought and philosophy – but no explicit conceptual connection between his understanding of homeopathy and his ideas concerning Islamic theology, legal arguments and practice of Islam is provided.[11] The editor of Burhanuddin's *Pengantar Falsafah Perubatan Homeopati*, Muhamed Ahmed Abu Bakar, quoting from Burhanuddin Al-Helmy's speech delivered during the first general meeting of the Malaysian Homeopathy Medical Association in 1962, mentions, among others, famous Muslim physicians from the tradition of medieval Islamicate medicine (e.g. Al-Razi, 864–925 CE), who used herbal drugs for 'soft' medical treatments. No explicit conceptual link between Islam and homeopathy, however, was claimed.[12] It should be remarked that 'soft' herbal drugs are often considered as an analogy to 'soft' medical treatments associated with the sayings and the so-called Medicine of the Prophet Muhammad, and are also used as a discursive link to homeopathy in an Islamic context. Keeping in mind the personal and ideological divisions in the developing lines of homeopathy in Malaysia and Singapore, such comments, abridgments and (selective) quotations should be read in the light of the later claims of Malaysian homeopaths, as they will be discussed in the analysis.

As far as the perspective of Islamic institutions on homeopathy is concerned, two sources of statements appear of particular interest. The first regards publications (in particular *fatwas*) by the Department of Islamic Development Malaysia. *Fatwas* concerning the relation between Islam and homeopathy will be discussed in the analysis.

The second type comprises publications and statements by Malaysian Islamic Academies or institutions and associations of practitioners of Islamic Medicine (i.e. officially recognised Islamic Medical Practice). These (rather rare) publications usually treat specific questions or problems; however, they open a larger Islamic perspective. This consists in proving or establishing the compatibility of a certain treatment in a medical context with the understanding of a possible Islamic background (see e.g. Ariffin *et al.* 2015 on the question of compatibility of Islamic medicine and '*jinn* therapy', i.e. therapy in which the spiritual influence of *jinns* is evoked). These sources differ from the *fatwas* in that they provide more or less reliable statistical information on the practitioners of Islamic medicine and their various methods of treatment. In the text by Ariffin *et al.*, mentioned above, the authors expose the main features and claims of Islamic medicine, and despise medical practitioners evoking the action or influence of *jinns*. Homeopathy is mentioned as one of the alternative medical treatments; however, no explicitly mentioned link between Islamic medical practices and homeopathy practice could be traced.

A further type of source comprises numerous individual blogs and Facebook sites in Malay in which links between homeopathy and Islam are proclaimed. These links are rather of an apologetic character focusing on quotations from the Qur'an or *hadith*, in which 'soft' (e.g. herbal) medical treatments are mentioned, which is interpreted as a recommendation for homeopathy. They can be seen as indicators of public discourses on Islam-explains-everything – including theory and practice of homeopathy.

Finally, it should be remarked that P.C.Y. Chen's reports, even when touching on the differences between rival traditional medical practices inspired by religious traditions, neither stress nor analyse explicitly religious issues – regardless of the fact that he has served as a senior pastor and ordained minister at the Christian River of Life Sanctuary in Selangor, Western Malaysia.

Analysis

On the level of methodology, the analysis basically follows a historical-hermeneutical approach along a political-historical thread in order to overcome the colonial-orientalist ideological bias of the 1940s–1950s, mentioned above, as well as in order to explain the emerging and specific development of some categories and perspectives in approaches to medical anthropology from the 1970s onward. The hypothesis to be checked claims that the encounters of homeopathy practices and Islam, as depicted in the corresponding discourses in Malaysia, are due to the specific context of the Malaysian social and political history and the shifts in the balance of the relations among the ethnically connoted medical traditions. In this perspective, the claim of the present study is that these encounters are rather forms of appropriating certain homeopathic approaches by the more or less dominant discourses of Malaysian political Islam, even when the actors (leading Muslim homeopaths) were or were not themselves politically active figures (as e.g., in the case of the leaders of homeopathy schools and associations, who succeeded Burhanuddin Al-Helmy).

The political and social developments in Malaysia since the end of the 1950s make it necessary to re-assess these encounters and, at the same time, yield frameworks for new interpretations. These developments are characterised by the emergence of political Islam in the form of the Pan-Malaysian Islamic Party (PAS), which considered itself as a Malay-Islamic nationalist party combining modernist-reformist Islam and populist Malay ethnic nationalism. PAS emerged as a radical religious wing of UMNO and claims that Malaysia is an Islamic state, whereas UMNO officials distinguish between an Islamic state and a state with Islam as the official religion of the state (Liow 2009: 103–5). Mahathir Mohamed, a physician who became the longest-serving Prime Minister of Malaysia (1981–2003 and later 2018–2020) under the governing UMNO party, adopted Islamisation measures as a strategic compromise in opposition to PAS. Liow (2009) shows how this strategy has become dominant across the borders of the major political parties and actors, thus forming an Islamic mainstream in the ethnic (Malay) and national (Malaysian) self-representation and the corresponding identity discourse:

> Tellingly, the increasing visibility of Islam in Malaysian society and politics is being driven not only by the Islamist opposition party or PAS, as one should anticipate, but also by the UMNO, whose members were presumably the architects of Malaysia's brand of

> progressive, moderate Islam. In addition, alternative actors such as NGOs and civil society groups are increasingly weighing on the discursive emergence of political Islam in Malaysia today. In certain respects, this active engagement in Islamic discourse and counter-discourse is eclipsing mainstream political parties in terms of intensity. (Liow 2009: 4)

Ellen (1983) comments on these developments from the perspective of historical anthropology: 'Islam in traditional Malay states was partial, idiomatic and syncretic'. Islam in Malay states 'often served to legitimate relations of exploitation, centralisation, and class hegemony…' (1983: 74). 'In Malaysia Islam was used to articulate anticolonial feeling' (1983: 76). In this sense Islam served historically as a distinctive element to distinguish Malays from Chinese and Indian immigrants whose settlement in British Malaya was supported by the British colonial administration. On the other hand, it was precisely the British colonial administration which institutionally reinforced the association between Islam and *adat* (local Malay customs), thus bringing ethnic Malays closer to Islamic institutions (1983: 83).

That was the political-ideological background of the activities of Burhanuddin Al-Helmy. In the context of the legally prescribed ethnic confinement and the tendencies to identify 'Malay' with:

(a) adherence to Islam,
(b) use of the Malay language,
(c) knowledge and practice of *adat*,

Burhanuddin represented a particular position, which deviated from the mainstream during the formative period of Malaysian identities. His father, Haji Muhammad Nor, a Malay *ṣūfī* of the Naqshabandī *ṭariqah*, may have accounted for Burhanuddin's future positioning in the Islamic discourses, in which he became known for his treatises on sufism. His mother, Sharifah Zahrah bint Habib Osman, was a Malay-Indian Muslim of mixed parentage (Omar 2005: 290). In 1928, Burhanuddin went to study in (British) India. At the Aligarh Muslim University, where he obtained his PhD, he met leading Indian political figures such as Mohammed Ali Jinnah (the future founder of Pakistan). At the Ismaeliah Medical College in New Delhi he obtained his degree of Medical Doctor of Homeopathy. After travelling to the Middle East, he returned to

Malaya in 1935. In 1937, he founded the first association of homeopathy in Malaya (Bach 1991: 164). With the support of an Indian physician, Dr. Rajah, he opened homeopathy clinics in Singapore and Johor Bahru in 1939, which lasted till the Japanese invasion in 1942.

Significant in our context is Burhanuddin' political commitment after the colonial period (Omar 2005). As president of the Pan-Malaysian Islamic Party (PAS) from 1956 to 1969, he said: 'PAS and I are in content, character and orientation, "Malay nationalists" with "Islamic aspiration"' (Eppenich 1998: 154, n. 31). The assessments of his engagement for a Great Malay Federation (including Indonesia and the Philippines) and of his assessing the potential of Islam as a unifying factor (unavoidably excluding non-Muslims) are controversial. Malay authors try to harmonise the Muslim-Malay equation by evoking the term Muslim patriotism, instead of Malay nationalism (Omar 2005). Even when they demonstrate the conflicts between Burhanuddin and his Malay adversaries, a holistic view of Malayan affairs (both economic and religious-cultural) is attributed to the immaculate activist (Haji Ismail 2015). Western scholars insist on characterising Burhanuddin's position as deviating from the dominant convention according to which being Muslim is a necessary constituent of Malay identity. They reconstruct a more elaborate picture of Burhanuddin claiming the implementation of procedures that would allow Chinese-Malaysians and Indian-Malaysians (whether Muslims or not) to join the *bangsa Melayu* (Milner 2011: 234). Being himself affiliated to Muslim Indians through his mother, Burhanuddin could understand well the exclusionary function of ethnicity and religion in the process of building the multi-ethnic Malaysian society. More elaborate studies on Burhanuddin's role in shaping PAS underline the importance attributed by Burhanuddin to the three anticolonial forces: Islam, nationalism (in this particular case: Malay nationalism) and socialism/communism (Noor 2014: 52) – an aspect that places Burhanuddin in the specific political frame of the 1950s–60s.

What kind of relationships can be traced between this historically enacted frame of religious-ethnic ideology with the Muslim-Malay reference on one side, and homeopathy, Burhanuddin's medical affiliation, as medical theory and healing practice on the other? It should be remarked firstly that the homeopathy introduced and practised in British Malaya (later Malaysia) by Burhanuddin from the 1930s onwards was strongly related to Indian Ayurveda practices, rather than to a European tradition in the spirit of Hahnemann. Certainly, we can pose the question concerning possible *structural* parallelisms, or analogies, between the introduction of homeopathy into the Malayan Peninsula and Hahnemann's movement in Europe. Historically, Hahnemann opposed his contemporary physicians on epistemological premises insisting on practical experience and using as a guide line the *similis similibus* concept (Jütte 2011: 125–9). In the Malayan/Malaysian case there exist several narratives referring to Islam and to the Malay ethnicity or 'spirit' – all of them embedded in the historical context of the political developments in the Peninsula.

Comparing the links between homeopathy and Islam or politics in the reports of Burhanuddin's speeches we find general formulations, e.g. on applying the principles of homeopathy (in line with the will of nature) in order to cure the state. Leow (2014) has analysed several speeches and writings of Burhanuddin and has elaborated on the claim that Burhanuddin considered homeopathy as an alternative medical system analogous to Malaysia conceived as an alternative nation. In line with his political engagement, Burhanuddin considered his activities as a homeopathic physician as another kind of national service: 'I believe that homeopathy as a medical science is a national asset (*milik bangsa*), one which I proffer as an eternal legacy for our nation's independent future'.[13] For sure, medical metaphors for political governance (as in the case of Burhanuddin), as well as governance metaphors for medical practice, are well-attested in several cultural frames: in Europe and South Asia, as well as in China and Southeast Asia (e.g. in connection with Buddhist concepts of salvation).[14]

Explicit references linking the theory and practice of homeopathy in Malaysia to Islam date to the 1990s and 2000s; it must be noted that they are provided by the next generations of Malaysian practitioners of homeopathy – even when referring to Burhanuddin himself. Mohamed Hatta Abu Bakar (2011), for example, reports that Burhanuddin linked homeopathy to Islam in a way that distinguishes the Malaysian tradition from the history of early homeopathy and the homeopathy practice in other countries. As evidence for this linkage he considered the *similis similibus* concept 'as purported to the hadith of the Prophet about the fall of the flies into the drink (narrated by Bukhari and Abu Daud), and, further, the names of several homeopathic remedies as being already mentioned in the Qur'an' (Abu Bakar 2011). In a similar tone, the Malaysian Homoeopathic Medical Bumiputra Association (founded in 1979) vaguely claims Islamic roots for homeopathy (Eppenich: 1998).

The apologetic claims of compatibility between Islam and homeopathy correspond to a general, world-wide pattern of Muslim discourses of the last decades engaged in a tireless effort to find an implicit allusion to any modern scientific knowledge or invention within the Islamic tradition – written or oral. Significant for the Malaysian context are also the political developments *after* Burhanuddin's death (25 October 1969). The student riots in the name of militant Islam (*dakwah*, i.e. 'summon' or 'call' to renew Muslim faith) in May 1969 led to a political crisis, and triggered, together with other factors, the proclamation of Emergency Rule. The decade that followed the Emergency Rule, the 1970s, was marked by the strengthening of social groups challenging the UMNO-dominated government in the name of Islam, such as the Islamic Youth League of Malaysia (ABIM) under the leadership of Anwar Ibrahim. It is the decade during which the charismatic figure, who would later dominate the Malaysian political stage for five decades, Mahathir bin Mohamad, developed his ideas and his tactics. After being expelled from UMNO in 1970 he published *The Malay Dilemma*, a book demonstrating how Malays should attain the hegemony they deserve, which had very few mentions of Islam. After returning to politics in 1973, he utilised a large police contingent in 1974 to arrest thousands of militant students protesting with an Islamic rhetoric, including the ABIM leader, Anwar Ibrahim. Considering the increasing Islamic influence of PAS as the major threat for the fragile intra-ethnic, Malay-dominated coalition under UMNO, he persuaded ABIM's president, Anwar Ibrahim, to stand as a candidate for UMNO in 1982, and inaugurated as elected prime minister an unprecedented policy of supporting Islamic issues – including the organisation of the Department of the Advancement of Islam (JAKIM), a federal authority responsible for defining and controlling Islamic Orthodoxy. A series of accusations and organised trials against his rival, Anwar Ibrahim, ongoing since 1998, eventually led in 2002 to the climax of affirming that Malaysia – statistically a country with c. 40% non-Muslims – had indeed attained the status of an Islamic state (Means 2009: 75–90, 119–48). It is precisely this climate that is reflected in the report of Eppenich (1998) in which the apologetic Islam-explains-everything trend is accompanied and enforced by the omnipresence of Islamic symbols and the strengthening of Islamic discourses in Malaysia during the long Mahathir era. Homeopathy as an alternative healing treatment for Malays (a soft medicine for soft people), its alleged compliance with Islam, its potential to be combined with popular Islamic practices, its adaptability to the local (popular) perceptions of health and illness etc. – all these claims are entirely affiliated not to Burhanuddin himself, but to his disciples and successors in the organisations of homeopathy during the Mahathir era.

A contrapuntal perception of homeopathy practice in highly urbanised, Chinese-dominated, Singapore is reported by Bach (1991). In the description of perceptions of homeopathy documented in interviews we find allusions to traditional indigenous Malay medical practice, called in a pejorative manner '*bomopathy*' (from the central healer figure, the *bomoh*), as well as to popular Islamic (Prophetic) medicine. Both links show the capacity of homeopathy practice in the Malaysia–Singapore context to absorb elements from other TACM practices.

Following a comment by Schreiber (2017: 184) on Malay lifeworlds, we may claim that the role of homeopathy in Malaysia and Singapore can be traced as a repercussion of the negotiations between the discourses about Islam, medical science and modernity at specific historical situations. Whether homeopathy would stand for scientific rationality, for identification with Malay tradition (Burhanuddin's option), or rather with an Islamic cosmological view (the choice of Burhanuddin's disciples) is a question of negotiating the balances of the epistemological framework under the given political boundary conditions.

If one looks for evidence on the perception of homeopathy from a scholarly Muslim perspective, beyond the limit of the homeopathy practitioners, possible references could be found in *fatwas* (the opinions of the most senior Muslims) upon questions on the subject. Of particular interest in this context is one *fatwa* judging that 'traditional, cultural and artistic performances that contain elements of mysticism, superstitions and imaginary beliefs are prohibited by Islam as it can undermine the creed of a Muslim' (Department of Islamic Development Malaysia 2010: 27), as well another one on yoga exercise judging that, if yoga is accompanied 'by religious elements and worship to obtain certain objectives, it is not appropriate and can damage the creed of a Muslim. [...] However, mere physical movements not accompanied by the aforementioned elements do not constitute an offence' (Department of Islamic Development Malaysia 2010: 29). Both were released by the Conference of the Fatwa Committee of the National Council for Islamic Religious Affairs Malaysia. They do not touch homeopathy proper; however, they express the 'conservative' mainstreaming attitude, according to which practices outside Islamic prescriptions are accepted only under the condition they do not constitute a danger to the creed of a Muslim. In this sense the acceptance (or the support) of homeopathy would depend on the narrative and the terminology employed – a concern that is obvious in the formulations provided by the Burhanuddin's disciples as discussed above. It should be remarked, however, that 'where religion is invoked, it may well be in the guise of *sufi* [mystical] precepts or the words of a popular preacher, rather than an official fatwa' (Brockopp and Eich 2008: 7). Such shifts or misunderstandings are especially common during turbulences in the historical framing of the relations between Islam, political authority and popular medicine (Federspiel 2007).

Further thoughts on the relations between homeopathy and the various Islamic framings of healing practice are given below. Syncretism forms between Malay and Islamic medicine (spiritual Islamic medicine, medicine of the Prophet, practices of Unani medicine)[15] on one side, and homeopathy on the other, are certainly a challenging frame for an approach in the horizon of medical anthropology. This framing should include evidence on theoretical concepts, as well as on forms of medical practice. On the other hand, it should also consider behaviour patterns of patients seeking practitioners both in the area of homeopathy as well as in those of Malay and Islamic medicine mentioned above. Both approaches demand evidence that was not considered in the present study. Indeed, Bach (1991) conducted field research, including interviews, on forms of medical cross-over in Singapore. The concept of 'medical pluralism', however, is an object of detailed research and multi-layer debates that go far beyond the scope of the present study.[16]

Yet in order to assess the singularity or regularity ('normality') of the relationship between homeopathy and Islam in Malaysia, one is tempted to compare it with the alternative pairing, mentioned above, the (possible) relationship between homeopathy and Ayurveda. The latter is often associated with Hinduism, although several historical works distinguish deliberately between a religious discourse and a populist-nationalist appropriation of the Ayurveda as the 'authentic Hindu medical tradition' in India (Das 2012: 453, n. 5). Indeed, Ayurveda is neither practised exclusively in Hindu communities in India, nor exclusively in Indian communities in Malaysia. Such considerations would lead inevitably to a stronger challenge, which would be a comparative study of the development of such relations in South Asia and Malaysia. Hinduism and Islam would be the religious references, the British colonial past would be in both cases the historical framework that conditioned the entering of homeopathy in both geographical areas. In the case of South Asia, the history of homeopathy as an initially 'imported' (nineteenth century), but very quickly locally appropriated, medical practice has been extensively studied from several perspectives (Jütte 1996b; Dinges 2014; Das 2019). Of particular interest for the 'religious link' are certainly the early claims of local leading homeopaths, such as Mahendrae Lal Sircar (1833–1904) in 1868, associating the homeopathy theory of Hahnemann to Hinduism (Jütte 1996b: 356). It has been often showcased how the institutionalisation of traditional medical systems (AYUSH)[17] in India as an integral part of the national health system in 1973 enhanced the diffusion of homeopathy (e.g. Jütte 1996b).[18] Similar processes – with different priorities – took place in Pakistan, where the institutionalisation was already established in 1965.[19] In Malaysia this diffusion was enhanced – as has been shown above – mainly by Muslim actors under a different set of historical conditions. The institutionalisation act came much later (2001/2004) than in India and Pakistan.

The claims of an (alleged) intrinsic affinity of homeopathy with the principles of Islam or the 'essence' of Muslims in Malaysia, as reported by some medical anthropologists (Eppenich; Bach) and encountered in the homeopathy discourse of leading homeopathic practitioners in Malaysia were approached in the present study by contextualising these claims and the evidence of medical anthropology in the specific historical framework of the region, from the colonial era through independence up to the present. In this approach the question on the validity of the claims concerning the relationship between homeopathy and Islam in Malaysia was re-framed in the specific historical context – a 'general' or fundamental answer beyond the specific context would appear artificial, arbitrary or with limited validity. In this sense, the present study weaves together existent intrinsic narratives of Malaysian homeopathy with critical studies on Malaysian history and Malay anthropology. It cannot, however, undertake or substitute a theological approach in an Islamic frame. The mentioned *fatwas* are legal opinions of authoritative Muslims on particular questions: they do not themselves constitute a fundamental theological analysis on the relationship between homeopathy and Islam.

A quite new set of questions arise if one looks for patterns or traces of possible influence of homeopathy on religion itself – in our case: Islam in Malaysia. For an anthropological approach – e.g. in order to check the question of whether Muslims practising homeopathy (as healers or patients) perceive Islam in a different way – specific evidence would be necessary, evidence unknown to the author. The same unavailability regards theological evidence for assessing the influence of homeopathy on Muslim scholars. Regarding the Islamic legal framework, the Malaysian *fatwas* mentioned above do not deviate from those delivered in India, or in the more or less globalised Muslim communities, on the same questions concerning the permissibility of homeopathic treatment for Muslims. The posed questions are commonly formulated as follows: 'Should a Muslim use complementary therapies (homeopathy)?' Or: 'Is it *harām* (forbidden) or *halāl* (allowed) to use homeopathic drugs that contain alcohol?' The answers and the comments refer to the classical fundaments of such Islamic legal opinions (especially in the Hanafi school): If the dilution is very high or the alcohol has gone through change (*istihala*) in the process of treatment, the drug (or the treatment) is beneficial, and the Muslim patient is not tempted to deviate from his or her trusting on Allah, then homeopathic treatment is permissible for Muslims. (Rassool and Morris 2019: 5–8)

Indeed, the perception of an all-encompassing Islam capable of complying (without any change or adaption) with any beneficial scientific development is characteristic of a trend of apologetic modernisation in the Islamic world since the end of the nineteenth century and has nothing specific to do with homeopathy or the Malay Muslim community.

Conclusions

The first step of the present study was to identify evidence on the types of relationship between homeopathy and other TACM concepts and practices inside and across the borders of ethnic or religion-based groups in the case of Malaysia. The recognisable degree of syncretism of TACM practices depends on the patterns used to distinguish between the various ethnic groups in Malaysia and their medical practices. The interweaving, since the creation of Malaysia, of TACM practices and ethnic identities in the multi-ethnic nation has developed its own dynamics depending on the changes in the relations of power inside the political constellation, as well as on the historically conditioned modes of influence of the (Indian, Chinese, Malay) cultural environment. Currently, these relations of power are strongly conditioned (if not dominated) by the discourses of, and about, political Islam.

In the field of political controversies and negotiations, homeopathy enters as an epistemic issue within various discourses about popular healing practices, public health and religious links. Further, the practice of homeopathy seems capable of incorporating not only 'Western' alternative medical traditions, but also indigenous practices that are not compatible with biomedical rationality ('homeopathic magic'). Whereas Burhanuddin Al-Helmy claimed homeopathy to be 'soft therapy for peaceful people' (implying a broader, dynamic understanding of 'Malayness'), his disciples position the homeopathic model in discourses dominated by both religious (Islamic) and ethnic (Malay) symbols.

Notes

1 The category of Orang Asli has been used in different ways by the authorities – colonial or, later, Malaysian – and various scholar disciplines to refer to indigenous groups in the country. Despite the state designation as 'Orang Asli', these groups might self-identify with different sub-ethnic categories. Anthropologists and physicians concerned with medical traditions in the various ethnic groups would occasionally differentiate them in various ways. Paul C.Y. Chen, for example, uses the term Orang Asli exclusively for the indigenous groups of Peninsular Malaysia. He refers to the people living on Borneo (Sarawak and Sabah) either under the group name Iban in the state of Sarawak, or Kadazan in the state of Sabah (Chen 1975: 171). Uncareful re-categorisations can lead to misunderstandings or misperceptions, especially when scholars generalise their observations concerning medical practices from the specific focused group to the broader category – Orang Asli or even Malay.

2 For several discussions on the peculiarities of the Chinese minority in Malaysia (in a Southeast Asian context), such as its role in politics and the economic life in a historical perspective, see Somers Heidhues (1974), Reid (1996) and Lee and Ackerman (1997: 58–82).

3 In spite of the official census, reliable absolute figures are rather difficult to obtain. Comparing statistical data becomes additionally complicated through the separate listings referring to the peninsular population. Lee and Ackerman (1997: 15) report a population of about 15 million on the Peninsula (1980 census) comprising approximately 55% Malays, 34% Chinese, 10% Indians, and less than 1% Orang Asli, Europeans and Eurasians. Peninsular statistics alone should not be regarded as representative for the whole country, since insular East Malaysia (on Borneo) has a particularly high percentage of indigenous groups. The quantitative figures reported depend further on the particular focus of the specific study: Milner (2011) e.g., focusing on the Malay group, quotes a number of 12 million Malays in Peninsular Malaysia (with more than 300,000 in Sabah and some 500,000 in Sarawak) from a source published in 2007 (Lee and Ackerman 1997: 1).

4 For a comparison: On the basis of the 1980 census (since the statistics of the 1990 census were not available when their book was written) Lee and Ackerman report 56% Muslims, 32% Buddhists-Daoists, 8% Hindus, 2% Christians and 2% others on the peninsula, i.e. without considering Borneo (Lee and Ackerman 1997: 15).

5 During the 2010s, P. C. Y. Chen served as a senior pastor and ordained minister at the Christian River of Life Sanctuary in the Peninsular state of Selangor, Western Malaysia.

6 The relations between Ayurveda and homeopathy in the Malaysian context are certainly beyond the scope of the present study. However, the various links and perceived similarities demand a closer comparative study. Some remarks accompanied by literature and sources will be presented below at the end of the analysis.

7 www.persatuanmrhp.freehomepage.com and www.similima.com/scope-of-homoeopathy-in-malaysia, accessed 4 June 2022.

8 Omar (2005: 292), with reference to Wan (1997: 63), lists the following writings by Burhanuddin on homeopathy without further bibliographical data: *Falsafah Perubatan Homeopathy* (The Philosophy of Medical Homeopathy); *Asas Pamakopia Homeopathy* (The Foundation of Pamachopic Homeopathy); *Mutiara Homeopathy* (The Valuable Homeopathy). These writings could not be verified or accessed for the present study.

9 Burhanuddin Al-Helmy died on 25 October 1969, aged 58. Unfortunately, this edition of *Pengantar Falsafah Perubatan Homeopathy* (Introduction to the Philosophy of Medical Homeopathy) could not be made available and, therefore, could not be considered in the present study.

10 The Malay spelling *homeopati* is widely used in parallel with the English term 'homeopathy' – even when referring to the same treatise or compilation published in Malaysia.

11 www.homeolibrary.com/NewHomeo_2011/FalsafahPerubatan/KataPenyunting.htm, accessed 20 July 2019.

12 www.homeolibrary.com/NewHomeo_2011/FalsafahPerubatan/Indekskuliah.htm, accessed 20 July 2019.

13 Leow (2014: 10) quotes from Burhanuddin's inaugural speech at the opening of the Homeopathic Association of Malaysia in 1961 – i.e. during the period of decolonisation between the independence of the Federation of Malaya (1957) and the creation of Malaysia (1963). See also Abu Bakar (1977).

14 I am grateful to Michael Stanley-Baker and Pierce Salguero for drawing my attention to the specific connection between Buddhism and medicine regarded as expression of compassion and metaphor for salvation – aspects that in the public sphere constitute goals of social engagement and political practice.

15 Unani medicine has been transmitted and practised initially in Muslim societies in South and Central Asia. Its links to Ayurveda and its geographical reference have probably motivated its occasional

classification as 'Indian traditional medical practice' in official Malaysian documents.

16 See the elucidating introduction by Dinges (2014: 7–19) on medical pluralism; see also the chapters on medical relativism in Leslie (1976: 322–82).

17 The acronym AYUSH is built from the initials of the terms Ayurveda, Yoga (and Naturopathy), Unani, Siddha (medical tradition among Tamil tribes), and Homoeopathy.

18 As has been pointed out in the literature overview (e.g. in the works of C.Y.P. Chen), the 1970s were internationally marked by focusing on TACM practices and the possibilities of their integration in national health systems.

19 Homeopathy was officially recognised by the Government of Pakistan in 1965. The Board of Homeopathic System of Medicine, Pakistan, as well as the National Council of Homeopathy were established under the Unani, Ayurvedic and Homeopathic Practitioners' Act 1965, II, www.nchpakistan.gov.pk/, accessed 17 July 2020.

Bibliography

Abu Bakar, M.H. (1977) *Perubatan* Homeopathy. Banting: HBI Health & Homoeopathy Centre.

Abu Bakar, M.H. (2011) *The Development of Homeopathy in Malaysia*, www.homeolibrary.com/NewHomeo_2011/NEWS_HOMEOPATHY; also published in Malay under the title *Perkembakngan homeopati di Malaysia* (The Spread of Homoeopathy in Malaysia) in 2002, www.homeoint.org/articles/malay/malaysia.htm, accessed 7 July 2018.

Amin, W. M. A. M. (1997) *Antara'asabiyyah dan nasionalisme: menurut pandangan Dr. Burhanuddin Al-Helmy*. Kuala Lumpur: Jabatan Pengajian Media Universiti Malaya.

Ariff, K.M. and Beng, K.S. (2006) 'Cultural Health Beliefs in a Rural Family Practice: A Malaysian Perspective', *Australian Journal of Rural Health*, 14: 2–8.

Ariffin, M.F.M. *et al.* (2015) 'Pusat Perubatan Alternative Islam di Malaysia: Persepsi perawat terhadap aplikasi jin dalam rawatan (Islamic Medical Centre in Malaysia: Perceptions of Evoking Jinns in Treatments)', *Jurnal Islam dan Masyarakat Kontemporari*, Bil. 9 Januari: 61–86.

Bach, G. (1991) *Zwischen Staatsideologie und Islam: Malaiische Medizin in Singapore*. Münster: Lit.

Bandel, K. (2004) *Medizin und Magie in der Modernen Indonesischen Prosa*. Norderstedt: Books on Demand.

Bianco, L. (1969) *Das moderne Asien*, Fischer Weltgeschichte Bd. 33. Frankfurt/M.: Fischer.

Brockopp, J. and Eich Th. (eds) (2008) *Muslim Medical Ethics: From Theory to Practice*. Columbia, SC: The University of South Carolina Press.
Chen, P.C.Y. (1972) 'An Analysis of Customs related to Childbirth in Rural Malay Culture', *Tropical and Geographical Medicine*, 25: 197–204.
Chen, P.C.Y. (1975) 'Medical Systems in Malaysia: Cultural Bases and Differential Use', *Social Science and Medicine*, 9: 171–80.
Chen, P.C.Y. (1979) 'Traditional and Modern Medicine in Malaysia', *The American Journal of Chinese Medicine*, 7.3: 259–75.
Chen, P.C.Y. (1981) 'Traditional and Modern Medicine in Malaysia', *Social Science and Medicine*, 15A: 127–36.
Colley, F. (1978) 'Traditional Indian Medicine in Malaysia', *Journal of the Malaysian Branch of the Royal Asiatic Society*, 51: 1.
Daniels, T. (2013) 'Introduction: Performance, Popular Culture, and Piety in Muslim Southeast Asia', in T. Daniels (ed.) *Performance, Popular Culture, and Piety in Muslim Southeast Asia*. New York: Palgrave Macmillan, 1–12.
Daniels, T. (ed.) (2013) *Performance, Popular Culture, and Piety in Muslim Southeast Asia*. New York: Palgrave Macmillan.
Dannaud, Ch. (2013) 'Malaien und Malaysier', *Le Monde Diplomatique* (German edition), Nov. 2013, 7.
Das, S. (2012) 'Debating Scientific Medicine: Homoeopathy and Allopathy in Late Nineteenth-century Medical Print in Bengal', *Med. Hist.*, 56.4: 463–80, https://doi.org/10.1017/mdh.2012.28, accessed 11 July 2020.
Das, S. (2019) *Vernacular Medicine in Colonial India: Family, Market and Homeopathy*. Cambridge: Cambridge University Press.
Department of Islamic Development Malaysia (ed.) (2010) *Decisions of the Fatwa Committee of the National Council for Islamic Religious Affairs Malaysia*. Putrajaya: Department of Islamic Development Malaysia.
Department of Statistics, Malaysia (ed.) (2011) *Population Distribution and Basic Demographic Characteristics 2010*. Putrajaya: Department of Statistics Malaysia.
Dinges, M. (ed.) (2014) *Medical Pluralism and Homeopathy in India and Germany (1810–2010)*. Stuttgart: Franz Steiner.
Edman, J.L. and Koon, T.Y. (2000) 'Mental Illness Beliefs in Malaysia: Ethnic and Intergenerational Comparisons', *International Journal of Social Psychiatry*, 46.2: 101–9.
Ellen, R.F. (1983) 'Social Theory, Ethnography and the Understanding of Practical Islam in South-East Asia', in M.B. Hooker (ed.) *Islam in South-East Asia*. Leiden: Brill, 50–90.
Eppenich, H. (1998) 'Malaiische Identität und Islamisierung der Homöopathie in Malaysia', in R. Jütte (ed.) *Medizin, Gesellschaft und Geschichte. Jahrbuch des Instituts für Geschichte der Medizin der Robert-Bosch-Stiftung*, 17. Stuttgart: Franz Steiner, pp. 149–75.
Federspiel, H. (2007) *Sultans, Shamans, and Saints. Islam and Muslims in Southeast Asia*. Honolulu: University of Hawai'i Press.

Foong-San, S. (1972) 'Some Beliefs and Practices Affecting the Health of the Aborigines (Orang Asli) of Bukit Lanjian, West Malaysia', *The Southeast Asian Journal of Tropical Medicine and Public Health*, 3.2: 267–76.

Haji Ismail, Z. (2015) 'Pemikiran dan perjuangan politik: Dr. Burhanuddin Al–Helmi (Thought and Political Struggle: Dr. Burhanuddin Al-Helmi)', *Jurnal Peradaban Melayu Jilid*, 10.

Hamidah, A. *et al.* (2009) 'Prevalence and Parental Perceptions of Complementary and Alternative Medicine Use by Children with Cancer in a Multi-ethnic Southeast Asian Population', *Pediatr. Blood Cancer*, 52: 70–4.

Harper, T. and Amrith, S.S. (eds) (2014) *Histories of Health in Southeast Asia: Perspectives on the Long Twentieth Century*. Bloomington, IN: Indiana University Press.

Hoffstaedter, G. (2011) *Modern Muslim Identities – Negotiating Religion and Ethnicity in Malaysia*. Copenhagen: NIAS Press.

Hooker, M.B. (ed.) (1983) *Islam in South-East Asia*. Leiden: Brill.

Institute for Public Health (2015) *National Health and Morbidity Survey 2015 (NHMS 2015). Vol. IV: Traditional & Complementary Medicine*. Kuala Lumpur: Ministry of Health, Malaysia.

Jelonek, A.W. (2004) 'Islamic Political Movement in Malaysia', *Studia Arabistyczne*, 12: 125–57.

Jütte, R. (1996a) *Geschichte der alternativen Medizin*. München: C. H. Beck.

Jütte, R. (1996b) 'Eine Späte Homöopathische Macht: Indien', in M. Dinges (ed.) *Weltgeschichte der Homöopathie*. München: C. H. Beck, 355–81.

Jütte, R. (2011) 'Homöopathie – Eine Alt-neue Heilkunst', in D. Stederoth and T. Hoyer (eds) *Der Mensch in der Medizin*. Freiburg/München: Karl Alber.

Kausar, Z. (ed.) (2005) *Contemporary Islamic Political Thought – A study of Eleven Islamic Thinkers*. Kuala Lumpur: Ampang Press.

Kehl-Bodrogi, K. (2012) 'Amulettwesen, Krankenheilung und Heiligenverehrung: Religiöse Alltagspraktiken unter Muslimen', in I. Pfluger-Schindlbeck (ed.) *Welten der Muslime*. Berlin: Reimer & Staatliche Museen zu Berlin, 89–122.

Lee, H.G. and Suryadinata, L. (eds) (2012) *Malaysian Chinese: Recent Developments and Prospects*. Singapore: Institute of Southeast Asian Studies.

Lee, R.L.M. and Ackerman, S.S.E. (1997) *Sacred Tensions: Modernity and Religious Transformation in Malaysia*. Columbia: University of South Carolina Press.

Leow, R. (2014) 'Healing the Nation: Politics, Medicine, and Analogies of Health in Southeast Asia', in T. Harper and S.S. Amrith (eds) *Histories of Health in Southeast Asia: Perspectives on the Long Twentieth Century*. Bloomington, IN: Indiana University Press, 202–9.

Leslie, C. (ed.) (1976) *Asian Medical Systems: A Comparative Study*. Berkeley, CA: University of California Press.

Liow, C.J. (2009) *Piety and Politics: Islamism in Contemporary Malaysia*. Oxford: Oxford University Press.

Ma, R. (2012) 'Being Muslim and Chinese in Malaysia', in H.G. Lee and L. Suryadinata. (eds) *Malaysian Chinese: Recent Developments and Prospects*. Singapore: Institute of Southeast Asian Studies, 26–44.

Mahathir, M. (1970) *The Malay Dilemma*. Singapore: Asia Pacific Press.

McAmis, R.D. (2002) *Malay Muslims*. Cambridge: William B. Eerdmans.

Means, G.P. (2009) *Political Islam in Southeast Asia*. Boulder, CO: Lynne Rienner.

Merican, I. (2002) 'Traditional/Complementary Medicine: The Way Ahead', *Medical Journal of Malaysia*, 57.3: 261–5.

Milner, A. (2011) *The Malays*. Chichester: Wiley-Blackwell.

Mo, B. (1984) 'Black Magic and Illness in a Malaysian Chinese Community', *Social Science & Medicine*, 18.2: 147–57.

Noor, F. (2014) *The Malaysian Islamic party PAS 1951–2013: Islamism in a Mottled Nation*. Amsterdam: Amsterdam University Press.

Omar, M.F. (2005) 'Burhanuddin Al-Halmy: Political activities and ideas', in Z. Kausar (ed.) *Contemporary Islamic Political Thought – A study of Eleven Islamic Thinkers*. Kuala Lumpur: Ampang Press, pp. 289–310.

Rassool, H.G. and Morris, H. (2019) 'Should a Muslim Use Complementary Therapies: Halal or Haram?', Islamic Online University: *Journal of Integrated Sciences*, 1: 1–24.

Reid, A. (1993) *The Making of an Islamic Political Discourse in Southeast Asia*. Clayton/Victoria (Australia): Aristoc Press, Monash Papers on Southeast Asia.

Reid, A. (1996) *Sojourners and Settlers: Histories of Southeast Asia and the Chinese*. St. Leonards (Aus.): Allen & Unwin.

Reid, A. (2010) *Imperial Alchemy: Nationalism and Political Identity in Southeast Asia*. Cambridge: Cambridge University Press.

Schreiber, J. (2017) *Politics, Piety, and Biomedicine: The Malaysian Transplant Venture*. Bielefeld: Transcript.

Siti, Z.M. *et al.* (2009) 'Use of Traditional and Complementary Medicine in Malaysia: A Baseline Study', *Complementary Therapies in Medicine*, 17: 292–9.

Somers Heidhues, M. (1974) *Southeast Asia's Chinese Minorities*. Melbourne: Longman Australia.

Somers Heidhues, M. (2000) *Southeast Asia: A Concise History*. London: Thames & Hudson.

Talib, N. (2006) 'Alternative, Complementary and Traditional Medicine in Malaysia', *Medicine and Law*, 25: 445–62.

Wan, M. A. M. A. (1997). *Antara 'Asabiyyah dan Nasionalisme: Menurut Pandangan Dr. Burhanuddin Al-Helmy (Between 'Asabiyyah and Nationalism: According to the View of Dr. Burhanuddin Al-Helmy)*. Kuala Lumpur: Penerbitan Baiduri.

Wan, F. and Wan, Y. (2018) 'Nature manifestation in philosophy, diagnosis and treatment of disease based on Ayurvedic and Malay traditional medicine: A comparative study', *SHS Web of Conferences 45*,

05001: 1–5, https://doi.org/10.1051/shsconf/20184505001, accessed 20 July 2019.
Weintraub, A.N. (ed.) (2011) *Islam and Popular Culture in Indonesia and Malaysia*. London: Routledge.
Werner, R. (1986) *Bomoh/Dukun: The Practices and Philosophies of the Traditional Malay Healer*. Berne: The University of Berne, Institute of Ethnology.
Winstedt, R. (1951; quoted from the revised edition1982) *The Malay Magician: Being Shaman, Shaiva and Sufi*. Kuala Lumpur: Oxford University Press.
Winstedt, R. (1948) *Malaya and its History*. London: Hutchinson University Library.

9

Questioning the boundaries between medicine and religion in contemporary Myanmar

Céline Coderey

Background

The ethnography I conducted among Buddhist communities in Rakhine State, Western Myanmar, over a period of 15 years starting in 2005 shows the diversity of conceptions and practices people use to deal – cognitively, emotionally and pragmatically – with health and illness, and which make up what I call the 'therapeutic field', is extreme. They draw from a variety of traditions locally referred to as indigenous medicine (*taing-yin hsay pyinnya*),[1] *weikza*[2] (Pāli, *vijaā*, meaning 'knowledge') or exorcist knowledge (*payawga pynnya*) including alchemy, remedies, recitation of mantra and esoteric diagrams, Western biomedicine (*ingaleik hsay pyinnya*), divination and astrology (*baydin pyinnya*), spirit cult (*nat pwe*) and Buddhism (*Buda bada*). Elements from different traditions are often combined within the same aetiological explanation or therapeutic practice to the extent that it is hard to say to which category they belong. The hybridity is further increased by the fact that the majority of healers combine a plurality of techniques, and even training, thus blurring the boundaries between therapeutic figures. In contrast to this, in their narratives people often associate a certain conception or practice to a certain tradition; in particular, they stress what belongs to Buddhism (*Buda bada*, the 'language/religion of the Buddha') and what does not, and what belongs to medicine (*hsay pyinnya*) and what does not, as a reflection of the fact that they attribute to Buddhism and medicine higher legitimacy and respectability. This hierarchisation is often reflected also in the aetiological system and therapeutic practices themselves, where elements associated with

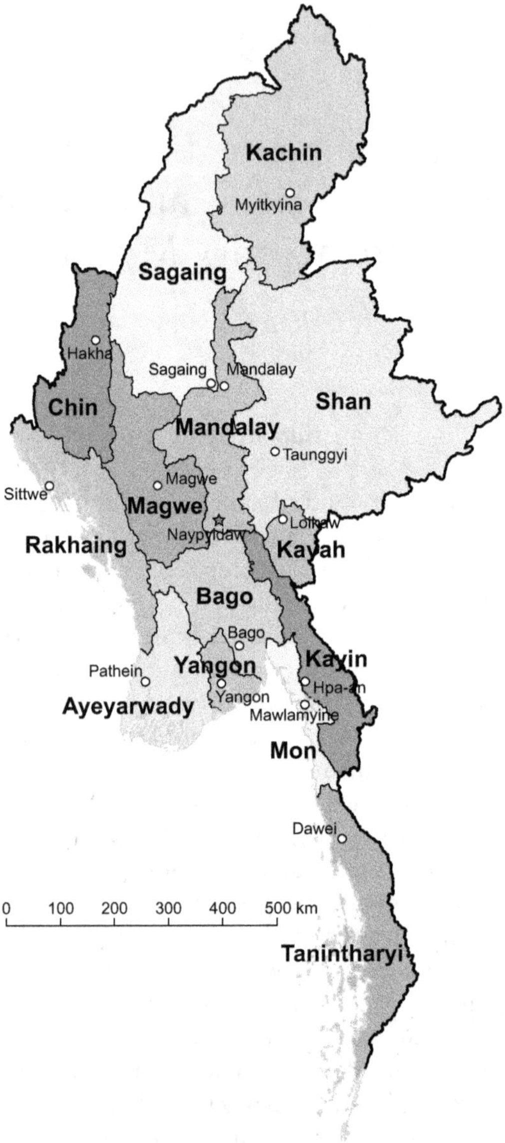

Map 9.1 Map of Myanmar and its divisions

Buddhism or medicine are attributed more legitimacy as well as a higher explanatory and therapeutic power.

Although this plurality is part of people's everyday life, it is seldom studied as such in the literature, leaving the dynamics underpinning it yet to be understood. This is true both for Myanmar and for other Theravāda countries which share a similar panorama in terms of health and healing (Golomb 1985; Monnais 2007; Pottier 2007; Guillou 2009). The main reason for this failure is that the conceptions and practices forming this whole have always been considered by scholars as belonging to different fields – mainly religion and medicine – and thus as objects of different disciplinary attention, these being, on the one side, religious studies, religious anthropology and history of religions and, on the other side, medical anthropology and history of medicine.[3] Scholars belonging to these disciplines have thus usually looked only at a limited number of traditions – the ones deemed to belong to their own discipline.

Such an approach is problematic because it separates what is connected in practice, missing the chance to show important links between the different components of the therapeutic field, and the overlapping of the religious and the medical. Moreover, this perspective is tacitly based on underlying assumptions grounded in Western categories, with little effort to interrogate their relevance in the local context. Do scholarly (etic) categories of religion and medicine bear any relation to the (emic) categories held by Rakhine, Burmese or other Buddhist people? How are these two different kinds of categories correlated, and what losses or misrepresentations occur when scholars assume an etic analytic stance with little reflection on emic categories?

In contrast to this literature, which filters the reality through pre-determined categories created by the observer, I adopt a comprehensive approach which looks at a wide, inclusive spectrum of conceptions and practices that Rakhine Buddhists use to apprehend health and illness and examine the coexistence and tension between hybridity and categorisation, hierarchisation and complementarity. I want, in particular, to examine the socio-political origin of categories of Buddhism and medicine and of their positioning above other traditions and the implication this configuration has on people's process of health seeking and on the therapeutic efficacy.

My analysis is developed in reference to Rakhine State but can be generalised to many other Buddhist regions of the country. Rakhine represents one of the seven minority ethnic states of Myanmar, which are located at the periphery of the central region that is predominantly Burmese. Historical works (Phayre 1883; Charney 1999; Leider 2004) show that before its conquest by the Burmese king Bodawhpaya in 1784, Rakhine was a highly Indianised independent kingdom. Since that time, though, it has shared the same destiny as the rest of the country, first experiencing British colonisation (from 1824 to 1948), and then fifty years of military dictatorship from 1962 to 2011, during which the centre always tried to control and dominate the peripheral states. After ten years of partial democratisation, starting in 2011, the country returned in 2021 to military rule.

This political history has deeply affected the religious and the medical landscapes of the country. Local authorities have played a significant role in introducing, spreading and then regulating specific religious and medical traditions: Theravāda Buddhism, Western medicine and a modernised version of traditional medicine. The symbolic power in which these three traditions have been invested has largely affected the other components of the 'therapeutic field' forcing them to adjust in order to fit the new values and norms in place.

The history of Buddhism in Myanmar probably extends more than two thousand years. Historians affirm that Rakhine, like the rest of Myanmar, received Buddhism in its different forms – Theravāda, Mahāyāna, and Tantric – from India at different times (Gutman and Zaw Min Yu 2001: 26; Bernot 1967: 129). According to the *Mahavamsa*, a fifth- or sixth-century Pāli chronicle of Sri Lanka, Ashoka sent two monks, Sona and Uttara, to Suvarnabhumi around 228 BCE with other monks and sacred texts. In 1057, the Burmese king Anawrahta, who reigned in Pagan between 1044 and 1077, sent an army to conquer the Mon city of Thaton and obtain the *Tipiṭāka* or Pāli canon. Having been converted to Theravāda Buddhism by the Mon monk Shin Arahan, Anawrahta implanted Theravāda Buddhism in Pagan. As a result, all other religious and ritual expressions were marginalised or incorporated into the new mainstream religion. Even the cult of tutelary spirits (*nat*), which Anawratha had previously unsuccessfully tried to eradicate, was then submitted to the hegemony of Buddhism.[4] Later, during the colonial era, British authorities didn't interfere with local religion, afterwards, however, with independence, the tradition of rulers supporting Buddhism was re-established. Indeed, military rulers continued patronising the religion – thus inscribing themselves in symbolic continuity with the royal tradition – and sponsoring the construction of pagodas and other religious buildings, in an attempt to garner some moral legitimacy (Brac de la Perrière 2009).

The state's control over religious practices was particularly marked by the nationalisation and 'purification' (*tan shin yay*, 'cleaning', 'purification') of Buddhism first with U Nu[5] (1948–1958, 1960–1962) and then with Ne Win (1974–1981) and Than Shwe (1992–2011). They indeed enacted a series of measures aimed at gaining control over the entire population, including the ethnic minorities living in the peripheral states and not necessarily embracing the Buddhism religion. Embodying the role of the righteous monarch, in 1950, 'U Nu created a Buddhist Sasana Council whose purpose was to propagate Buddhism and supervise monks [...]. In the manner of King Asoka and later Southeast Asian Buddhist monarchs, he called a sangha council to purify the dhamma and produce a new redaction of the Pali canon. [...] In August 1961, U Nu introduced an amendment in the Burmese Parliament to establish Buddhism as the state religion' (Swearer 1995: 111). Ne Win (1974–1981) held the Buddhist reform council ('the Congregation of the Sangha of All Orders for Purification, Perpetuation and Propagation of the Sasana') (Hayami 2011: 1091) and started a purification campaign intended to divorce Buddhism from these 'worldly practices' (astrology, *weikza*, spirit cults and medicines) so as to bring Buddhism back to its supposed original purity and original focus on 'otherworldly goals' (progression towards nirvana) (Tosa 2005).[6] This purification process operates according to the principles described by Latour (1993), who sees purification as a process separating the hybrids and forcing them into dichotomic categories. Ne Win also significantly tightened the control over monks and monastic organisations to make sure they did not engage in 'non-Buddhist practices'. It is noteworthy that the elements the state attempted to suppress were the more esoteric practices and notably the *weikza* practices, which it perceived as potentially threating for its power because they were transmitted and practised within semi-secret groups with millenaristic or messianic goals (Ferguson and Mendelson 1981). They (1981: 74) pointed out that under Ne Win, the state tried to limit the *weikza* by censoring all books related to them, and forbidding the members of these groups from naming the future king. In 1979, the regime had outlawed the rising Shwei Yin Kyaw Gaing, a popular esoteric sect, and arrested its leader, who had gained a large following including politicians and merchants (Hayami 2011: 1096). This process exemplifies what Brac de la Perrière (2009: 202–3) suggests, that in Myanmar the religious field is constituted through the incessant delineation of pure Buddhism against a diversity of practices and conceptions, and that it is through this process that the Burmese build their – dominant – position in their social world.

In the last few decades, the purification of Buddhism has acquired an additional meaning: projecting towards the outside world an idea of a modern Buddhist nation, freed from backward superstitions (Sadan 2005), something that became particularly relevant with the economic opening of the country and the promotion of tourism from 1996, and most notably from 2011, demonstrating how spiritual capital can be translated into, and manifest itself as, economic capital (Yew-Foong *et al.* 2017: 4).[7]

As for medicine, even though some Western medical practices were introduced to the country around the seventeenth century by Christian missionaries, the formal introduction of Western medicine dates to the latter half of the nineteenth century (Richell 2006; Naono 2009). At that time the country was a province of India and the British government organised medical services to provide facilities for medical relief and improvement of public health (Edwards 2010). The locals referred to this medicine (as they still do nowadays) as *ingaleik hsay*, 'medicine of the English', to mark its foreign origin. The establishment of biomedicine introduced for the first time the idea of medicine as something distinct and separate from religion and from other healing traditions.[8] It also brought forth the idea of medicine as a system of knowledge and practice, alongside a distinction between formal and informal, licit and illicit. Indeed, before the introduction of Western medicine, there was no such thing as a 'medical system' or a 'medical institution'. What people had was a kaleidoscope of knowledge and techniques of different natures and origins that they would use to deal with health issues and other misfortunes. Everything which had the power (*swan*) to prevent or cure natural or supernatural disorders and other misfortunes was considered medical and thus referred to as 'medicine' (*hsay*). This included remedies made of natural ingredients, *weikza* practices such as alchemy and esoteric diagrams, amulets, water empowered by uttering Buddhist formulae, and so on. Although basic forms of these practices could be easily learned by anybody, a more in-depth knowledge of these practices, allowing one to be recognised as 'medicine master' (*hsay hsaya*) was accessible only through a training from a master. The main training was in traditional medicine (herbal medicine, *beyndaw*, combined with astrology and recitation of mantra) to cure natural disorders, *weikza* knowledge (alchemy, esoteric diagrams, mantra, remedies) to cure natural but especially supernatural disorders, divination and *nat* mediumism. If some techniques (herbal medicine, exorcist practices) were specific to one or another training, others (astrology and mantra recitation) were common to many or all of them. This complex healing universe still exists nowadays beside the formalised and official health care system.

Even though Western medicine came with Western domination, the Burmese authorities who took power after independence in 1948 continued to support and expand it, certainly motivated by the desire to get legitimacy and recognition – at the local and global level. Nevertheless, they also gave formal recognition to traditional medicine by integrating it into the health care system. This initiative was not only meant to compensate and neutralise the Western presence/power, but more specifically, as I have shown elsewhere (Coderey 2020), to contribute to the postcolonial agenda of nation building, consisting in the creation of an independent country, autonomous from the West, united despite the ethnic diversity, modern and yet holding strongly to its Buddhist tradition. Even though this medicine has been promoted as the national traditional medicine, it has actually been crafted by selecting only medical traditions from the Buddhist, mainly Burmese, areas. It has also been stripped of all elements the state perceived as a threat to its authority and/or which did not conform to the Western idea of medicine and science. Natural products and massage to cure physical illness have been kept, while astrology as well as mantra, esoteric diagrams and alchemy (the so-called *weikza* path), used to deal with supernatural aggressions, have been excluded.[9] The formal exclusion of *weikza* practices from medicine came to strengthen the marginalisation of these practices that was happening concurrently as a tool of domination and control, as described above. An analogous selection motivated by analogous reasons had been previously enacted by the British when they were planning to integrate traditional medicine into the health system. As Aung-Thwin (2010) tells us, this project though was never realised because the medicine started to be strongly associated with the anticolonial movement led by Saya San, who claimed he would restore the authority of the Burmese monarchy, revitalise the Buddhist religion, and expel the British. He also assured his followers that they would be protected by his magical charms and tattoos.

Interestingly, in the shaping of this formalised version of traditional medicine, the connection to Buddhism – in terms of aetiological concepts and some curing principles – has instead been kept, I claim, for the sake of legitimacy and respectability. This Buddhisation of medicine stands in contrast to the separation of Buddhism from worldly practices, including medicine, which was the object of the above-mentioned Buddhism purification campaigns conducted by the state's authorities. To ensure further control – from the Burmese – over this medicine, the transmission of its knowledge – in the form of university teaching – has been centralised in Mandalay, the last Burmese capital and core of the Burmese and Buddhist tradition.

Even though Western and local medicine are now both part of the official health system, they remain institutionally separated and biomedicine occupies the dominant and favoured position, as visible in policy, economic support and legislative influence. That being said, both sectors remain highly lacking. Indeed, although the state has for a long time seen in medicine an important symbolic tool to achieve its nationalistic goals, it has never invested in it as much as it has done in other sectors, such as military defence and control of border areas. This long-lasting condition of financial neglect has decimated the health care system, which is lacking in quality services, medical professionals, medication and equipment, especially in remote areas (Skidmore 2008; Coderey 2016). Despite the low quality of services, the cost is often very high, especially because patients are expected to pay almost in full for health expenses (Saw *et al.* 2013).

Literature

Religious studies

The largest group of studies of Myanmar are those related to Buddhism. Moving away from the works of the first orientalists who studied Buddhism from texts and generally considered it as being purely otherworldly oriented, consecutive works, especially those of anthropologists, have looked at Buddhism as practised in daily village life. One of the main concerns they faced initially was to understand how to conceive the relationship between Buddhism and the other traditions embraced by local populations, mainly spirit cults, that they – unlike local people – considered a form of religion. The majority of scholars working on Burma (Mendelson 1961; Nash 1963; Brohm 1963; Pfanner 1966), like scholars working on other Theravāda societies (Obeyesekere 1963; Kirsch 1977; Tambiah 1970, 1984, 1985; Terwiel [1975] 1994), have understood Buddhism and spirit cults as part of a single religious system that is dominated by Buddhism, which provides the conceptual framework and system of values within which the other practices are integrated. If Obeyesekere and Kirsch stress the difference in functionality between Buddhism, dedicated to other-worldly aims, and spirit cults, concerned with worldly aims, Nash and Tambiah recognise that Buddhism itself is used for both aims. The latter's approach is particularly interesting and relevant to this work because they both include in their reflections not only Buddhism and spirit cults but other traditions as well. They both argue, moreover, for a coherence of the 'system' and tried to provide an explanation for it. Nash (1965: 65) affirms that *nat* (spirits) cult, divinatory and medical systems are analytical categories divided by the recording anthropologist. In the eyes of local people, they form a coherent whole of which Buddhism is also part. The coherence stems from the fact that all practices – medicine, astrology, alchemy – aim at modifying the 'magical balance' of the body. Even though, unfortunately, none of these authors provided substantial data to prove their important statements, the very fact that they started to think in terms of a 'coherent whole' represents an inestimable progression towards a more comprehensive and articulated approach to the reality.

It is nevertheless Spiro's works that dominated Burmese studies for a long while. Spiro, in strong opposition to others, considered Buddhism and what he called supernaturalism (including 'spirit cult', 'exorcism' and 'magic') as representing two different religious systems and consecrated a volume to each (1967 and 1971). A major concern of Spiro's was to understand how much the practices he observed represented a 'deviation' from the Buddhist 'Great Tradition' inscribed in the texts. It is on this basis that he produced the distinction between nibbanic, kammatic and apotropaic Buddhism. Spiro also defended the idea that, canonically, Buddhism is a religion of salvation but that, while becoming a religion of the masses, it started to be used also for worldly concerns. This use of supernatural-related practices was, in Spiro's opinion, often incongruous with the Buddhist doctrine, which was modified as a consequence. More generally, Spiro looked in detail at how specific Buddhist and non-Buddhist concepts and practices have been adapted to align with one another and to avoid cognitive dissonance, in a similar way to the work Gombrich (1971) did in Sri Lanka.

A further generation of scholars such as Houtman (1999), Swearer (1995) and Brac de la Perrière (2009) argued that the differentiation between Buddhism and non-Buddhism is not only a construct created by scholars but also a process actually occurring on the ground orchestrated by the central government for political, nationalistic, goals, as previously discussed.

Other recent works on Myanmar, but also on other Theravāda countries (Swearer 1995; Schopen 1997; Collins 1998; Patton 2010), question the validity of both the idea of an 'original pure Buddhism' and the categorisation between Buddhism and non-Buddhism held by other scholars and local authorities, and argue that apotropaic practices, such as astrology, amulets, etc., were part of Buddhism since the origin and were also sanctioned in the canon.

Medical studies

Few humanistic scholars of Myanmar have studied aspects of what they, like many people, see as medicine, mostly 'Western medicine' and in a minor way 'traditional' or 'indigenous' medicine. The historians Edwards (2010) and Naono (2009) have written on

Western medicine in the colonial era, the former highlighting nationalistic aspects of this medicine, the latter describing vaccination propaganda and obstacles to its acceptance from the local population. Except for my own works, which I will discuss later, the only anthropological work of which I am aware on medicine in contemporary Myanmar is Skidmore (2008). Although the title of the piece is 'Contemporary Medical Pluralism in Burma', its focus is on biomedical health care facilities, their uneven geographical distribution and their inadequacy resulting from the military regime's neglect of the health sector, especially among ethnic minorities. A mention of other alternative approaches, such as traditional medicine and alchemy, is made, but no detail of these practices is given, and the argument is made that people still resort to them because of the low quality of biomedical health care. Skidmore's approach reflects a trend common in the 1990s among anthropologists working in Asia (Kleinman, Das and Lock 1997; Ferzacca 2002; Lock and Nichter 2002). Pointing out that biomedicine, which usually represents the main if not the only component of the official health system, is generally accessible only to a tiny – rich and educated – part of the population, those scholars considered medical pluralism as the expression of hierarchical social relations and inequalities in access to health services.

Aung-Thwin (2010) is, to my knowledge, the only other scholar who has written on traditional medicine in Myanmar. Aung-Thwin describes how British colonisers envisioned the possibility of integrating traditional medicine – or at least the aspects they considered medical – into the health system. This project though was never realised because the medicine started to be strongly associated with the anticolonial movement led by Saya San, who claimed he would restore the authority of the Burmese monarchy, revitalise the Buddhist religion, and expel the British. He also assured his followers that they would be protected by his magical charms and tattoos.

In Myanmar studies there is no work on medical pluralism in the sense intended by Leslie (1980), who was interested in how people navigate and make use of the different medical options available to them and in the question of the cognitive and conceptual coherence between the different medical traditions at stake. Nash (1965) and Spiro (1967) represent the only exception in this sense as they provided a detailed description of health and healing-related concepts and practices, though their focus was more on those dealing with the supernatural and much less attention (or not at all for Spiro) was paid to traditional and Western medicine. More studies of this kind exist for other Theravāda countries. The works of Guillou (2009) on Cambodia, of Golomb (1985) and Salguero (2016) on Thailand and Pottier (2007) on Laos, have looked at biomedical doctors, herbalists and exorcists and questioned if and how they form a coherent whole. Golomb is to my knowledge the only one who sees them as forming a coherent whole and explains this by arguing that all these therapies rely on 'magical' practices that manipulate the supernatural forces responsible for the problems. This conclusion is reminiscent of Nash's interpretation presented above about how Buddhism, medicine, alchemy, astrology, etc. form a coherent whole.

If important reflections on pluralism have been developed both in Buddhist studies and in medical studies, none provides a comprehensive reflection of local realities. Firstly, they look only at (what they consider as) medicine or religion and, secondly, they considered only one dimension – conceptual, functional or structural/political. Relations of complementarity or hierarchy between the components of the plurality are understood in only one of these terms.

Sources

I have been conducting ethnographic research among Buddhist communities living in the coastal but rural area of Thandwe in the centre of Rakhine State since 2005. The aim of the research has been to discover how local people understand health and what they do to maintain it or restore it when it is lost. Arthur Kleinman (1980: 24) states that, 'in every culture, illness, the responses to it, individuals experiencing, and treating it, and the social institutions relating to it are all systematically interconnected [...]' and that, for this reason, the 'health care system' must be studied in its integrity as a whole. Following his approach, I have included in my study every concept, practice, object and type of specialist that I have encountered that is used locally in the apprehension of health and illness.

The range of healers is particularly wide but they can be divided into two categories. Firstly, the specialists in Western medicine and the institutionalised version of traditional medicine, forming the national health care system. For this sector, Thandwe area is provided with a public hospital of Western medicine located in Thandwe town and, under it, a network of rural health centres located in the surrounding villages. The private sector is represented by services started by professionals who also work in the public service, most of which were based in Thandwe city. There are also one public and three private clinics of traditional medicine all based in Thandwe town. All these services are under-resourced, lacking in staff, equipment and medicine, and they are able to provide only very basic services. The area is provided, in addition, with several medicine shops and generic outlets selling medical products of both the Western and the local pharmacopeia.

Beside these healers belonging to the official health system, there are monks, diviners, astrologers, spirit mediums, specialists in indigenous medicine in its more traditional, non-institutional, form, masseurs and bone setters. These healers not only deal with health and illness but more generally with fortune and misfortune. They are widespread across the territory and easily accessible to the local population.

Through my research I have realised that the different conceptions, practices, actors and the traditions they relate to, together form what I have called a 'therapeutic field'. 'Field', in the sense given by Bourdieu (1971), stresses the relative positioning of the different actors depending on their habitus, their social, cultural and economic capitals and the rules of the field. Following Dozon and Sindzingre (1986), I use the qualifier 'therapeutic' to refer to this field, as well as to the plurality of conceptions and practices, because this term can integrate elements of different nature and not only those commonly qualified as 'medical', which is actually the word often chosen in medical anthropology.

On the basis of data collected through my fieldwork and the existing literature, I intend to show in this chapter that the way people understand and deal with health issues is strongly related to the way the state has, across time, regulated the therapeutic field and notably the way it has defined and treated the categories 'religion' (*bada*) – meaning Buddhism (*buda bada*) – and 'medicine' (*hsay pyinnya*) thus reshaping the relationship these have with the other traditions, astrology, alchemy, divination and so on. I argue that on the one hand their recognition as the national religion and the national medicine, respectively, have bestowed upon them visibility, legitimacy and authority, in that they come to dictate what is valuable, acceptable and what is not. On the other hand, the purification they went through has reduced their content and thus space of action – Buddhism having been reduced to address only otherworldly aims – and medicine having being reduced to the use of herbal or chemically produced remedies for the cure of physical illness. The capacity of medicine – whether Western or traditional – to deal successfully with illness has been further reduced by the weakness of the state support it has received in terms of logistics and finance. Moreover the promotion, but also redefinition, of the boundaries of religion and medicine has not only affected their field of action but has caused a shift in their relationship with the other components of the therapeutic field, which are now officially downgraded to superstitions, lower forms of medicine or simply 'non-pertaining to medicine nor religion', and are thus forced to adjust to the new definitions and values in place in order to preserve their legitimacy. They, however, become even more important as they come to fill the gaps left by purifications, thus bringing an element of complementarity despite the hierarchy. Hence, the hybridity remains.

Explaining health and illness

When asked about what illness is and what can cause it, the majority of my informants replied that illness (*yawga*) is a physical or mental disorder produced by an imbalance among the elements of the body: air, fire, earth and water. They explained that, although these elements were intrinsically unstable according to the Buddhist principle of impermanence (Pāli *thinkhaya*), they mainly went out of balance because of the effect of other factors: *kan*, the karma, meaning the demeritorious (*akutho*) deeds people accomplished during their successive life cycles; *seik*, the mind, which could face a shock or excessive stress; the climate and the seasonal change (*utu*); the ingestion of food (*ahara*) that is not suitable for the person as too hot or too cold.[10] People said that the four factors could act alone or in combination with each other thus reinforcing each other and that this was particularly true in the case of karma. As explained by an old man from Lintha during a conversation in February of 2007, 'a person's good karma acts as a barrier against the other factors, while a negative karma with its corresponding planetary influence gives free rein to the other factors to harm the individual'.

While illustrating this view of health and illness, my informants usually commented that it corresponded to the theory of traditional medicine, which they said largely draws from the Buddhist doctrine, in particular in what concerns the four elements and the opposition between hot and cold.

When invited to elaborate more extensively about illness causalities, as well as when discussing specific cases, most villagers would also recognise the possible involvement of other factors which they saw as external to indigenous medicine and Buddhism. These factors are *hpon*, a spiritual, psychical and physical essence (Nash 1963: 289, Spiro 1977: 236, Kawanami 2009: 224), and *gyo*, the planets. Interestingly, despite these exclusions, when discussing these factors my informants did relate them to those they see as part of the authoritative traditions and notably to karma. The amount of *hpon* a person possessed depends on the status of his or her karma. Similarly, the influence of the planets on one person reflected their karma.

Fully embracing a standardised and purified reading of medicine and of Buddhism some people refused to recognise the role of those factors discussed above, because that they did not see them as part of those traditions. This is particularly true for planetary influences, regarding which people said, 'astrology is not part of Myanmar traditional medicine; it is a later addition from India' and 'it is not relevant'. Some claimed, 'this doesn't concern Buddhism', according to the Buddha there is nothing but karma… one collects the fruits of one's own karma… our fate is not affected by the planets'. Now, this opinion seems to contradict the fact that astronomy and astrology have been part of all Southeast Asian medical traditions (Skorupsky 1999: 153) in the same way as they are part of the subjects studied by Buddhist monks. That being said, literature on this matter (Fiordalis 2014; Salguero 2018) shows that the relationship between Buddhism and astrology, and between Buddhism and medicine, has long been a source of conflicts, especially because of the lasting association of astrology and medicine with worldly concerns, and the association of Buddhism with otherworldly goals. The relationship has thus shifted back and forth from unity to incompatibility. I believe that the dichotomised understanding conveyed by my informants – and the categorisation and hierarchisation of practices it reflects – built on these existing fractures that were present but not well-defined in the prior culture, but that have been reified through the postcolonial government propaganda against what the state perceives as non-scientific and non-modern practices, and especially its efforts to separate them from both Buddhism and medicine through the institutionalisation, regulation and standardisation of the latter.

Although often initially a bit reluctant to talk about it, most villagers acknowledged the existence of a second kind of illness in addition to *yawga*. This type of illness is *payawga*, literally 'external disturbance', troubles caused by aggression (*ahpan*) from vindictive and malevolent beings, such as witches, sorcerers and spirits. This explanatory model is attributed to 'local traditions' (*yoya*) disassociated from both traditional medicine and Buddhism and yet, once again, the reasons for these illnesses were thought to be related and coherent with causal factors associated with the orthodox traditional medicine and Buddhist cosmology. Indeed, even though anybody could be 'attacked', one could be harmed only if the victim's karma was negative. The reluctance to talk about *payawga*, I encountered, seemed to be related to a certain fear of the powers of the occult, but also to the fact that they were speaking to a (foreigner) ethnographer who, in their eyes, represented modernist-positivist discourses that categorised these 'beliefs' as 'superstitions'. It is also very likely that they themselves had at least partially embraced this modernist-positivist thought through the wide spread of rational materialism through education, adoption of technology, sciences and media and through the state's anti-superstition campaigns.

Villagers' understanding of illness rarely included biomedical concepts and this despite, or perhaps because of, the fact that biomedicine is officially presented as *the* medicine and that it epitomises science, modernity and positivist thought – and therefore was also seen to be the measure of other notions and practices. Biomedical conceptions were known and embraced primarily by biomedical specialists. As for the rest of the local population, even though many were familiar with some biomedical terms, very few understood the principles of this medicine. Most of them articulated these conceptions as coherent with the more traditional ones drawn from traditional medicine, Buddhism or astrology. Instead of defining HIV as an immunodeficiency virus, for instance, they defined it as a hot disease, because the body became skinny and the skin dried. A woman from Lintha reported that her heart disease, previously diagnosed by a doctor, lasted a very long time because of the negative influence of a planet.[11]

The weak integration of biomedical idioms of illness within the local etiological system has less to do with a conceptual incompatibility between the two systems (indeed, the aetiological framework that existed before the introduction of biomedicine does admit the existence of strictly physiological illnesses that have nothing to do with karma, planets and the supernatural) than with the weak implementation of public health and health education programmes, as well as with the social gap and problematic relationship between medical professionals and patients. Because of the poor working conditions in which they operated, the medical staff was often unable and unmotivated to carry out their duty – including the health education programmes – in an effective way. They also tended to compensate for the low salary they received by charging extra fees and focusing on their private practice, thus giving the impression they cared more about the money than the patient's wellbeing. This created a situation of mistrust that hindered the communication, and hence the transmission of, biomedical knowledge (Coderey 2016, 2017).

Maintaining and restoring health

Asked about how they prevented illnesses and other unpleasant events, most villagers replied: 'practising *dana*, *thila*, *bawana*' (generosity, morality and meditation), the three practices forming the core of the Buddha's teaching, whereas to the question 'what do you do in case of illness?' they generally answered: 'I go to buy some medicines or see an 'English' (biomedical) doctor'. Interestingly, these answers placed prevention and cure at two different levels – the first one pertaining to religion and more precisely to Buddhism – with *dana*, *thila*, *bawana* protecting from illness by virtue of the improvement of the karma and the spiritual progression they are deemed to grant – and the second one to medicine, which cured by acting on the biological, physical aspect of the disease.

When observing people's everyday practices, one realises how much these answers are actually only a partial reflection of the reality in that the therapeutic repertoire enacted is way richer and less clear-cut. Not only were 'biomedical' practices and 'Buddhist' practices often combined within preventive and curative processes but they were also, and especially, complemented with a plurality of other recourses. Heterogeneity of resources is not just common among health seekers but also among healers. With the exception of biomedical doctors and specialists of traditional medicine operating in the official sector, most healers combined a plurality of teachings and roles and their techniques usually included components associated with different traditions.

Although inaccurate, the answers I received from my informants are interesting as they revealed the system of values which largely shape people's choices. Indeed, they reflected the hierarchisation of traditions that made Buddhism and medicine higher than the other traditions in terms of legitimacy, respectability and therapeutic efficacy; in this sense they were what one could see as the 'right answers', which it was assumed the interlocutor wanted to hear. Similarly to the aetiology presented to me that often hid or downgraded the conceptions that had come to be classified as external to Buddhism or medicine, the narratives about the practices tend to hide non-Buddhist and non-medical practices. The main difference is that they considered the aetiological system of traditional medicine more authoritative, but in practice they would turn first and more often to Western medicine to meet their needs. I will return to this later. By illustrating in this section what people actually did in order to protect and restore health, I intend to show that even though Buddhist and medical practices are far from being the only resources people relied upon, they were actually given a predominant position by lay people and specialists alike.

I also suggest that my informants' answers expressed an ideal situation that cannot be achieved and that this impossibility has to do with the reduced capacity Buddhism and medicine have to deal with health issues as a result of their institutionalisation and purification; a situation which has made the resort to other practices even more necessary.

Preventive practices

A very important component of daily life was religious activity. First, devotional gestures were made at the Buddha's domestic altar – the offering of food, water, flowers, candles and incense to the Buddha, the recitation of the formula of taking refuge (in the Three Gems), the recitation of the precepts, protective formula (*payeik*) and prayers, the practice of meditation.[12] Second, the offering of food to monks, and listening to their chants. These gestures are understood as the core of Buddhist life in that they are a way to pay homage to the Buddha and his teaching, but also as a powerful means to improve one's present life – including one's health – and to prepare for an even better future existence. They do so by increasing the person's karma and power (*hpon*), purifying the mind and inducing the help of deities and powerful beings. Villagers stated that Buddha himself suggested his disciples resorted to this technique in order to prevent dangers from the social, natural and supernatural world.

Another important aspect of the maintenance of individuals' wellbeing was the preservation of good relationships with the tutelary spirits (*nat*), who oversee places where people live – the house, the village, the city – or which they cross during their daily activities – the sea, the rice fields, the forest. By regularly honouring them with food and drink, and through possession ceremonies led by professional mediums, people tried to maintain a harmonious relationship with them in order to benefit from their support and prevent their vengeance, which would arise from neglect. Although scholars tend to look at this practice as a form of religion (*bada*), locals do not. They reserve the label of religion for Buddhism only, to which they accord higher respect. The distinction is mainly conceptual because though, in terms of practice, the two are often interconnected – a connection that the military government has consistently tried to dissolve through its anti-superstition/purification campaigns (Sadan 2005; Brac de la Perrière 2009). Due to the effectiveness of these campaigns, as much as to modernistic positivistic thought, which was gaining acceptance, many people have started abandoning these practices or denying their involvement in them.[13]

Beside the *nat*, a second category of supernatural beings has to be dealt with: the one of wandering spirits, who haunt the streets' corners, old houses and big trees; hungry ghosts; witches and sorcerers. People protected themselves from these beings by reciting protective formula (notably the *payeik*) hoping in this way to produce an 'emergency karma' (Nash 1965) or get protection from some deities or from Buddha himself (Spiro 1967), as well as by wearing amulets and tattoos. The main amulets were the *payeik gyo*, and the *lethpwe*, a special protection provided by exorcists (*payawga hsaya*). It consisted of a sheet of paper or metal inscribed with esoteric diagrams (*in* and *sama*),[14] combinations of letters or numbers referring to Buddhist and astrological concepts further empowered by the recitation of mantra or Buddhist formula.[15] This object was believed to neutralise the planetary, and thus karmic, negative influence and keep the harmful beings away thanks to the power of the Buddhist authority embedded in it. People stressed that exorcist practices 'have nothing to do with traditional medicine' (*taing-yin hsay pyinnya*). This idea was very possibly related to the spread of a Western conception of medicine as dealing only with physical illness and – related to it – the exclusion of exorcistic techniques from the institutionalised version of traditional medicine. In a similar way, people also said that 'exorcist practices have nothing to do with Buddhism', because 'Buddhism only deals with the otherworldly'. If the involvement of Buddhism in worldly matters and its entanglement with other practices has often been a source of tensions in the history of Buddhism (Swearer 1995; Schopen 1997; Collins 1998; Patton 2010; Hayami 2011), the separation of Buddhism as originally pure has certainly been made stronger as a result of the Buddhism purification campaigns and the anti-*weikza* persecutions conducted by the government. Yet, paradoxically, they acknowledged that Buddhism is crucial in exorcisms because it represents the superior, higher, forces cosmologically opposed to the ones that are the object of exorcisms (Hayashi 2003; Spiro 1967). The efficacy of exorcism, indeed, mainly stems from the power issuing from Buddhist symbols and recitations, itself conditioned by the power of the exorcist himself, which is the result of the practice of meditation and respect for the precepts.

Another practice, which played a crucial role in maintaining wellbeing and preventing illness and other misfortunes, was divination (*baydin pyinnya*). The most common divinatory practices in the region were astrology and divination through the *weikza* (individuals released from the cycle of reincarnation), or the deities of the Hindu-Buddhist pantheon (*daywa, nat*) whom diviners were able to contact with their minds. Diviners read a person's astrological chart, which is supposed to reflect the condition of the karma and advise strategies to benefit from positive moments and prevent negative ones.[16] Besides amulets, *payeik gyo* and *lethpwe*, the most common technique used by diviners was the *yadaya*, a process which neutralises negative planetary forces and improves the karma to prevent, or release one from, harm and misfortune.[17] The most common consisted of the offering to the pagoda of objects (flowers, candles, etc.) chosen according to astrological calculations and on the basis of the symbolic association between days of the week, planets, letters, objects and cardinal points.[18]

Despite the popularity of divination and astrology among villagers, most were reticent to admit that they resorted to them and often initially denied that they did so: 'I only follow the Buddha's way, this does not concern Buddhism; this is a worldly practice while Buddhism's only concern is with otherworldly aims', 'according to the Buddha the only thing that counts is your action; you act and you collect the fruits of your actions; *yadaya* and planets cannot help'. Very aware of this system of values, diviners and astrologers tended to stress the Buddhist components in their practice – both in the way they enacted it and in the explanation they provide. They would, for example, give more visibility to the interaction with the *weikza* or the deities of the Hindu-Buddhist pantheon, while concealing the astrological calculations. They might also say that they practised out of *mytta* (compassion) and seldom asked overtly for monetary compensation.

The only two practices that strictly focus on the physical body and its elements, aiming to preserve the balance between hot and cold, are rules for diet and for the appropriate time for taking showers and baths. According to these rules, which people attributed to traditional medicine, one should avoid eating food which is too hot or too cold but should suit it to one's own physique state of health.[19] They should also refrain from having showers at the coldest time of the day. Interestingly, at the prevention level, there was no recourse to specialists in traditional medicine, as people were not used to taking medicines if there were no sign of a problem.

Similarly there was a very minimal use of preventive methods promoted by biomedical public health programmes (immunisation programmes, consumption of vitamins, use of condoms, and so on). Several factors explain this lack of uptake in the community. The main one is a conceptual difference. Most people understood health and illness in traditional terms – an imbalance in the body elements due to karma, the mind, the weather, the planetary influence, or as a supernatural aggression. Prevention thus consisted of actions addressing these factors. Moreover, the biomedical idea of acting on the body for the prevention of a single disorder only was something quite alien to local people. Their preference was for a more generic and inclusive approach. Both the people's general lack of understanding of, and unwillingness to accept, such important disease prevention methods were, however, largely related to the shortcomings of Rakhine's health system and to the problematic relationship between its staff and the villagers. For instance, one woman explained that, 'the nurses rarely go to look for those who do not come to get the vaccination, and if they do, they scold [the villagers] for not coming'. This attitude certainly increased resistance against vaccinations and reinforced people's mistrust in public health programmes. Indeed these programmes had long been considered instruments of control and an expression of false paternalism on the part of the Myanmar government and, before it, the British colonisers (Naono 2009).

Curative practices

When symptoms appeared in one's body, they were, most of the time, taken as signs of a natural disease and addressed as such. In cases of minor problems and chronic diseases, whenever a specialist was not available or accessible, or simply when recourse to him was not deemed necessary, people resorted to self-medication. Self-medication included following a special diet and the use of home-made remedies, which, people stressed, represented the basis for and popular versions of traditional medicine. They also purchased medicines in shops. Most people first had recourse to biomedical products, which, differently from herbal products, were considered to appease the symptoms very quickly. Yet indigenous medicine was preferred for certain ailments, notably chronic disorders for which it was considered most effective. When symptoms did not diminish through self-medication, or when more serious illnesses, such as acute diarrhoea or strong abdominal pain occurred, or when surgery was needed, people usually went to a biomedical specialist, be they a doctor or a nurse. This being said, the deficiencies of these services, their high cost and the problematic relationship with specialists, hindered this recourse (Skidmore 2008; Coderey 2016, 2017). As for specialists of indigenous medicine, they were usually appealed to in cases of chronic diseases, menstrual disorders, paralysis and some forms of cancer, for which this medicine was considered particularly effective, in addition to instances where biomedical practices failed. Most people, regardless of social status and education background, still preferred to resort to the traditional doctors, who operated outside the government's system, than to the 'modernised', state-trained doctors. The former were seen as possessing greater knowledge and experience and being more respectable, also because they usually saw their following of Buddhist morality as the *sine qua non* condition of the efficaciousness of their practice. The latter, very much like Western doctors, were usually seen as the embodiment of a system which was both lacking and unreliable.

If the patient's symptoms did not disappear after a certain period of treatment, or if the person encountered other difficulties in addition to the disease, they would start considering the possibility that some karmic, planetary or supernatural factors were involved, which prevented the medical treatments from being effective. As a result, the person turned to practices and healers who dealt with misfortune. Most people would generally resort first to a diviner or an astrologer to know the state of their karma and, if needed, to prescribe some *yadaya* or deliver some protective amulets. Yet, if the aggressor was a witch or a sorcerer, the patient would then consult an exorcist (*payawga hsaya*), who would perform an exorcism[20] by using particular techniques, such as esoteric diagrams and mantra, and by appealing to Buddhist spiritual forces (Spiro 1967; Coderey 2011).

Even though diviners and exorcists were not difficult to find – as most villages had at least one of each – people considered several criteria when making their choice about which one they would appeal to. They would prefer those who followed the Buddha's way – respecting the main Buddhist precepts and regularly practising meditation – and who operated out of *mytta* (loving-kindness) and *saydana* (generosity) – meaning without asking for money – which are signs of authenticity and honesty and increased efficacity.

Depending on the nature and gravity of the disease, and on the availability and accessibility of the resources, health-seeking processes could become very complex. And yet choices were always made according to a certain logic which, as pragmatic as it could be, was seldom incoherent as Skidmore (2008: 196) suggests in her essay on medical pluralism in Myanmar: by acting on different causal factors, all actions are understood as contributing – at least potentially – to healing as observed by Golomb (1985: 277) in Thailand and Pottier (2007: 141) in Laos. When a person has recovered he/she generally thinks that all recourses have contributed to that outcome. In the event the illness turns out to be incurable or a person dies from it, karmic actions are considered to be the cause. Karma represents the origin but also the limits of the space of freedom (Gombrich 1971).

Analysis

The fieldwork shows that different notions and practices occupy different positions in the therapeutic field. These positions were complementary and yet hierarchical in the sense that some notions and practices – and mainly those associated with Buddhism and medicine – were attributed higher legitimacy, respectability and, often, therapeutic power, and yet remained unable to cover the entire field of health, thus making recourse to other resources necessary.

Looking at the representations of health and illness, one sees that factors identified as coming from Buddhism and traditional medicine were the main causalities people had in mind. Buddhism in particular was accorded a higher status in these epistemic relations as reflected in the fact that the main theory of traditional medicine was identified as coming from Buddhism. Karma, the notion locally understood as key to Buddhism, was given an encompassing role: it was karma which determined the weight of other factors' actions and which decided the gravity of the disease.

Other conceptions, which were categorised as 'non-belonging to Buddhism' and 'traditional medicine', were either reinterpreted in a way which made them coherent with other factors, discredited or hidden. That said, they seldom disappeared, bringing their own contribution to the understanding of health and illness.

If traditional medicine was attributed high legitimacy in the aetiological system, the same could not be said for Western medicine as its conceptions remained relatively unknown to most people. On the one hand, this failure of biomedical education to penetrate the hinterlands of Myanmar, speaks to the limited resources of biomedicine in Myanmar, which had led to insufficient biomedical staffing, resources and education. In the face of this, the strong rural reliance on traditional and Buddhist medical notions evinced the pervasive influence of Buddhism and traditional medicine, and spoke to local networks of knowledge exchange, social support and therapeutic care in the hinterland, tangential to biomedicine, and in which monastic communities played a powerful role as centres of knowledge dissemination, if not production as well.

A similar relationship of complementarity and hierarchy between the components of the therapeutic field was attested in the practices people relied on for prevention and cure. As for prevention, we have seen that Rakhine villagers constantly engaged in a plurality of practices and rituals, which contributed in one way or another to maintaining health and preventing illness, and to improving the general wellbeing in both the current and future lives. Buddhism and medicine – both traditional and Western – played a dominant and yet inadequate role in this mission. The insufficient contribution of Buddhism was particularly noteworthy, since it came to contradict people's statements that Buddhism was their sole resource for prevention. Such claims suggested the idea that if one followed the Buddha's law, one would be fully protected. And yet, as my informants explained to me, nobody was able to follow strictly and constantly the Buddha's teaching, and even if one did, one was never free from the past lives' karma which could hit suddenly, and increase one's vulnerability to other factors: the climate, the diet, the mind, malevolent beings. Moreover, while individual karma moderated the intensity of these factors, karma did not govern how they operated, which made it important to address the factors directly. This was mainly done through practices villagers identified as external to Buddhism – divination, exorcism, traditional and Western medicine. Buddhist practices had another limit. If it were true that they promised a wide range of protection in the short and long term by improving the person's karma and personal power and granting the preservation of positive relationships with human and supernatural entities, they were limited in their capacity to master specific problems and uncertainty related to the near future. Hence the necessity to resort to other practices, which were more focused on short-term and specific protections. The different divinatory techniques, including astrology, were particularly appreciated in this sense because of their ability to reveal the causal factors involved and, more importantly, to determine the status of the karma and the planets, and whether one should act on them, providing people with a sense of control and agency. Although para-Buddhist practices were necessary, however, as they accomplished functions that were out of reach to Buddhist practices, they remained submitted to Buddhist practices, as their efficacy depended on the status of the person's karma generated through Buddhist practices in the past and current life, and in the Buddhist power of the healer her/himself granted by respect for Buddhist morality and meditation practice. They always, moreover, included Buddhist dimensions (symbols, recitation of mantra or else), which were seen as playing a crucial role in determining the efficacy of the practice.

When it came to curing, it was Western medicine that played a dominant, and yet never exclusive, role. Because of the local availability of biomedical products and other technologies in village shops and clinics and the efficacy attributed to them, biomedicine tended often to be used as a first resort. Yet due to the inadequacy of services and the several obstacles – mainly social and economic – hindering their accessibility, people often avoided appealing to it or failed to find in it the solution to their problems. While this certainly contributed to people's continued recourse to all kinds of more traditional practices, other reasons played a role in this. For a large number of ailments, indigenous medicine remained the most popular choice because it was considered the more effective. In any form it took locally – self-medication, medical consultation or surgical intervention – biomedicine failed, moreover, to address the non-biological factors of an illness (Dozon 1987: 17), which were extremely important for local people. It also tended to put patients in a passive position, failing to provide them with a sense of agency and control over their health. This gap left by biomedicine, and by traditional medicine in its institutionalised form as it operated according to the same principles, was actually filled by the more traditional healing traditions and notably divination and exorcism. The fact that Buddhist practices played a minor role here, compared to the prevention process, made sense because, in this case, the treatment of unease concerned an ad hoc kind of intervention, while prevention was also oriented towards a distant future, including future lives. Nevertheless, Buddhist practices remained important in a healer's practice, as they provided it with more efficacy and respectability. Finally, Buddhist cosmology enacted a hegemonic force on what was considered possible, in the sense that it was karma which fixed the limits of what could be managed.

The fact that Theravada Buddhism had come to occupy a dominant position in the social and therapeutic sphere certainly stemmed from the fact that as a religion it provided the cosmography, the system of values orienting people's action, and determined the directions and the limits within which one could shape one's destiny. It was also of an integrative nature which favoured the accommodation of other systems of beliefs. The fact that it had benefitted from state support and had been made the national religion by U Nu further contributed to the strengthening of its social and epistemic power.

This expansion and strengthening of Buddhism, coexisted and contrasted with the process of purification led by the State, the attempt to separate it from all components it was being related to and which had been labelled as backward superstitions. If this process had only a limited impact on the practices, it affected people's representations, which now often presented Buddhism as an otherworldly religion separated from other worldly practices. Buddhism was seen as highly respectable, while the other practices were something several people sat uncomfortably with and sometimes even rejected or hid. Ironically, this purification process had helped to sustain the hybridity of the therapeutic field, making both Buddhist and non-Buddhist components even more necessary. Reducing

Buddhism to the otherworldly realm meant limiting its ability to deal with worldly matters and thus creating the necessity for other resources able to fill the gap. Yet by being separated from the rest and elevated to a purely otherworldly realm, it acquired even more legitimacy, respectability and epistemic authority. This superiority of Buddhism was replicated in the therapeutic field and translated into a superior explicatory and therapeutic power. Similarly, practices, forces and symbols associated to Buddhism – meditation, respect of precepts, auspicious formulas, Buddha images – were seen as increasing, when they did not condition, the efficacy of other, para-Buddhist, practices, forces, symbols, etc. All other notions and practices had been reinterpreted in a way that made them fit the Buddhist logic in order to preserve their legitimacy. And practices officially presented as non-Buddhist had been more and more often combined with, and complemented by, Buddhist practices in order to increase their respectability and efficacy.

Something similar and yet different happened with the category of medicine. The institutionalisation and development of medicine, Western and local alike, contributed to give them visibility and legitimacy. The case of traditional medicine was particularly interesting because, rather than simply redefining a pre-existing category (of medicine in this case) as was the case with Buddhism, the state actually created a medical system which was non-existent before. It did so by combining knowledge and practices before disconnected, and eliminating or modernising the more esoteric, spiritual elements, of local medical knowledge. These the state perceived as a potential threat to its own authority. At the same time, they did not fit the Western conception of medicine. If the health care system created by juxtaposing Western and traditional medicine was meant to replace 'old, superstitious' practices, this did not happen. Indeed, the possibility for medicine to provide satisfying care was considerably reduced by the limitations placed on it by the long-term economic neglect from the state and the numerous regulations, which had reduced what medicine was and was allowed to do. This situation kept alive the need people had to look for other resources. Overall, traditional medicine, in its non-institutionalised version, remained the most legitimised and legitimising form of medicine, challenged only by certain biomedical technologies and medicines holding a more sophisticated diagnostic and/or therapeutic power.

Therapeutic efficacy had thus been built and shaped through this epistemic and conceptual hierarchisation strictly related to politics of governance to assert control over all threatening forces, either esoteric, millenaristic or related to ethnic minorities. In a sense then, the maintenance of hierarchy within practices confirmed and reproduced categories and hierarchies on which political authority relied. Yet the persistence – despite exclusion and purification – of the other components, sheds light on the limits of state policies and on the fluid and resilient nature of the therapeutic field and the people relying on it.

Conclusions

In this chapter I have examined the different conceptions and practices Buddhist Rakhine villagers used to deal with health and illness. In so doing, I have reunited what has often been kept separate in Southeast Asian studies – medicine and religion. Health-related conceptions and practices used in Rakhine included those that scholars through the twentieth century had understood as medical (scientifically provable remedies to cure natural disorders), as well as those they understood as religious (complex of symbols, rituals and beliefs that connect human experience to the essential nature of the universe; provide cosmology and rules of behaviour, supernatural).

By removing *etic* categories of religion and medicine from the ethnographic approach, the epistemic force of *emic* categories is regained in its entirety, not as defined by scholars, but as crafted and recrafted by local people in their everyday life as part of the country's specific social, political and religious history. I have argued that the definition of these categories, as well as their relative positioning in the social space, were largely related to the way the Myanmar state authorities have defined and treated the plurality of health-related conceptions and practices through their politics of governance and the way people have responded to these politics. The state's intervention, indeed, affected the way the different components of the therapeutic field were implemented, made more or less visible, accessible, and the field they were able, and allowed to cover; it also shaped the way people valued and engaged with the components of the field and hence the very outcome of the health-seeking process.

This complex process of categorisations and redefinition of relations, coexists and contrasts with the persistent hybridity of health-related notions and practices that keep cutting across all categories. The coexistence of, and tension between, the clear categories in people's representations, and the blurriness of these categories in practice, reflected the complex interplay between biological, cultural, social and political forces. This also contributed to shape therapeutic efficacy in ways which reproduced political interests and power.

Notes

1 Appearing in the postcolonial period to refer to the institutionalised version of traditional medicine, this expression is intended to mark the difference from the medicine introduced by the British.
2 The term *weikza* refers to the practices, the knowledge acquired through those practices and the individuals who, through those practices and knowledge, acquired extraordinary powers including the one of extending one's life and being released from the cycle of rebirths. *Weikza* are now in a limbo waiting for the Future Buddha; by paying homage to him they will automatically enter nirvana.
3 The same division between medicine and religion was shown in the literature on South Asia by Zupanov and Guenzi (2008).
4 This hybridisation was identified by early scholars who regarded it as a form of folk Buddhism (as opposed to formal) or as a small tradition embraced by a particular society or community (as opposed to the great tradition proper to doctrinal Buddhism) (Redfield 1965).
5 Even today Theravāda Buddhism is by far the main religion of Myanmar, and yet a large number of Muslims live scattered around the country with large pockets in Yangon and Rakhine State; Christians are largely predominant in Chin, Kachin and Karen States.
6 This purification process is not specific to Myanmar, but is actually a common phenomenon among Theravada countries, and detailed descriptions exist for Thailand and Cambodia, with scholars referring to it as a 'modernisation process'. That being said, the extent to which reforms and purifications were carried out has been uneven between countries and the standardisation and centralisation has rarely been as strong as in Myanmar.

7 At the same time, one should not forget that building a strong Burmese national identity was not only important for the government in order to maintain its grip on the country, but also to protect it from the external threat from 'neo-colonialists' and 'cultural imperialists', and to preserve its 'Asian' values (Philp and Mercer 2002: 1592).

8 A similar statement is made by Lambert (see Chapter 5 in this volume) regarding India where 'medicine' has not existed as a separate institution fully distinct from 'religion'. The author suggests that what is considered as 'medicine' has been constructed through a combination of enacted practice, official authorisation and scholarly representation, assuming that an 'interface' between 'medicine' and 'religion' can exist only where these have been constituted as discrete domains.

9 To be precise, astrology and alchemy are taught in the university but only in a basic form and only for the cure of natural illness; their practice is prohibited in the public services (Coderey 2020).

10 Similar aetiologies have been found elsewhere in Southeast Asia and South Asia where Buddhist medicine and Ayurvedic medicine are widespread (Monnais 2007; Salguero 2016).

11 The same phenomenon is apparent in other southeast Asian countries as well (Owen 1987: 21). Golomb (1985: 765), for instance, reports that in Thailand some people thought that germs need to be activated by sorcerers in order to be pathogenic. All these examples are manifestations of a hybridisation of knowledge, which expresses the integrative capacity of the system.

12 Meditation practised by laymen was usually the *thamahta* (Pāli *samatha,* 'concentration') meditation practised by concentrating on the breath. For studies on meditation practices see King (1980), Houtman (1990), Jordt (2005) and Rozenberg (2001).

13 The only *nat* which is still very much and openly worshipped locally is U Shin Gyi, the *nat* of the sea. The cult of this *nat* was already attested by Delachet-Guillon (2000 [1978]: 144), who conducted her research in the region in the seventies.

14 The same technique is attested elsewhere in Myanmar (Sangermano 1966 [1833]: 148); Shway Yoe 1910: 43; Brohm 1957: 33; Spiro 1967: 36; Tosa 2005: 160; Patton 2010) and in Southeast Asia where they are known as *yantra* (Skrt.) (Heisenbruch 1992: 299; Hayashi 2003: 179; Renou 1968). Meanings and uses of diagrams have been studied in detail by Bizot (1981), Rosu (1986) and Olivier de Bernon (1998).

15 This kind of amulet has been described by Sangermano (1966 [1833]: 148), Shway Yoe (1910: 44), Bernot (1967: 413–15), Brac de la Perrière (1989: 92) and de Mersan (2005: 106).

16 References to astrology and astrologers are very common in the literature while diviners are seldom mentioned apart from *natkadaw* (*nat*'s wives) acting as diviners (Spiro 1967; Brac de la Perrière 1989; de Mersan 2005), who are studied more for their social functions and their own characteristics than for their divinatory skills. According to historians the first astrologers operating in the country were Indian Brahmins known as *ponna*, who were working at the royal court (Bernot 1967; Shway Yoe 1910; Leider 2004). Although *ponna* probably still exist nowadays they are largely outnumbered by Buddhist astrologers who have inherited their knowledge. A detailed description of diviners and astrologers can be found in Coderey (2011, 2012). Robinne (1998: 95), Tosa (2005) and Rozenberg (2007) give some details about astrologers and their techniques.

17 *Yadaya* have been described by Tosa (2005), Rozenberg (2007) and myself (Coderey 2011: 172–4).

18 These associations and use in astrological practices come from Hinduism and have been described in detail by Guenzi (2004) in her work on the astrologers from Benares.

19 See also Robinne (1995).

20 Exorcism is here understood in the broad sense used in anthropology as liberation from malefic forces that had taken control over one's mind and body either from a distance, often through an object, or directly via possession of the person.

Bibliography

Aung-Thwin, M. (2010) 'Healing, Rebellion, and the Law: Ethnologies of Medicine in Colonial Burma', *Journal of Burma Studies*, 14: 151–85.

Aotearoa (2006) 'Map of Myanmar and its divisions, including Shan State, Kachin State, Rakhine State and Karen State', *Wikipedia*, CC BY-SA 3.0 https://commons.wikimedia.org/w/index.php?curid=1234889

Bernon, O. de (1998) *Yantra et Mantra*. Phnom Penh: Centre Culturel et de Coopération Linguistique.

Bernot, L. (1967) *Les Paysans Arakanais du Pakistan Oriental: L'histoire, le Monde Végétal et l'Organisation Sociale des Réfugiés Marma (Mog)*. Paris, La Haye: Mouton.

Bizot, F. (1981) 'Notes sur les Yantra Bouddhiques d'Indochine', in M. Strickman (ed.) *Tantric and Taoist Studies in Honour of R. A. Stein*, vol. 1. Brussels: Institut Belge des Hautes Études Chinoises, pp. 155–91.

Bourdieu, P. (1971) 'Champ du Pouvoir, Champ Intellectuel et Habitus de Classe', *Scolies*, 1: 7–26.

Brac de la Perrière, B. (1989) *Les Rituels de Possession en Birmanie: Du Culte d'État aux Cérémonies Privées*. Paris: Éditions Recherche sur les Civilisations.

Brac de la Perrière, B. (2009) 'An Overview of the Field in Burmese Studies', *Asian Ethnology*, 68. 2: 185–210.

Brohm, J.F. (1957) 'Burmese Religion and the Burmese Religious Revival'. PhD thesis, Cornell University.

Brohm, J.F. (1963) 'Buddhism and Animism in a Burmese Village', *Journal of Asian Studies*, 22.2: 155–67.

Bynum, W.F. and Bynum, H. (eds) (2007) *Dictionary of Medical Biography*, vol. 5. Westport, CT; London: Greenwood Press.

Charney, M.W. (1999) 'Where Jambudipa and Islamdom Converged: Religious Change and the Emergence of Buddhist Communalism in Early Modern Arakan (Fifteenth to Nineteenth Centuries)'. PhD thesis, University of Michigan.

Coderey, C. (2011) 'Les Maîtres du "Reste": La Quête d'Équilibre dans les Conceptions et les Pratiques Thérapeutiques en Arakan (Burma)'. PhD thesis, University of Aix-Marseille.

Coderey, C. (2012) 'The *Eeikza's* Role in Arakanese Healing Practices', *Journal of Burma Studies*, 16.2: 181–211.

Coderey, C. (2016) 'Accessibility to Biomedicine in Contemporary Rakhine State', in R. Egreteau and F. Robinne (eds) *Metamorphosis. Studies in Social and Political Change in Myanmar*. Singapore: NUS Press, pp. 260–87.

Coderey, C. (2017) 'Health', in A. Simpson, N. Farrelly and I. Halliday (eds) *Routledge Handbook on Contemporary Myanmar*. London: Routledge, pp. 279–88.

Coderey, C. (2020) 'Myanmar Traditional Medicine: the Making of a National Heritage', *Modern Asian Studies*, 55.2: 514–51.

Collins, S. (1998) *Nirvana and other Buddhist Felicities: Utopias of the Pali Imaginaire*. Cambridge: Cambridge University Press.

Delachet-Guillon, C. (1973) 'La Maternité, la Naissance et leurs Rituels en Birmanie. Contribution à l'étude de la Maternité en Asie du Sud-Est'. PhD thesis, Musée de l'Homme, Paris.

Delachet-Guillon, C. (2000 [1978]) *Daw Sein, les Dix Mille Vies d'une Femme Birmane*. Paris: Editions Kailash.

Dozon, J-P. (1987) 'Ce que Valoriser la Médecine Traditionnelle Veut Dire', *Politique Africaine*, 28: 9–20.

Dozon, J-P. and Sindzingre, N. (1986) 'Pluralisme Thérapeutique et Médicine Traditionnelle en Afrique Contemporaine', *Prévenir*, 12: 43–52.

Edwards, P. (2010) 'Bitter Pills: Colonialism, Medicine and Nationalism in Burma', *Journal of Burma Studies*, 14: 1870–940.

Egreteau, R. and Robinne, F. (eds) (2016) *Metamorphosis. Studies in Social and Political Change in Myanmar*. Singapore: NUS Press.

Eisenbruch, M. (1992) 'The Ritual Space of Patients and Traditional Healers in Cambodia', *Bulletin de l'École française d'Extrême-Orient*, 79.2: 283–316.

Ferguson, J.P. and Mendelson, E.M. (1981) 'Masters of the Buddhist Occult: The Burmese *Weikzas*', *Contributions to Asian Studies*, 16: 62–80.

Ferzacca, S. (2002) 'Governing Bodies in New Order Indonesia', in M. Lock and M. Nichter (eds) *New Horizons in Medical Anthropology. Essays in Honour of Charles Leslie*. London and New York: Routledge, pp. 35–57.

Fiordalis, D. (2014) 'On Buddhism, Divination and the Worldly Arts: Textual Evidence from the Therav da Tradition', *The Indian International Journal of Buddhist Studies*, 15: 79–108.

Golomb, L. (1985) *Anthropology of Curing in Multiethnic Thailand*. Urbana: University of Illinois Press.

Gombrich, R. (1971) *Precept and Practice: Traditional Buddhism in the Rural Highlands of Ceylon*. Oxford: Clarendon Press.

Guenzi, C. (2004) 'Destin et Divination: Le Travail des Astrologues de Benares'. PhD thesis, École de Hautes Études en Sciences Sociales, Paris.

Guillou, A.Y. (2009) *Cambodge, Soigner dans les Fracas de l'Histoire*. Paris: Les Indes savantes.

Gutman, P. and Zaw Min Yu (2001) *Burma's Lost Kingdoms*. Bangkok: Orchid Press.

Hayami, Y. (2011) 'Pagodas and Prophets: Contesting Sacred Space and Power among Buddhist Karen in Karen State', *The Journal of Asian Studies*, 70.4: 1083–105.

Hayashi, Y. (2003) *Practical Buddhism among the Thai-Lao: Religion in the Making of a Region*. Kyoto; Melbourne: Kyoto University Press.

Hinnells, J.R. and Porter, R. (eds) (1999) *Religion, Health and Suffering*. London; New York: Kegan Paul International.

Hla Pe (2004) *The Myanmar Buddhist: His Life from the Cradle to the Grave*, [bilingual version Burmese-English of a series of conferences given at the Collège de France in May 1984, trans. T. Hlaing]. Yango: Daung Books.

Houtman, G. (1990) 'Traditions of Buddhist Practice in Burma'. PhD thesis, School of Oriental and African Studies, London.

Houtman, G. (1999) *Mental Culture in Burmese Crisis Politics: Aung San Suu Kyi and the National League for Democracy*, ILCAA, Study of Languages and Cultures of Asia and Africa Monograph Series, 33. Tokyo: Institute for the Study of Languages and Cultures of Asia and Africa, Tokyo University of Foreign Studies.

Hui Yew-Foong, Hsiao, H.M. and Peycam, P. (eds) (2017) *Citizens, Civil Society and Heritage-Making in Asia*. Singapore: ISEAS Publishing.

Jordt, I. (2005) 'Women's Practices of Renunciation in the Age of Sāsana Revival', in M. Skidmore (ed.) *Burma at the Turn of the 21st Century*. Honolulu: University of Hawai'i Press, pp. 41–64.

Kawanami, H. (2009) 'Charisma, Power(s), and the *Arahant* Ideal in Burmese-Myanmar Buddhism', *Asian Ethnology*, 68.2: 211–37.
King, W.L. (1980) *Theravāda Meditation: The Buddhist Transformation of Yoga*. University Park, PA: Pensylvania State University Press.
Kirsch, T.A. (1977) 'Complexity in the Thai Religious System: An Interpretation', *The Journal of Asian Studies*, 36.2: 241–66.
Kleinman, A. (1980) *Patients and Healers in the Context of Culture: An Exploration of the Borderland between Anthropology, Medicine, and Psychiatry*. Berkeley, CA: University of California Press.
Kleinman, A., Das, V. and Lock, M. (1997) *Social Suffering*. Berkeley, CA: University of California Press.
Latour, B. (1993) *We Have Never Been Modern*. Hemel Hempstead: Harvester Wheatsheaf.
Leider, J. (2004) *Le Royaume d'Arakan, Birmanie. Son Histoire Politique entre le Début du XVe et la fin du XVIIe siècle*. Paris: École française d'Extrême-Orient.
Leslie, C. (ed.) (1980) 'Medical Pluralism in World Perspective', *Social Science and Medicine*, 14b.4: 190–6.
Lock, M. and Nichter, M. (2002) *New Horizons in Medical Anthropology: Essays in Honour of Charles Leslie*. London; New York: Routledge.
Lopez, D.S. (ed.) (1995) *Buddhism in Practice*. Princeton: Princeton University Press.
Mendelson, E.M. (1961) 'A Messianic Buddhist Association in Upper Burma', *Bulletin of the School of Oriental and African Studies*, 24.3: 560–80.
Mersan, A. de (2005) *Espace Rituel et Construction de la Localité. Contribution à l'Étude Ethnographique d'une Population de la Birmanie Contemporaine: Les Arakanais*, PhD thesis, École de Hautes Études en Sciences Sociales, Paris.
Mi Mi Khaing (1984) *The World of Burmese Women*. London: Zed Books.
Monnais, L. (2007) 'Medical Traditions in Southeast Asia: From Syncretism to Pluralism', in W.F. Bynum and H. Bynum (eds) *Dictionary of Medical Biography*, vol. 5. Westport, CT; London: Greenwood Press, pp. 67–77.
Naono, A. (2009) *State of Vaccination: The Fight against Smallpox in Colonial Burma*. Hyderabad: Orient Black Swan.
Nash, M. (1963) 'Burmese Buddhism in Everyday Life', *American Anthropologist*, 65.2: 285–95.
Nash, M. (1965) *The Golden Road to Modernity; Village Life in Contemporary Burma*. New York: John Wiley & Sons.
Nash, M. (ed.) (1966) *Anthropological Studies in Theravāda Buddhism*. New Haven: Yale University.
Obeyesekere, G. (1963) 'The Great Tradition and the Little in the Perspective of Sinhalese Buddhism', *Journal of Asian Studies*, 22.2: 139–54.

Owen, N.G. (1987) *Death and Disease in Southeast Asia: Explorations in Social, Medical, and Demographic History*. Singapore; New York: Oxford University Press.
Patton, T. (2010) 'By the Power of All the *Weikzas*: Technologies of *Inn/Sama* as Practices of Potency', paper presented at the International Burma Studies Conference, *Burma in the Era of Globalization*, 6–9 July 2010, Marseille.
Phayre, A.P. (1883) *History of Burma including Burma Proper, Pegu, Taungu, Tenasserim, and Arakan from the Earliest Time to the End of the First War with British India*. London: Susil Gupta.
Philp, J. and Mercer, D. (2002) 'Politicised Pagodas and Veiled Resistance: Contested Urban Space in Burma', *Urban Studies*, 39.9: 1587–610.
Pfanner, D.E. (1966) 'The Buddhist Monk in Rural Burmese Society', in M. Nash (ed.) *Anthropological Studies in Theravāda Buddhism*. New Haven: Yale University Press, pp. 77–96.
Pottier, R. (2007) *Yû dî mî hèng*: *'Être Bien, Avoir de la Force'*. *Essai sur les Pratiques Thérapeutiques Lao*. Paris: École française d'Extrême-Orient.
Redfield, R. (1965) *Peasant Society and Culture: An Anthropological Approach to Civilisation*. Chicago: University of Chicago Press.
Renou, L. (1968) *L'Hindouisme*. Genève: Edito-service.
Richell, J.L. (2006) *Disease and Demography in Colonial Burma*. Singapore: NUS Press; Copenhagen: NIAS Press.
Robinne, F. (1995) *Savoirs et Saveurs: L'identité Culinaire des Birmans*. Paris: Presses de l'École Française d'Extrême-Orient.
Robinne, F. (1998) 'La Notion de "Reste" dans le Choix du Nom Personnel en Birmanie (Myanmar)', *Aséanie*, 1: 91–105.
Robinne, F. (2000) *Fils et Maîtres du Lac. Relations Interethniques dans l'État Shan de Birmanie*. Paris: Centre national de la recherche scientifique/MSH.
Rosu, A. (1986) 'Mantra et Yantra dans la Médecine et l'Alchimie Indiennes', in *Mantras et Diagrammes Rituels dans l'Hindouisme*, Paris: Éditions du Centre national de la recherche scientifique: 117–26.
Rozenberg, G. (2001) 'Thamanya: Enquête sur la Sainteté dans la Birmanie Contemporaine'. PhD thesis, École des Hautes Études en Sciences Sociales, Paris.
Rozenberg, G. (2007) 'Le Saint qui ne Voulait pas Mourir. Hommage à Robert Hertz', *L'Homme*, 182: 97–130.
Sadan, M. (2005) 'Respected Grandfather, Bless this Nissan: Benevolent and Politically Neutral Bi Bo Gyi', in M. Skidmore (ed.) *Burma at the Turn of the 21st Century*. Honolulu: University of Hawai'i Press, pp. 90–111.
Salguero, P. (2016) *Traditional Thai Medicine: Buddhism, Animism, Yoga, Ayurveda*. Bangkok: Lotus Press.
Salguero, P. (2018) 'Healing and/or Salvation? The Relationship Between Religion and Medicine in Medieval Chinese Buddhism', Working Paper

4, *Working Paper of the HCAS Multiple Secularities – Beyond the West, Beyond Modernities*. Leipzig.

Sangermano (1966 [1833]) *A Description of the Burmese Empire*. London: Susil Gupta.

Saw, Y.M., Win, K.L., Shiao, L.W.S., Thandar, M.M., Amiya, R.M., Shibanuma, A., Tun, S. and Jimba, M. (2013) 'Taking Stock of Myanmar's Progress toward the Health-related Millennium Development Goals: Current Roadblocks, Paths Ahead', *International Journal for Equity in Health*, 12.1: 1–7.

Schopen, G. (1997) *Bones, Stones and Buddhist Monks. Collected Papers on the Archaeology, Epigraphy and Texts of Monastic Buddhism in India. Studies in the Buddhist Traditions*. Honolulu: University of Hawai'i Press.

Shway Yoe U (1910) *The Burman: His Life and Notions*. London: Macmillan.

Simpson, A., Farrelly, N. and Halliday, I. (eds) (2017) *Routledge Handbook on Contemporary Myanmar*. London: Routledge.

Skidmore, M. (ed.) (2005) *Burma at the Turn of the 21st Century*. Honolulu: University of Hawai'i Press.

Skidmore, M. (2008) 'Contemporary Medical Pluralism in Burma', in M. Skidmore and T. Wilson (eds) *Dictatorship, Disorder and Decline in Myanmar*. Canberra: Australian National University Press, pp. 193–207.

Skidmore, M and Wilson, T. (eds) (2008) *Dictatorship, Disorder and Decline in Myanmar*. Canberra: Australian National University Press.

Skorupski, T. (1999) 'Health and Suffering in Buddhism: Doctrinal and Existential Considerations', in J.R. Hinnells and R. Porter (eds) *Religion, Health and Suffering*. London; New York: Kegan Paul International, pp. 139–65.

Spiro, M.E. (1967) *Burmese Supernaturalism. A Study in the Explanation of Reduction of Suffering*. New York: Prentice-Hall.

Spiro, M.E. (1971) *Buddhism and Society. A Great Tradition and its Burmese Vicissitudes*. London: George Allen & Unwin.

Spiro, M.E. (1977) *Kinship and Marriage in Burma: A Cultural and Psychodynamic Analysis*. Berkley, CA: University of California Press.

Strickman, M (ed.) (1981) *Tantric and Taoist Studies in Honour of R. A. Stein*, vol. 1. Brussels: Institut Belge des Hautes Études Chinoises.

Swearer, D.K. (1995) 'The Way to Meditation', in D.S. Lopez (ed.) *Buddhism in Practice*. Princeton: Princeton University Press, pp. 207–15.

Tambiah, S.J. (1970) *Buddhism and Spirit Cults in Northeast Thailand*. London: Cambridge University Press.

Tambiah, S.J. (1984) *The Buddhist Saints of the Forest and the Cult of Amulets: A Study in Charisma, Hagiography, Sectarianism, and Millennial Buddhism*. New York: Cambridge University Press.

Tambiah, S.J. (1985) *Culture, Thought, and Social Action: An Anthropological Perspective*. Cambridge, MA: Harvard University Press.

Terwiel, B.J. ([1975] 1994) *Monks and Magic; an Analysis of Religious Ceremonies in Central Thailand*. Bangkok: Cheney, White Lotus.

Tosa, K. (2005) 'The Chicken and the Scorpion: Rumor, Counternarratives, and the Political Uses of Buddhism', in M. Skidmore (ed.) *Burma at the Turn of the Twenty-first Century*. Honolulu: University of Hawai'i Press, pp. 154–74.

Yew-Foong, H., Hsin-Huang M., Peycam, P. (2017) 'Introduction: Finding the Grain of Heritage Politics', in Hui Yew-Foong, H.M. Hsiao and P. Peycam (eds) *Citizens, Civil Society and Heritage-Making in Asia*. Singapore: ISEAS Publishing, pp. 1–14.

Zupanov, I. and Guenzi, C. (2008) 'Introduction', in I. Zupanov and C. Guenzi (eds) *Divins Remèdes. Médecine et Religions en Asie du Sud*. Paris: Éditions de l'École des Hautes Études en Sciences Sociales, coll. 'Purusārtha', pp. 10–38.

Zupanov, I. and Guenzi, C. (eds) (2008) *Divins Remèdes. Médecine et Religions en Asie du Sud*. Paris: Éditions de l'École des Hautes Études en Sciences Sociales, coll. 'Purusārtha'.

Index

Adams, Vincanne 268, 278, 279
aetiology 17, 113, 225, 358
ailment 64, 72, 75, 79, 80, 113, 140, 144, 145, 147, 191n.9, 207, 363, 366
  see also illness; suffering
Alauddin Hussain Shah 222
alchemy 19, 23, 42, 144, 149, 150, 260, 341, 347, 349, 351, 352, 354, 371n9
  divine origins of 34
  nandan 男丹 (male alchemy) 34, 132, 149
  neidan 内丹 (inner alchemy) 33, 128–38, 141, 143–6, 150, 152, 156n.2, 156n.6
  nüdan 女丹 (female alchemy) 33–4, 128, 131–5, 137–41, 144–55, 157n.18
  Tantric alchemy 260–261
  waidan 外丹 (external alchemy) 128–129, 131
allopathic biomedical model 306
anachronism 27, 240
Andreeva, Anna 23–5
anthropology 15, 25, 66, 67, 312, 320, 325, 343, 372
  applied anthropology 15
  history of 5
  medical anthropology 15, 17, 41, 203, 267, 279, 291, 305, 313–15, 320, 324, 330, 332, 343, 353
  social anthropology 37, 44, 211
anticolonialism 38, 228, 325, 326, 348, 351
  see also colonialism, postcolonialism
applied clinical psychology, 15
appropriation, 9, 75–6, 82, 331
Arai, Paula, 16
Ardener, Edwin, 37, 44, 211
Aschoff, Jürgen C., 264, 291
Aṣṭāṅgahṛdaya, 167, 192n.20
Aṣṭāṅgahṛdayasa, 264
Aṣṭāṅgahṛdayasaṃhitā, 266, 267, 271, 272, 274, 292n.6
astrology, 42, 43, 62, 167, 341, 345, 347, 349, 350, 352, 354–7, 361, 366, 371n.9, 372n.16
Aung-Thwin, M. 348, 351
authority 3, 7, 9, 12, 27, 28, 33, 44, 64, 75, 97, 102, 115, 147, 172, 199, 222–3, 228, 229, 258, 284
  'Authority of Empiricism' 280–1
  Buddhist authority 75, 285–7
  Daoist authority 75, 78, 80
  epistemic authority 13, 25, 36, 40, 41
  government authority 198
  religious authority 81, 286
  textual authority 204
Ayodhyā 170, 171, 175, 178, 181, 187

Ayurveda (Āyurveda) 152, 167, 171–2, 183, 186, 187, 190, 204, 208, 210, 212, 226, 230, 258, 259, 272, 311, 314, 316, 320–1, 327, 331
ayurvedic literature 17, 34
Ayurveda's *materia medica* 181
Ayurvedic medicines 41, 205, 209, 228, 371n.10
deity of Ayurveda 182
study of Ayurveda 225, 321
'the age of Ayurveda' 228
traditions of Ayurveda 202
doṣa 169, 261, 274–275
AYUSH (Āyurveda, Yoga, Naturopathy, Unani, Siddha, Sowa-Rigpa and Homoeopathy) 8–9, 36–7, 210–13, 279, 331, 336n.17

Babri Masjid 187, 194n.35
Barnes, Linda 15
belief 9, 36, 37, 41, 105, 134, 141, 147, 152, 166, 171, 190, 202, 211, 231, 240, 244, 310, 313, 315, 330, 356, 367, 369
Bell, Catherine 63, 68, 84n.24
Bengal 29, 37–8, 220–47, 257
Illyas Shahi dynasty 221–2
Sultanate in Bengal 221
bhakti (devotion) 167, 173, 176, 178, 180–2, 190, 202
binaries 13, 18, 32, 36, 37, 40
healers vs. physicians 65
medicine and religion 3, 6, 12, 15, 17–18, 24, 30, 32–3, 35, 39, 41, 45, 109, 117, 165–7, 170, 178, 186, 189, 201, 212, 369
sccience and religion 18
religion vs. secular 24, 33, 36, 98, 108, 113–15, 277
biomedicine 13, 36, 37, 40
in Bengal 229
in China 85n35
in India 187, 194n34, 201–3, 208–9, 212
in Japan 99, 118n8
in Myanmar 341, 346, 351, 357, 365–7
in Tibet 260–3, 275, 278–80, 286
blood 25, 132–5, 138–49, 151–2, 174–5, 222
blood-letting 208
blood pressure 261
menstrual blood 34, 133, 139–41, 144, 153
and pollution 133, 140–1
body 8, 12, 21, 32, 33–4, 39, 41, 69, 72, 73, 77, 80, 83, 86, 96, 105, 115, 128–31, 165–70, 175, 177, 184, 229, 271, 283, 286, 316, 349, 354, 357, 361–2
body *dharma*, 178, 181
female body 34, 45, 131–55
as gendered 154, 155
as non–gendered 34, 45, 137, 140
as singular 13
subtle body 4, 274, 275
see also embodiment
Bokenkamp, Stephen 65
botanical medicines 35
boundary formation 26, 36, 280, 329
Bourdieu, Pierre 14, 27, 28, 353
social fields 14, 27, 95, 116
Brac de la Perrière, Éloïse 345, 346, 350, 359, 371n.15, 372n.16
Buddhisation of medicine 348
Buddhism 23
Amitābha 100, 114, 119n9
Buddhist Canon 70
see also Tripiṭaka
Buddhist clerics 65, 78, 98

Buddhist scriptures 97
Buddhist temples 62, 78, 98, 114, 120n.28
Buddhist tradition 106, 261, 347, 348
deities of 361
esoteric Buddhism 106, 111, 117–18
in Bengal 221, 223, 228
in China 66, 70, 73, 75, 82n.1, 84n.23
in Japan 25, 33, 67, 68, 83n.15, 101–29
in Myanmar 42, 43, 341, 343, 345–70
in Tibet 257, 261, 267, 280, 283, 285, 287, 290
intellectual history of 43
Pure Land 106, 111, 114, 119n.9
Rakhine Buddhists 343
Rinzai Zen 110
Tantric Buddhism 287–288
Theravāda Buddhism 343–4, 349–50, 352, 367, 370n.5
Vajrayāna Buddhism 118
Buddhist cosmology 356, 367
Buddhist medicine 27–8, 102, 103, 111, 265, 371n.10
Buddhist ritual 108, 114, 259, 261, 269
Buddhist texts 95, 96–7, 103–4
Burhanuddin Al-Hemy 42, 44, 317, 320–30, 333, 335nn.8, 9
Burma *see* Myanmar

Cadden 34, 153
Campany, Robert 6
Camus, Albert 8
Canavas, Constantin 41
canon 107, 150, 279, 344
formation 31
Caraka–saṃhitā 228
Cartesian pure consciousness 11
categorisation 39, 43, 146, 208, 237, 306, 308, 317, 343, 350, 356, 370
as knowledge production 9, 31
see also knowledge
biomedical categories 68
Cerulli, Anthony 17, 35, 169, 178, 182, 192n.16, 194n.32
Chakrabarty, Dipesh 229
charisma 27, 33, 115
charismatic figures 28, 32, 43
Chattopadhyaya, Debiprasad 228, 229
Chen Kuang-Hsing 5, 6
China 1, 7, 9–10, 13, 18, 22–3, 24, 95–6, 103, 105, 108–11, 135–6, 153, 263, 282, 288, 327
early imperial China 6
Han dynasty 23, 128, 129
imperial period 23, 63, 139, 142, 143, 147
medieval China 25, 28, 43
middle-period China 31, 35, 62–85
Ming dynasty 142, 143–147
Northern Song period 78, 83n.11
People's Republic of China (PRC), 260, 263
Qing dynasty 34, 131, 135, 139
Republican period 34, 135, 150–1
Shang dynasty 62
Six Dynasties 24
Song dynasty 22, 78, 79, 81, 83nn.9, 11, 12, 128, 135, 137, 138–9, 141, 143, 146
Sui dynasty 24
Tang dynasty 128
wu 巫 (wizard) 62, 66, 80
Zhou period 62, 83n.5, 129

Chinese medicine 9, 14, 17, 18, 24, 41, 66, 95, 99, 139, 260, 266
 Traditional Chinese Medicine (TCM) 10, 16, 311, 313, 314, 320
classification 104, 213, 271, 307, 336n.15
 as fluid 7
 scholarly categories 30, 42, 343
Coderey, Celine 41–3, 44, 347, 348, 357, 363, 371n.9, 372nn.16, 17
Cohen, Daniel 17
colonialism 220, 242
 British colonial administration 308, 325
 decolonisation 41
 colonial accounts 205–8, 212
 colonial period 198, 205–6, 212, 226, 332, 345, 351
 postcolonial 28, 29, 42–3, 44, 190, 200, 207, 235, 247, 317, 347, 356, 370n.1
 precolonial 181, 194n.33, 219, 232–4, 240, 245
 see also anticolonialism, postcolonialism
comparative categories of action 15
Confucianism 66, 102, 129, 310
 Confucian healers 104
 Neo-Confucianism 98, 110
corporeality 152, 154
correspondence theory 9
cosmology 32, 34, 41, 136–7, 140, 143, 148, 152, 154, 369
 Buddhist cosmology, 356, 367
 as folk, 36
 doctors as applied cosmologists, 69
curing 33, 36, 64, 68–71, 77, 80, 82, 83nn.5, 6, 111, 149, 203, 316, 348, 366
 popular curing 75–6
 religious curing 32, 61, 66, 70, 71
Daoism 22, 23, 63, 66, 68, 70, 73, 75, 82, 84nn.22, 23, 85n31, 116, 118n.4, 135, 142, 150, 152, 156n.2, 310
 Celestial Masters 64, 77, 81
 Daoist liturgy 67, 70
 Daoist ritual 24, 86n.54, 96
 Daoist temples 74
 Daoist texts 131, 135
 deities 118n.4
 folk Daoism 73
 histories of 22
 and medicine 22
 monastic life of 67
 Rectifying Rites of of the Heart of Heaven 78, 80–2, 86n.62
 study of 67–8, 84n.22, 136
Daoist Canon (*Daozang* 道藏) 67, 70, 132 135, 141, 142, 156n.12
definitions 4, 7, 44, 85n.35, 154, 155, 211, 213, 216, 307, 369
Dharamsala 44, 258, 261–2, 265–6, 276
dharma 167, 172, 176, 178, 181, 182, 190, 192n.14
discourse 14, 15, 18, 37, 45, 72, 99, 132, 133, 137, 147, 148, 155, 165, 187, 190, 275, 306, 308, 310, 312, 313, 317–18, 321, 323, 324, 325, 328, 329, 331, 332, 333, 356
 cosmological discourse 131
 medical discourse 118n.6, 290
 neidan discourse 141
divination 21, 42, 129, 260–1, 341, 354, 361, 366, 367
du 毒 25
Duden, B. 34, 152, 153, 154

efficacy 16, 20, 45, 64, 70, 72, 78, 135, 168, 207, 208, 211, 245, 269, 279, 287, 290, 358, 366, 368
biomedical 40 140
therapeutic 343, 369–70
of exorcism 360
of religious ritual 82n.3
of spiritual therapy 32, 71
of Tibetan practice, 288
embodiment 12–14, 18, 169, 363
embryology 21, 23, 34, 152
emic and etic 26, 45, 343, 369
Emmerick, Ronald 264, 266, 272
epistemes 26, 27, 33, 113, 115, 165
epistemic authority 13, 25, 36, 40, 368
epistemological control 24
epistemic frameworks 228
epistemic landscape 42
epistemic practices 24
epistemic structures 26, 120n.27
epistemology 3, 11, 20, 333, 16, 11, 14, 114, 228
as empirical approach 286
Evans-Pritchard, E. E. 201
experience 7, 12, 16, 44, 71, 72n.2, 73, 101, 145, 153, 168, 203, 269, 273, 280–4, 309, 319, 327, 363, 369
female experience 34
lived experience 20
as subjective 40, 279
of physicians 61, 66
explanatory models 13, 14, 17, 28, 32, 41

Farquhar, Judith 14, 17, 18, 31
fashi 法師 (master of arts) 64, 73, 75, 81
Felski, R. 189
female body 34, 45, 131–55
illness of *see* illness, as gendered
Foucault, Michel 13
Fujikawa Yū 100–1, 104, 112

g.Yu thog pa 265, 267, 272, 275–6, 284, 287, 289, 292n.6
Gangetic valley (Indian sub–continent) 220, 222, 224
Garrett, Frances 21, 23, 263, 267, 270, 276
Geertz, Clifford 188–9
gender 33, 34, 132, 136, 142, 145, 147, 152
gender difference 137, 140, 154, 155
gender equality 150–1
non–gendered body 45, 140
genealogy 5, 8, 201, 243
Sanskrit genealogies 36
Gerke, Barbara 25, 260, 268, 272
Goldman, Robert 170, 172, 173, 180, 192n.13, 193n.25
Gorai Shigeru 五来重 106
governance 7, 24, 36, 41, 211, 327, 369
Gyatso, Janet 20, 21, 27, 29, 40, 267, 275, 277, 280–91, 292n.10
gynaecology 138, 139, 144, 152

Haeckel, Ernst 100, 119n.10
Hanson, Marta 292n.10
Hanumān 166, 170–90
Haraway, Donna 10, 11, 30
Haṭha Yoga Project 19
Hattori Toshirō 101–4, 112
healing, 15, 18, 25, 27, 32, 33, 35, 37, 61, 83n.5, 94–5, 96, 104–17, 144–6, 149, 165, 189, 191, 202, 203, 208, 211, 212, 226–7, 311–17, 326, 329, 343, 346, 347, 364
categories of healing 191

healing (*continued*)
healers 15, 27, 31, 65, 66, 72, 76, 104, 115, 120n.29, 311, 316, 332, 341, 352, 358, 363
'Way of healing' 16
healing rituals 24, 33, 114, 259, 311, 316
healing practices 40, 106, 113, 305, 333
Tibetan healing 257–91
hegemony 35, 95, 171, 308, 325, 328, 345
of Western knowledge traditions 3
tacit Eurocentric assumptions 30
heritage 10, 20, 36, 38, 103, 306
hierarchy 42, 70, 352, 354, 365, 369
Hindu nationalism 38, 187, 228–9
see also Hindutva
Hinduism 171, 177, 223, 309, 331, 372n.18
deities of, 41, 361
Hindutva 187
see also Hindu nationalism
Hinrichs, TJ 78, 81
historiography 5, 20
as nationalist 31
history of Buddhism 344, 360
history of homeopathy 319, 331
history of religion 15, 107
history of religion and medicine 94, 110
homeopathy 5, 41–2, 44, 209–10, 212, 306–33, 335nn.6, 8, 9, 10, 336n.19
Tao Hongjing 陶弘景 65
Hsu, Elisabeth 25, 44, 266, 272

identity 6, 8, 9, 199, 241, 244, 257, 269, 277, 324, 326, 371n.7
construction, 8, 2, 69, 277, 307, 324–6
illness 15, 27, 62, 72, 74, 78, 106, 111, 119, 134, 135, 137, 138, 139, 140, 142, 143–55, 157, 168, 183, 194n34, 201, 202, 205, 261, 269, 274, 277, 279, 341, 343, 347, 352, 369, 371n.9
diagnosis of 74, 113
vs. disease 36, 40, 85n.34
as gendered 134–5, 138–40, 144–7, 149, 151, 155–6
mental illnesses 113, 311, 314
as sin 64
as spirit-related 261
incantations 12, 28, 75, 86n.48, 173, 208
India 6, 7, 9, 10, 13, 18, 26, 34, 69, 95, 103, 170, 171, 174, 176–7, 183, 186–9, 198–201, 204–13, 220, 221, 223–48, 257–63, 272, 275, 276, 325, 331, 332, 344, 346, 355
Bharatiya Janata Party (BJP) 9, 187
Indian medicine 35, 37, 102–3, 188, 204, 209, 213, 227, 260, 314, 320
Indic knowledge 228
Siddhaṃ 97
indigenous groups 189, 309, 311, 314, 311, 333, 334n1
indigenous *materia medica*, 111
indigenous medicine 25, 84, 190, 201, 203–4, 208, 209, 307–11, 314, 329, 341, 355, 363, 366
individual 12, 22, 308, 355
interpretation 33, 38, 94, 113, 120n.27, 147, 267, 272, 275, 283, 352
Islam 29, 41–2, 220, 223, 247n1, 305–35
Islamic medicine 29, 41, 311, 316, 320, 323, 330

Qur'an 42, 316, 323, 328
as political 42, 310, 317, 324, 325, 333
sunna 41, 316
Sunni Muslims 309
as tolerant 41, 313
ISM&H (Department of Indian Systems of Medicine & Homeopathy), 210

Japan 6, 16, 23–6, 32–3, 43, 67, 68, 94–118
Catholic missionaries in 98
Nara period 102–3, 104
Taishō period 104
Japanese medicine 95, 104–5, 109
Lee Jen-der 137
jhara (ritual sweeping) 205
jharas (exorcism) 208
jing 精 (essence) 33, 130, 139, 140, 142–3
jinn 41, 313, 323

Kampo 99, 105
karma 354–67
Katsumi, Fukunaga 68, 104
Katz, Paul 68, 84n.24
Kleine, Christoph 6, 26, 104, 115, 120n.29
Kleinman, Arthur 13, 17, 204, 279, 351, 352
knowledge 30–2, 43–4, 117, 211, 225, 228, 232, 241, 258, 264, 266, 274, 280, 282, 286, 287, 290, 325, 341, 351–2, 363, 365
and power 7
and meaning response 72
as archaic modernity 38, 228–30
embodied 148
knowledge production 9, 31
local 35
medical 4, 5, 9, 13, 32, 98, 105, 109, 114, 154, 271, 278, 368
scientific 5, 11, 101, 328
situated 10–12, 35
Asian 18–23
in Chinese textual tradition 96
guidelines for recognising 31
male 34, 155
of taboos 75
organisation of 44, 45
South Asian 35, 38, 103, 167
suppression of 105
systems of 5, 19, 114, 115, 204, 346
translation of 27
Western tradition of 3
transmission of 5, 26, 31, 95, 209, 348, 357
in Japan 98, 107–11

Lackner, Michael 23
Lambert, Helen 17, 36–7, 39, 44, 202, 204, 205, 207, 210, 213, 219, 227, 371n.8
Latour, Bruno 11, 19, 345
Leslie, Charles 9, 203, 204, 336n.16, 351
Lévi-Strauss, Claude 12
Li Lian 李濂 63
liturgy 67, 70, 82
as vernacular 75
Luhmann, Niklas 27, 113
Lutgendorf, Philip 177, 180, 181, 182

magic 29, 104, 116, 117, 208, 236, 237, 316, 333, 350
black magic 236, 237, 240, 314
Malaysia 5, 41, 42, 43, 305–36
Malayness 307–9, 333
and Muslim patriotism 326
PAS (Islamic Party of Malaysia) 310, 324, 326, 328
Mandal, Panchanan 234, 237–9
mantra 35–9, 42, 44, 97, 168, 191n.9, 205, 208, 219–48, 341, 347, 360, 363, 366
Bengali mantra 5, 38, 246
as 'low-brow' 39

mantra (*continued*)
mantric therapies 39, 219, 227, 229–48
power of 236
recitation of 42, 341, 347, 360, 366
marketplace 28, 190
religio-medical marketplace 28
wellness market 1, 7, 10, 35
Marxism 38, 228
materia medica 22, 25, 33, 65, 77, 98, 109, 111, 114, 176, 181, 187, 208, 269, 271
material culture 95, 116
meaning 7, 8, 37, 41, 97, 129, 165, 166, 184, 185, 203, 237, 245, 246, 269, 270, 284, 286, 287, 289, 307, 354
medicine
Asian medicine 7, 14, 26, 236
category of 11, 17, 31, 100, 104, 115, 165–6, 199, 201–3, 206–7, 211–13, 346–7, 353, 368
herbal 28, 347
history of 32, 99, 100–2, 106, 197, 108, 116, 117, 119n.19, 224
ingaleik hsay (English medicine) 42, 341, 346
langauge of 151
medical pluralism 36, 37, 41, 203, 212, 313, 314, 320, 331, 351, 364
medical practice 37, 101, 113–14, 140, 257, 258, 263, 269, 273, 282, 290, 314, 323, 329–31, 336
medical system 37, 99, 105, 313, 315, 318, 327, 346, 368
medical theory 16, 45, 326
medical traditions 4, 27, 29, 36, 42, 155, 204, 209, 220, 227, 258, 259, 277, 291, 306, 312, 324, 333, 334n.1, 344, 347, 351, 355
mental illness 311, 314, 315, 354
as a system of knowledge 346
value of 32, 71
women's medicine 136, 137–41
Men-Tsee-Kang 265, 276
Moerman, Daniel 32, 45, 71–2, 76
Mol, Annemarie 7, 14
MPIWG (Max Planck Institute for the History of Science)
Department III 11, 22
Mughals 187, 194, 222–3, 232
Mukharji, Projit 29, 36–9, 44, 220, 224, 226, 235, 244, 246, 247n3, 248n6
Myanmar (Burma) 42–3, 341–70
Rakhine State 341, 344, 352, 370
mysticism 22, 38, 228, 309, 330

Nash, M. 349, 351, 352, 355, 360
nation-states 25, 41
Ne Win 345–6
Needham, Joseph 9, 18, 22, 288
Negi, Surendra Singh 183–90
Nickerson, Peter 68, 84n.25
nomadology 38, 219–47

Ojha 219–20, 236
ontology 11, 13, 24, 211
orientalism 8, 10, 11, 324, 349
origins 10, 69, 106, 111, 116, 136, 292n.6, 343, 346, 350, 364
otherness 8, 285

Pakistan 198, 223, 227, 325, 331, 336n.19
pharmacology 96, 187, 264, 274
philology 25, 67
critical philology 25
methods of 112, 117
pluralism (medical) 36, 37, 41, 203, 212, 313, 314, 320, 331, 351, 364

Pollock, Sheldon 5, 20, 29, 187, 192n13
postcolonialism 28, 29, 42, 43, 44, 207, 370n.1
  see also anticolonialism, colonialism
power 7, 10, 12, 14, 28, 33, 38, 39, 44, 62, 72, 74, 81, 100, 115, 116, 119n9, 138, 140–1, 155, 168, 184, 189, 221–3, 228, 236–9, 241, 244, 246, 247, 285, 310, 333, 343, 344, 345, 347, 359, 360, 366, 367, 370
  as colonial 220
  as gendered 154
  as hierarchy 42, 70, 352, 354, 365, 369
  as spiritual 70
  practice 13
prana 4
  see also qi
prayer 2, 63, 64, 96, 99, 106, 359
  as sincere 75

qi 4, 24, 33, 69–70, 76, 77, 78, 130, 133, 134, 135, 139, 143, 146, 148

Radcliffe-Brown, Alfred 200
Rajasthan 36–7, 186, 198, 200, 204, 205 206, 207–9
Rajputana 199, 200, 206, 208
Rakhine State 341, 344, 352, 370
Ram Setu controversy 187
Rāma 170–1, 173–86, 187, 194n.35
Ramanujan, A. K. 171, 178, 192n.15
Ramayan (TV series) 181, 238
Rāmāyaṇa 35, 167, 170–3, 176–93
religion
  affective power of 189
  as belief 9, 37, 72, 152, 231
  category of 1–3, 5–6, 12, 31, 42, 100, 104, 185, 202, 211–13, 354
  and gender 116–17
  folk religion 73
  material religion 37, 39, 231
  popular religion 32, 61, 63, 68, 69, 70, 71, 73, 75, 79, 82
  religious pluralism 108
religious studies 15, 40, 291, 343, 349–50
  as academic discipline 5
  category of 6
  Christo-centric frameworks of 6
  identity of 6
rGyud bzhi (Four Tantras) 40, 257–79, 282–85, 289–90, 292n.6, 292n.7, 292n.8
Ricoeur, Paul 189, 194n.36
ritual 2, 12, 17, 18, 20, 24, 27, 33, 35, 63, 65, 69, 73, 74, 78, 99, 105, 106, 110, 116, 128, 140, 141, 168, 203, 208, 211, 212, 235, 241, 259, 269, 276, 277, 288, 311, 313, 316, 344, 365, 369
  curing rituals 64
  popular 70, 78
  religious 82n3
  ritual documents 70
  ritual logics 37
  ritual studies 36
  Tantric ritual 279, 284
Rivers, W. H. R. 200

Sagar, Ramand 180–1
Salguero, Pierce 4, 27, 28, 29, 44, 69, 84n.28, 113, 119n.18, 119n.25, 335n.14, 352, 355, 371n.10
saṃjīvanī 35, 174, 179, 180–189
Samuel, Geoffrey 4, 21, 40, 41, 259, 261, 262, 268, 274, 275, 276, 278, 279, 288, 291n.3

Sangh Parivar 187
Sanskrit literature 35, 38, 165–99, 220, 224–5
canon 35, 230, 240
Mahābhārata 170, 174, 178, 192n.14
premodern Sanskrit texts 181, 186
Rāmāyana see *Rāmāyana*
Sartre, Jean-Paul 8
Schäfer, Dagmar 22, 45n.1
Schipper, K. M. 67, 84n.20, 85n.37, 156n.12, 156n.15
sDe srid (Regent) 40, 264, 273, 282–5, 287, 289, 290n.8
Seaman, G. 141
secularity 26, 112
multiple secularities 20, 26, 32, 120n.26
Selby, M. A. 34, 53, 152
self 1, 8, 15, 41, 130, 169, 281
self-cultivation 25, 34, 131, 132, 133, 134, 141–2, 143, 144, 151, 154
self-medication 362, 363, 366
sexuality 33, 136, 141
sexual practices 129, 136, 156n.7
Shakyamuni 102, 103, 112
shamanism 73, 82n1, 83n.16, 226
shen 神 (spirit) 9, 33, 130
Shennong (Shinnō) 96
Shinmura Taku 106, 110, 112, 119n.19
Shinran 100–1, 103, 119n.9, 119n.15
shūkyō 宗教 6, 100, 102, 103, 104
Siddha 8, 36, 37, 172, 202, 203, 204, 209, 210, 225, 226, 311, 314, 336n17
Singapore 22, 307, 308, 312, 315, 316, 322, 326, 329, 331
Sino-Japanese War 67
situating knowledge 10–12
Sivin, Nathan 73, 74, 78, 81, 82nn.2, 3, 83nn.10, 11, 13, 84nn.19, 22, 87n.64
siwu 司巫 (Director of Scorcery) 62
Slouber, Michael 227, 230, 242–243, 245, 247, 248n.4
snake-bites 219, 220, 224, 238, 240, 242, 243, 248n.6
sources 27, 30–2, 36, 43, 44, 61–2, 66, 68, 69–71, 94, 96, 97, 103, 106–8, 112, 115–17, 128, 135–6, 141–2, 147, 155, 167, 172, 173–4, 186, 204–6, 209, 220, 231, 232, 234, 236, 237, 238, 241, 242, 246, 247, 258, 266–7, 270, 272, 290, 317, 318, 322, 323, 352
Buddhist sources 102
Chinese sources 110, 307
Daoist sources 129, 141, 143, 152
primary sources 12, 22, 30, 41, 70, 100, 138, 142, 282, 321
secondary sources 204
Sowa Rigpa 40, 210, 225, 257–91
spirit cults 345, 349
spirits 16, 24, 33, 63, 64, 70, 74, 81, 128, 240, 242, 263, 344, 356, 359, 360, 369
as ancestors 69, 82, 95, 202
as evil 115, 202
hierarchy of 70
Spiro, M. E. 350, 351, 352, 355, 360, 363, 372n.16
Staal, Fritz 18, 20, 230, 231
state, the 25, 32–3, 40, 41–3, 61–3, 208, 324
and biopropspecting 182–5
interaction with health care practitioners 269, 274–5, 283–5, 289–90

precolonial Bengal 220–23
role in defining religion 31, 102, 208–209, 310–11, 313, 329, 345–6, 353–4
role in defining medicine 206–9, 211–13, 353–4, 356
state-building 40, 41, 96, 102, 290, 307–9, 347–8
state-defined authorities and institutions 198–200, 210–11, 305
training institutions 95
Steavu, Dominic 23, 24, 137
subaltern therapeutics 213, 220, 227, 231, 243–4
subjectivity 6, 7, 11, 12
formation of 6
Subramaniam, Banu 38, 39, 229
subtle body *see* body, subtle body
suffering 15, 16, 17, 72, 101, 113, 115, 153, 171, 175, 219
see also ailment; illness
Sun, Simiao 孫思邈, 22, 131, 271
superstition 11, 105, 212, 330, 346, 354, 356, 367
Suśrutasaṃhitā 167

T&CMD (Traditional & Complementary Medicine Division) 318–20
taboo 64, 75, 105, 141
TACM (Traditional, Alternative and Complementary Medicine) 41, 305–7, 311–20, 329, 333
Taiwan 67, 84n21, 85n37
Takeuchi, Yoshimi 5, 6
talismans 4, 42, 76, 80, 81, 85n45, 86n62, 87n63, 96, 104, 114, 116, 191n.9
Tambiah, S. J. 9, 349
Tamilnadu 185, 187
Tantra
Tantric healing 263
Tantric medicine 230
Tantric practice 275, 288–89
Teiser, Stephen F. 70, 84n24, 85n32
theory of traditional medicine 355, 364
therapy 2, 26, 62, 65, 66, 71–3, 74, 82, 113, 201, 203, 204, 212, 275, 311, 323, 333
approaches to 32
mantric therapy 37, 39, 219, 227, 229, 230–47
popular therapy 75, 76, 77
religious therapy 45, 71, 75
ritual therapy 69
secular therapy 64
spiritual therapy 32, 71, 227
therapeutic field 341, 343, 353, 354, 364, 365, 367–69
therapeutic power 343, 364, 368
thunder rites (*leifa* 雷法) 64, 69, 78, 79, 87n.64
Tibb 28–9, 225, 226
Tibet 16, 19, 26, 43, 118, 221, 224, 257–91
Lhasa 40, 258, 263, 273, 284
Tibetan Buddhism 257, 267, 290
Tibetan Buddhist practice 276
Tibetan healing practices 257, **259**, 260, 272, 278, 280, 285
Tibetan medicine 20–1, 40, 210, 226, 258, 264–70, 272, 277–8, 280, 286, 288, 290
tradition 39, 96, 97, 100, 102, 106, 108, 110, 114, 116, 118, 128, 131, 135, 136, 141, 151, 191, 202, 219, 226, 229, 239, 243, 244, 258, 266, 272, 277, 285, 290, 306, 322, 327, 341, 345, 350
as 'Great Traditions' 36, 37

tradition (*continued*)
folk tradition 212
medical tradition 155, 167, 172, 181, 186, 227, 257, 268, 273, 283, 312, 331, 336n.17
Traditional and Complementary Medicine (TCM) 319, 320, 321
Chinese tradition 96, 314
Indian tradition 170
Islamic tradition 316, 328
Malay tradition 329
Vedic tradition 230, 233, 246
traditional medicine 42, 105, 112, 226, 313, 318, 321, 347, 348, 351, 353, 355, 356, 357, 358, 362, 364–5, 367–8
translation 27, 31, 96, 100, 105, 177, 179, 264–7, 292nn.6, 7
Tripiṭaka (Pāli Canon) 35, 167, 344, 345
Triplett, Katja 24, 32–3, 45, 102, 105, 106, 108, 110, 115, 116, 118nn.1, 7, 119n.24, 120n.31, 120n.36

U Nu 345, 367
UMNO (United Malays National Organisation) 310, 324, 328
Unani 4, 8, 37, 172, 187, 202, 204, 207–10, 225, 311, 314, 330, 335n.15, 336n.17, 336n.19
Unschuld, Paul 24
Uttarakhand 173, 182, 183, 186

Valussi, Elena 33–4, 45, 135, 136, 156n8, 157n17
Vargas-O'Bryan, Ivette 16, 17, 260
Vedas 35, 38, 168
Atharva Veda 167, 168, 227, 228, 240, 244
Ṛg Veda 167, 168
Venkataraman, Ayesha 183–184
Verran, Helen 2

Wang, Jun 14
weikza 42, 341, 345–8, 360, 361, 370n.2
Wilms, S. 138, 156n.11
Wong Tai Sin 黃大仙 (temple) 16
wu 巫 (wizard) 62–63, 66, 81, 83n.5, 83n.7, 83n.8
Wujastyk, Dagmar 19, 226

Yakushi Nyorai 99, 106
Yangga Trarong 267
Yangsheng 養生 (nurturing life) 45, 83n.10, 129, 136, 143, 144
yin and *yang* 16, 69, 129, 137, 141
yoga 4, 8, 18, 19, 210, 226, 330, 336n.17
study of 19
Tantric yoga 23, 275
Tibetan yoga 21, 24

Zysk, Kenneth 167, 191n.5, 225, 227–30, 233, 239, 243

EU authorised representative for GPSR:
Easy Access System Europe, Mustamäe tee 50,
10621 Tallinn, Estonia
gpsr.requests@easproject.com

www.ingramcontent.com/pod-product-compliance
Lightning Source LLC
Chambersburg PA
CBHW051554230426
43668CB00013B/1849
9781526191120